The Burdens of Disease

The Burdens of Disease

Epidemics and Human Response in Western History

Revised Edition

J. N. Hays

Rutgers University Press

New Brunswick, New Jersey
and London

Library of Congress Cataloging-in-Publication Data

Hays, J. N., 1938–
    The burdens of disease : epidemics and human response in western
    history / J.N. Hays. — 2nd ed.
        p. ; cm.
    Includes bibliographical references and index.
    ISBN 978–0–8135–4612–4 (hardcover : alk. paper) —
ISBN 978–0–8135–4613–1 (pbk. : alk. paper)
    1. Epidemics—History. I. Title.
    [DNLM: 1. Disease Outbreaks—history—Americas. 2. Disease
Outbreaks—history—Europe. 3. Western World—history—Americas.
    4. Western World—history—Europe. WA 11 GA1 H425b 2009]
    RA649.H29 2009
    614.4—dc22

                                                        2008051487

A British Cataloging-in-Publication record for this book is available from the
British Library.

Visit our Web site: http://rutgerspress.rutgers.edu

Manufactured in the United States of America

For Roz

Contents

Tables

Acknowledgments

In this revised edition of *The Burdens of Disease* I remain deeply indebted to those historians and other scholars whose works continue to inform my ideas about the history of epidemic disease. Since the first edition was published in 1998 that scholarship has grown steadily richer, deeper, and more enlightening. The updated "Suggestions for Further Reading" reflect some of that wealth, and I hope that the readers of this book will make use of them and so derive the same pleasures from them that I have enjoyed.

Early in my historical training three distinguished scholars at the University of Chicago inspired me. Allen Debus introduced me to the history of science, still my bridge between C. P. Snow's two cultures. William McNeill's breadth of vision and imagination provided excitement and stimulus, even before his seminal *Plagues and Peoples* helped create interest in the history of disease. John Clive (later of Harvard University, and now deceased) constantly reminded me that history is a humanistic pursuit.

My students at Loyola University Chicago, including undergraduate, graduate, and medical students, persistently asked unanswerable and hence important questions. Loyola's Department of History has remained a genial and stimulating group of colleagues and friends; I could not have found a more congenial environment for my career. I must also thank Loyola University for the grants of two leaves of absence that facilitated the original conception and completion of the book.

Since the appearance of the first edition, I have gained both ideas and encouragement from a variety of readers and reviewers. And as have so many scholars, I have shamelessly exploited the professionalism and resources found in libraries, especially (in my case) those of the University of Chicago, Loyola

University Chicago, and the Wellcome Centre for the History of Medicine at University College London. At Rutgers University Press, senior editor Doreen Valentine has rendered invaluable professional counsel, and the whole Rutgers Press staff has made the production process a pleasure.

And to my wife, Rosalind Hays, I still owe more than I can properly express, and certainly more than I can ever repay. She shares whatever merits this book may possess. The flaws and errors that remain are mine, all mine.

The Burdens of Disease

Introduction

Disease and illness have obvious importance to human life. In recent years, popular awareness of them has sharpened with concerns about a new worldwide pandemic, perh aps of some form of Asian bird flu spreading to humans. More than ever some understanding of the workings of disease within Western (and world) history should inform our responses to present and future epidemic crises. This book, a second and revised version of the original, presents a view that emphasizes alike the individual reality of sickness and death, the social responses to such physical illness, and the changing ways in which Western societies have constructed the meaning of disease.

Disease is both a pathological reality and a social construction. Both material evidence for it and convictions about it exist; concentration on one to the exclusion of the other (as some earlier historical writing has done) has sometimes made a neater story, but an incomplete one. Especially during the period from the late nineteenth century through the mid-twentieth, disease seemed an objective biological phenomenon, and those who combated it were scientific physicians. A large literature in the history of medicine resulted, one that focused on those figures from the past whose actions and thoughts most closely foretold the model of modern Western biomedicine. That literature usually said little about the effects of disease on social structures or on individual, everyday lives. More recently two other conceptions of disease complicated this positivist picture. Many social scientists and historians came to consider disease above all as a cultural construct, rooted in mental habits and social relations rather than in objective biological conditions of pathology. Other writing saw disease as a force in its own right, an implacable product of a biological world in which humans are prey as well as predators. That view, associated with historians' concern with the

1

long-term conception of time and with environment rather than events, shifted attention from the medicine-centered approach to disease, but in doing so it may have reduced human responses to insignificance.

The rich volume of scholarship in the last three decades on the history of particular diseases and disease episodes has shown the connections between diseases and social and political changes, the role of disease in the uncovering of social tensions, and the interactions of disease and changes in medical practice. It has explored the complex role of governments in the provision of health care, and the even more complex factors of professionalization that lay behind modern scientific medicine. It has recovered both the variety and persistence of folk traditions and other responses to disease outside the realm of official medicine. This book aims to apply such approaches to the history of disease in Western civilization as a whole, while also insisting on the importance of the biological and pathological realities of disease and hence of the traditions of scientific medicine.

Disease has affected Western civilization in a number of ways in different times and places. Some of its most obvious effects have been demographic: disease has led to periods of stagnant or falling human population, for example, in Europe in the late fourteenth and early fifteenth centuries. In the last two centuries human responses (especially in the West) to disease have themselves affected demography, in ways still subject to historical argument. Disease has had social effects, as in the sharpening of class lines between immigrants and "natives" in nineteenth-century American cities. Its political effects have been numerous, and sometimes dramatic: it played a crucial role in the overwhelming of Native American polities by European invaders, and it has decided both battles and the fates of European dynasties. Disease has affected economies, both by demographic pressure that has changed the supply and hence the price of labor and by its effects on the productivity of a particular region or social group. Disease's intellectual and cultural effects have been far-reaching and profound; it has channeled (or blocked) individual creativity, and it may on occasion have set its stamp on the "optimism" or "pessimism" of an entire age.

In perhaps less obvious ways, civilization has also affected disease. Some civilizations, by their very restlessness, have increased disease's opportunities. European incursions in the tropics have meant contact with yellow fever; European contacts with Native Americans resulted in a complex interchange of microorganisms and diseases; the networks of medieval trade, both by sea and land, made the movement of plague easier, as did the steam transportation of the nineteenth century. Many cultures and civilizations, including the Western, have attempted to control disease or perhaps even eliminate it, although control and elimination are different goals that have been adopted for different reasons. And finally, civilizations have affected disease by their definitions of it. In the Western

#4

world, those definitions have most often been created by social, political, and intellectual elites, whose aim has been to separate themselves from the poor or the otherwise deviant. Here cultural constructions and material evidence feed each other: as this book argues, the poor get not only the blame, but also the disease.

Our uses of the word "disease" betray considerable uncertainty about its meaning. For many people disease has an objective reality, apart from human perceptions and social constructs. Henry Sigerist, writing in 1943, called disease a "material process," a "biological process," which was "no more than the sum total of abnormal reactions of the organism or its parts to abnormal stimuli."[1] In this view there is little doubt about whether a person is or is not "sick," and illness is a group of recognizable physical symptoms that may involve weakness, incapacity, organ failure, malformation, or death.

This ontological view of disease carries further implications. First, disease exists apart from human beings, because the "organism" in Sigerist's definition hardly has to be human. Disease may therefore have a separate history. Erwin Ackerknecht, in his influential and useful survey of the history of medicine (first published in 1955), tells us that "disease is very old, far older than mankind, in fact about as old as life on earth. Our evidence tells us that disease forms have remained essentially the same throughout the millions of years."[2] Second, disease is a *physical* abnormality and is hence a fit subject for study by biological, natural science. The extent to which we now think of the profession of medicine as a "scientific" vocation testifies to the strength of this definition of disease. And third, disease—at least in part and perhaps entirely—is produced by external stimuli, apart from the normal human body. That disease exists "out there," and that it invades us, is a view that first gained particular currency in the late nineteenth century, especially because the persuasive power of explanations involving bacteria and viruses made those organisms seem the very essence of disease itself. But even apart from the heavy criticism leveled at such positivism by the views of cultural relativists, popular usages have always remained uncertain, and the invasion model has never eliminated other conceptions. AIDS, some people believe, is a condition brought on less by the invasion of an infective agent than by internal *moral* degeneracy.

Nevertheless, it may be possible to accept Sigerist's "objective" view of disease, if we also understand the social construction argument as well. Robert Hudson (for example) puts the case: "Diseases are not immutable entities but dynamic social constructions that have biographies of their own."[3] Historians, especially those working in the long shadow of Michel Foucault, have found that view particularly persuasive, and have joined anthropologists and sociologists in awareness "that illness, health, and death could not be reduced to their 'physical,' 'natural,' or 'objective' evidence."[4]

In fact these views—both Sigerist's (that disease is a biological process) and Hudson's (that it is a social construct)—may overlap. For a start, we may imagine Hudson questioning Sigerist about his word "abnormal": abnormal by what standard? According to whom? And if Sigerist's objective view may have a relativist Achilles' heel, even Hudson would confess that some "diseases" so constructed by societies are in fact "benign"; a social construct may define a condition as a disease, but it may have more trouble making people die of it. To be sure, some past socially-constructed disease states have resulted in death, but has spirit possession been responsible, or some other unrecognized organic cause? But certainly social constructions of disease have led to the isolation and stigmatization of many people in many different times and places, and in that sense such constructions have had "real" effects.

Past realities reflect the ambiguous relations of these seemingly incompatible understandings of "disease." In this book I shall emphasize those diseases of the past which—regardless of what societies called them—caused social disruption by their biological processes that led to physical incapacitation and death. But I am also concerned with the ways in which societies define and conceive disease, and so I shall discuss responses (some intellectual, some not) to diseases as well. Cases in which human conceptions of disease result in social, political, or economic change fall legitimately within the scope of this study.

Because this book principally concerns itself with "physical" ailments, I will pay little attention to the role of mental illness in past societies. Modern historical writing has been especially sensitive to the social construction aspects of mental illness. Roy Porter quotes the seventeenth-century Englishman who, on being judged insane, exclaimed: "They said I was mad; and I said they were mad; damn them, they outvoted me!"[5]I recognize that such cultural relativism is an important aspect of "disease," and that by omitting discussion of mental illness I may lose the opportunity to provide some dramatic illustrations of social constructions. Different examples drawn from more plainly physical ailments may make the same points, however.

I am particularly concerned here with epidemic diseases. "Epidemic" is not a precise word. The *Oxford English Dictionary*, quoting the Sydenham Society's *Lexicon of Medicine and Allied Sciences*, defines an epidemic disease as "one prevalent among a people or community at a special time, and produced by some special causes and generally present in the affected locality." Most definitions agree that an epidemic is temporary, affecting a particular place, and resulting in mortality and/or morbidity in excess of normal expectancy. An epidemic is opposed to an "endemic" disease, present or prevalent in a population all the time. But the definitions contain no quantitative component. "Epidemiologists don't use the word 'epidemic' much, perhaps because they can't always agree on what constitutes a significant excess," one textbook said in 1974. Another text, in 1996, despaired of the word: "How do we know when we have an excess over what is expected? Indeed, how do we know how much to expect? There is no precise answer to either question."[6]

This uncertainty also characterizes the more general or less technical uses of the word. It has frequently been chosen to dramatize any problem, to convey notions of both severity and temporal emergency; in 1937 Franklin Roosevelt spoke of an "epidemic of world lawlessness." Charles Rosenberg has argued that those concerned with many different diseases have themselves bent the word out of its precise meaning to lend drama to any disease "problem." Thus another epidemiology text (in 1974) proposed: "It would perhaps be well to label as 'epidemic' the long-term increases such as that noted for lung cancer. If this term were applied, more action might be taken to investigate the causes and to institute control measures."[7] Long-term increases, not a temporary, exceptional statistical surge, could therefore be labeled "epidemic" if doing so would attract more attention to the phenomenon.

My use of "epidemic" shares some of these ambiguities. This book focuses on epidemics, but it includes other diseases that have had a marked effect on past societies. Especially difficult to categorize are those diseases, endemic to a society, that reached some unclear threshold of incidence that merited epidemic status, perhaps as a result of environmental change. Typhus in the war-stricken sixteenth century, tuberculosis in the industrial nineteenth, and AIDS in the globetrotting twentieth might all be so described.

Epidemic diseases are generally associated with the word "infections," and indeed they are generally the result of an invasion by infectious agents such as bacteria or viruses. Some—but not all—infectious diseases may also be called "contagions," in that they are communicated (directly or indirectly) from one person to another, but other infections (bubonic plague, for example) may arrive in other ways. Infectious, epidemic episodes (whether examples of contagion or not) have had the most marked effects on past societies; effects were greatest (especially in contemporary perceptions) when disease came as an unexpected physical blow. Three further terms may characterize many (though not all) infectious epidemics: "acute," and "high mortality," and "high morbidity." "Acute" diseases have rapid onsets, severe symptoms, and relatively short durations and are contrasted with "chronic" diseases. "Mortality" means death rate, and morbidity means rate of incidence of disease, both of which may soar in an epidemic.

In addition to infectious epidemics, the disease universe includes what William McNeill aptly calls the "background noise" of endemic, chronic, and degenerative ailments.[8] The distinction between background noise and sudden epidemic crashes has always been blurred; malaria, syphilis, and tuberculosis may all be chronic, and all have been endemic in different societies, but at times their mortality (whether real or perceived) justifies their inclusion here. As Western civilization has brought many traditionally important epidemic diseases under control, the background noise itself has become more audible. And the modern background noises (especially cardiovascular diseases and malignant neoplasms) deserve a separate treatment that this work makes no attempt to provide.

One other limitation: I concern myself with "Western" civilization, meaning that civilization which first emerged in western and central Europe between about 400 and 800 C.E., from a fusion of Greco-Roman, western Latin Christian, and Germanic-Slavic-Celtic roots, later spreading to the rest of Europe and to the Americas. This chronological and geographical limitation I adopt partly for convenience (to keep the book manageable) and partly in the belief that Western civilization's experiences with, and reactions to, disease and illness are important subjects in themselves.

Microorganisms have rarely been respectful of political and cultural frontiers, however, and in this edition I have been even less consistent about limiting the discussion to the West than I was in the first. The great twentieth-century pandemics can really only be understood in their world contexts, which now shape the ways in which Western society constructs them. On some level, Westerners long regarded the 1918–1919 influenza pandemic as "forgotten"; but as awareness of its colossal worldwide death tolls have spread, those facts have contributed to contemporary fears of a new Asian-based influenza on a similar scale. And as Europeans and North Americans gradually learned about the ravages of AIDS in Africa, their constructions of the disease belatedly shifted from a focus on deviant homosexuals toward more general heterosexual transmissions. Western civilization has been extraordinarily expansive in the last five hundred years, creating numerous give-and-take relationships between society and disease, as disease and concepts of it followed in the path of imperialism, diverted its course, and were diverted by it. And while the age of formal imperialism has largely passed, the world is more closely interlinked than ever, thanks to the combined pressures of aggressive commerce, swift transportation, and phenomenal contemporary communication and information technology. Disease history in the twenty-first century will be global.

Since the sixteenth century, the shrinking world has led to greater opportunities for the rapid movement of microbes to new populations; in the Western world previously dominant religious and magical paradigms of explanation for disease have been joined by others, adding new levels of complexity to human responses to disease; and Western civilization has experienced massive social change, many aspects of which have dramatically modified the human-disease relationship. The position of disease in Western society has therefore become more complicated than it has been in earlier centuries, and for that reason this book gives what may seem a disproportionate weight to the more recent period. In doing so I do not claim that disease played an unimportant role in the medieval world, or that the sufferings of medieval people have less meaning for us. Rather, I attempt to clarify the new complexities of the last several centuries.

This edition draws on the rich scholarship of the past decade. I have particularly revised the discussions of three great pandemics: the second plague pandemic, including the "Black Death" (in Chapter Three); the 1918–1919 influenza pandemic (in Chapter Eleven); and the contemporary AIDS pandemic (in Chapter Twelve). Controversies continue around the Black Death (and the larger second pandemic of which it was a part): about its total mortality, its points of origin, and (most vigorously) its causative organism. Chapter Three recognizes those arguments, although it still holds with *Yersinia pestis* and its resultant bubonic and pneumonic plague as the most likely—or perhaps the "least lousiest"— explanation of it. While total mortality from the Black Death remains disputed, historical estimates of the toll in the 1918–1919 influenza pandemic have steadily risen, as its horrific worldwide extent is more clearly documented; and historical and biological detection has recently (and triumphantly) traced its causative virus. Chapter Eleven now reflects those new points. In 1998 (the date of this book's first edition), the AIDS epidemic still seemed more a topic of current events than of historical analysis; Chapter Twelve now tries to take a current view of that subject, especially of its African origins and African effects. Readers will also discover other changes throughout that reflect new scholarship, and will especially notice that the "Suggestions for Further Reading" have been extensively updated.

The impact of disease on Western civilization, especially in particular episodes or periods in which one disease seemed unusually formidable, is the central theme of this book, the order of which is for the most part straightforwardly chronological. The first chapter presents Western civilization's intellectual inheritance: concepts about disease held by the ancient Greeks and Romans, and their responses, to disease that later Western people adopted. Subsequent chapters will include discussions of contemporary perceptions of a disease, its demographic, social, economic, political, and cultural/intellectual effects, and the ways in which opinions, preventive strategies, and remedies all shifted over time. More briefly, other sections will focus on the position of healers and general ideas of healing; though not a history of medicine per se, this book does notice the chronological evolutions of both the social positions of healers and the dominant—or contesting— paradigms of disease.

Much modern historical writing has been devoted to particular aspects of these topics; that body of scholarship has rightly emphasized the weaknesses of earlier "positivist" histories of disease and medicine. Historical writing that scorns the unlettered folk practitioner because she did not belong to a professional guild, or that employs the wisdom of the present to denounce past therapies, is simply not good history. I hope in this book to bring the views of modern historical scholarship, as they have been applied so fruitfully to particular topics in the history of disease and illness, to a broad synthesis of the subject. If at times this narrative is critical of past beliefs and practices, I hope that such criticism is tempered both by sensitivity to the underlying presuppositions of the past, and by an awareness of the all-too-human shortcomings of the most recent responses to disease.

One

The Western Inheritance

Greek and Roman Ideas about Disease

The ancient Greek and Roman civilizations, and the Jews, early Christians, and pagans who formed part of their populations, suffered from disease, saw their societies diverted by its effects, and developed a variety of ideas and beliefs to deal with it. Ancient Greek civilization was a predecessor of the West rather than an early stage of it, but extremely close intellectual and cultural links tie the two together; in those respects the Western tradition began in ancient Greece, and so some knowledge of ancient Mediterranean religious and intellectual traditions is important for understanding the West's general approaches to the meaning of disease.

Asclepios, Hippocrates, and Galen

The Greeks both received direct transmissions from older civilizations and had their own "prehistoric" cultural traditions and folklore. Many of their responses to disease were derived from earlier traditions, which employed divination, exorcism, pharmaceutical remedies, and invasive surgery. Greek attitudes and practices also illustrated that the border between "supernatural" and "natural" approaches could be very unclear, as it had been for the earlier Egyptians. At some point in the fifth century B.C.E., if not earlier, some Greeks may be said to have emphasized the natural approach, perhaps less ambiguously than earlier peoples; but the distinction between that approach and others remained one of degree, not absolute difference.

The best-known healing tradition of the early Greeks was associated with the cult of Asclepios, a mythic hero who emerged as a lesser god in the Greek pantheon of the sixth century B.C.E. The sick would repair to the temple of the god and perform ritual sacrifices and bathings, followed by a crucial "incubation sleep" in which dreams and visions appeared to the sufferer. Those dreams either healed directly, or gave directions (interpreted by the priests of the god) for an appropriate therapeutic regimen, which might include bathing, rest, the administration of drugs, and attention to diet. The cult of Asclepios gained a wide following in subsequent centuries, extending into the Greco-Roman world as the principal pagan religious response to disease. Particularly important centers of the cult were in Epidauros, Cos, and Pergamum, but Asclepian healing was carried on in many places, including some associated with hot springs and mineral waters. The cult's continuing vigor in the fourth century C.E. brought it into conflict with Christianity, as we shall see.

The Hippocratic tradition, named for the physician Hippocrates of Cos (c. 460–c. 360 B.C.E.), had some of its roots in Asclepian temple medicine, but it also included both older traditions of surgery and pharmacology and some newer conceptions about nature. The Hippocratic Corpus, the body of about seventy works on which our knowledge of the Hippocratic tradition depends, almost certainly had a number of different authors, who reflected differing emphases. But much of the Corpus repeated Asclepian advice and themes: an attention to rest, baths, and diet, combined with simple and gentle treatments and frequent expositions of the principle that "nature is the best healer." Hippocratic writings also illustrated careful observation and description of symptoms, notably in their discussion of the "fevers" that loomed large in ancient Mediterranean societies. Hippocratic authors evidently had particular familiarity with malaria, chronicled its intermittent ("tertian" or "quartan") effects, and constructed general interpretations of fevers around their "critical days."[1] In addition, Hippocratic authors also relied on older beliefs from Greek folklore or Egyptian writings, which may or may not have entered into Asclepian prognoses and therapeutics. Certainly some of the pharmacological and surgical remedies of the Corpus antedate the sixth-century emergence of the Asclepian cult.

Hippocrates and his colleagues, however, also lived in a vibrant period of Greek philosophy, initiated in the previous century by the "nature philosophers" such as Thales, Anaximander, and Anaximenes. Those thinkers had begun shifting the balance between "supernatural" and "natural" explanations in the direction of the latter, and "natural" explanations of disease make a clear appearance in the Hippocratic writings. A frequently cited Hippocratic passage proclaimed of epilepsy: "I do not believe that the 'Sacred Disease' is any more divine or sacred than any other," and presented instead an explanation based on human heredity for a disease that, involving as it may dramatic seizures, could easily be conceived as a product of supernatural forces, spirits, or demons.[2] At points the Corpus speculated about environmental causes: "Those [diseases] peculiar to a time of drought are consumption, ophthalmia, arthritis, strangury and dysentery." Heredity explained other (or even the same) disease states: "If a phlegmatic child is born of a phlegmatic parent, a bilious child of a bilious parent, a consumptive child of a consumptive parent [then heredity might also explain epilepsy]."[3] Some Greek attitudes toward disease came to include this strand of "rationalism," which de-emphasized the role of forces outside human control or understanding and urged instead that human disease could be comprehended in human terms. Such diseases might therefore be both understood and controlled by the exercise of human reason.

Of particular later importance in the West was the humoral theory to which Hippocratic authors contributed, which saw the health of the body dependent on the maintenance of a balance among the "humors": a surplus, or a deficiency, of one humor or another led to disease. The clearest exposition of this notion claimed:

> The human body contains blood, phlegm, yellow bile, and black bile. These are the things that make up its constitution and cause its pains and health. Health is primarily that state in which these constituent substances are in the correct proportion to each other, both in strength and quantity, and are well mixed. Pain occurs when one of the substances presents either a deficiency or an excess, or is separated from the body and not mixed with the others.[4]

Such humoral theories of disease, and indeed of physiology, grew out of Greek natural philosophy that both preceded the Hippocratic writings and existed contemporaneously with them. At the center of Greek natural philosophy in the fifth century B.C.E. was an interest in the basic substances (or "elements") that underlay all matter.

Of these element theories one of the most important, at least for later Western history, was that of Empedocles (fl. c. 450 B.C.E.). Empedocles proposed that four "elements" served as the fundamental constituents of all nature, and that those four elements were in turn manifestations of essential physical qualities. Water embodied wetness and coldness; earth, dryness and coldness; air, wetness and hotness; fire, dryness and hotness. Empedocles' element theory, and its association with human physiology, was adopted by Aristotle (384–322 B.C.E.) , which accounts for some of its later importance; Hippocratic authors also employed it, associating it with certain "temperaments" of individuals as well as with the humoral theory of disease. Much of the later influence of the humoral paradigm came through the writings of Galen, and the humoral theory may be best seen in them.

By the time of Galen (129–c. 210 C.E.) a unified Greco-Roman civilization had long been created across the Mediterranean, at least for the literate, prosperous ruling classes. Galen, a physician from Pergamum, spent some time in Rome as a physician to the emperor Marcus Aurelius. Galen was a very influential figure in his own time, and became yet more so in later centuries as his doctrines appealed to both medieval Christians and early Muslims. Galen stood at the intersection of two important traditions of Greek medicine and thought about disease and the human body. One was the Hippocratic and humoral approach; the other was anatomical study, which undoubtedly had its roots in the surgical practices of prehistory and (more especially) Egypt. Anatomy was pursued with particular seriousness in the early Hellenistic period, when the traditions of Greece and Egypt most clearly combined. Several "schools" of anatomy had subsequently arisen that used anatomical evidence to argue fundamentally different views of what went wrong with the human body. Some believed that specific solid tissues of the body became diseased and that therefore disease was *local* in character, restricted to one organ or set of organs. Others, following a line of reasoning consistent with the humoral theory, saw disease as a *systemic* problem: fluids carrying humors moved through the entire system of the body, and unbalanced humors affected the entire system.

Galen's picture of human physiology, derived from his anatomical ideas, was an impressively complex one that involved three largely independent systems conveying different fluids and "spirits" to the organs and tissues of the body. The channels of conveyance in the three systems were the veins, the arteries, and the nerves. The veins sprang from the liver, and were thus in turn associated with the digestive system; food entering the digestive tract led to the creation of "natural spirits" in the liver, and those spirits, the active principle of nutrition, moved to the rest of the body through the veins. The veins served (among other organs) the heart, wherein venous blood mixed with air, carried there from the lungs; "vital spirits" resulted from the combination of air and venous blood in the heart, and arterial blood carried these spirits, the breath of life, through the body in the arteries. Both venous and arterial blood fed the brain, the seat of the third system, that of the nerves. Nervous fluid carried "animal spirits," the active principle of animation, through the body.

Galen's beliefs about anatomy and physiology recognized, to a remarkable degree, that the definition of human "life" was a complex matter. Did the functioning of any single organ or system mark the difference between life and death? Aristotle had regarded the heart as the seat of life; when it stopped, life stopped. Galen was not so sure, and more recent thought, wrestling with "life" defined by electrical impulses, should see in him a sensitive forerunner of modern dilemmas.

Galen's three systems also involved the four humors, since he was heir to the Empedoclean and Hippocratic traditions. As such he believed in the theory of the four elements. Earth, water, air, and fire entered the body through food, drink, and the atmosphere, and the processes of digestion and respiration converted those elements into the four Hippocratic humors: fire into yellow bile, air into blood, water into phlegm, earth into black bile. The humors made up the body fluids, some of which (particularly blood, in its venous and arterial forms) carried the "spirits" or active principles that caused the body to function.

Galen's explanation of human physiology thus clearly descended from the "systemic" school, and may be seen as a sophisticated elaboration of it. If disease was a product of the imbalance of the humors carried by the different systems, the physician should restore the balance. And since ultimately the humors in the body derived from the four elements, from what we eat and drink and breathe, dietetic treatment played a major therapeutic role. For example, Galen reasoned, "those articles of food which are by nature warmer are more productive of bile, while those which are colder produce more phlegm."[5] This dietetic view of health, related to humoral explanations of disease, could assume a highly moral aspect.[6] In Galen's writings the moral emphasis was clear. Galen saw dietetic medicine as a branch of moral philosophy; errors in one's way of life, the individual's ignorance and/or intemperance, produced internal disease: ulcers, gout, digestive pain, arthritis, the "stone." Hence proper behavior—habits of life and diet—could avoid most disease. Although Galen may have emphasized the moral elements of medicine to legitimize the physician's social and intellectual position, many generations of later Muslim and Christian thinkers agreed with him about the connection between health and moral philosophy.[7]

Galen also represented the Hippocratic tradition in his professionalism as a physician. The Romans among whom Galen lived generally did not "practice medicine" as a profession. An extremely polytheistic people, the early Romans explained disease as the product of the many gods who superintended each household and indeed each part of the body. Heads of families performed the appropriate propitiary rites and sacrifices to preserve family health, just as the good Roman *pater familias* kept his tools and slaves in good working order. Medical practice as a vocation fell to foreigners, especially Greeks. Greek physicians throughout the Mediterranean lands had, over the centuries, found Hippocratic principles consistent with successful practice; Greek physicians originally lived as itinerant craftsmen who had to establish confidence through correct prognoses and who could ill afford therapeutic failures.[8] The careful empirical descriptions of Hippocratic writing offered a safer basis for diagnosis. The caution of the Hippocratic tradition, which (following Egyptian precedent) included frequent modest decisions that some ailments were beyond a physician's power to cure, safeguarded the practitioner from rash claims and dashed hopes, and hence from angry accusations of failure. By the late second century B.C.E., Greek medical practices had become influential in the expanding Roman world, and by Galen's time the Greek physician and the Asclepian temple were social fixtures throughout the Mediterranean world.

Within Greco-Roman medical society a number of professional demarcations remained unclear. Only the market determined the difference between a "legitimate" physician and a "quack." Further, the Greco-Romans made no attempt to delineate "medicine" (or "science") from "religion." Physicians often remained associated with Asclepian temples, and sacrifices and votive offerings remained essential parts of all healing, "not merely a negative response" (as Ralph Jackson neatly puts it) to the shortcomings and failures of medical treatment.[9] And Greco-Roman medical practice remained in most ways unspecialized. The later European gulf between physicians and surgeons, between theory and practice, did not come from Greco-Roman tradition; although (especially in the larger cities) some specialization did develop (care of the eye and obstetrics/gynecology, the latter often practiced by women), most surgical procedures simply remained part of a healer's general stock of remedies. Those remedies also included a formidable body of materia medica, swollen by the territorial expansion of the far-flung Roman Empire, which brought together many different peoples and their herbal traditions. The Romans were a remarkably adaptable people, who absorbed a wide range of beliefs and customs. But Christianity proved difficult for Greco-Roman medical practitioners to digest.

Christian Theory and Practice

Christianity, which began as a sect within Judaism in the first century C.E., soon broke away from its clannish parent and, in time, proclaimed itself a universal religion. By the third century C.E. the faith had diffused widely over the Roman Empire; although its followers remained a decided minority, its numbers increased steadily in that century. Among the many reasons for the appeal of Christianity was its radically different conception of healing, which deserves attention both as another version of health and illness in antiquity and as an important component of later Western beliefs.

From the start the early Christians formed a separate society in the ancient Roman world. They refused (as did the Jews) to worship the official gods of the polytheistic state, and so the orthodox Romans regarded them as "atheists"; and while Christians (at least by the third century) could be found at many levels of civil and economic society, they remained something of a world apart. Their conception of disease grew out of their different religious view, and at least on the surface their response to disease sharply contrasted with the ideas of high Greco-Roman culture.

Some (though not all) of the early Christian attitudes toward disease can be traced to the ideas of Judaism. The Old Testament contains many references to diseases and their causes, and they clearly show that Judaism shared with Mesopotamian cultures a supernatural view of the subject. Old Testament stories often relate disease to errant behavior that has angered the god Yahweh. For individuals, wanton conduct had consequences and adultery was especially serious.

Two other emphases of the Hebrews also had particular later importance. One was the notion that a god's wrath could be directed against an entire offending people as well as against errant individuals. Thus Phineas and his colleagues rebuked the Reubenites: "What is this treachery you have committed against the God of Israel? Are you ceasing to follow the Lord and building your own altar this day in defiance of the Lord? Remember our offence at Peor, for which a plague fell upon the community of the Lord. . . . If you deny the Lord today, then tomorrow he will be angry with the whole community of Israel."[10] From medieval plague epidemics to twentieth-century AIDS, diseases have been seen as divine judgments on subcultures or even on entire peoples who have strayed from the presumed paths of righteousness.

The other emphasis was the association of disease and the "unclean." Chapters 13–15 of the book of Leviticus provide a thorough discussion of impurities (including diseases) and the rituals required to atone for them. Those impurities are closely linked with skin diseases, and in some later ages the skin diseases of Leviticus were taken to be leprosy (see Chapter Two). Leviticus does not clearly associate those skin diseases with individual fault; rather, they are marks of ritual uncleanliness. But the god is clearly displeased by the uncleanliness. And further, the sufferer might be required to live in isolation: "So long as the sore persists, he shall be considered ritually unclean. The man is unclean; he shall live apart and must stay outside the settlement."[11] Did the unclean pose a danger to the others by their very proximity? If so, impurity and disease were contagious, and simple association with the impure might result in illness. Certainly the Hebrews were not the only Mediterranean people to emphasize cleanliness (however defined); but the Old Testament provided arguments that linked physical imperfections, God's anger, and disease, and thus suggested the isolation of the unclean for the protection of the godly (and healthy) community.

The Judaic tradition, then, connected disease and God's wrath, a wrath sometimes brought on by human misbehavior, a wrath that might be propitiated by rituals. While the early Christians shared many of the ideas of the Jews, they also lived in the expectation of the imminent end of the world, when Christ the Redeemer would reappear and usher in a new kingdom. Perhaps because things of the body therefore seemed transiently insignificant, perhaps because pagan learning was not to be trusted, some Christians scorned the orthodox healing routines of the Greeks and Romans. Perhaps the traditions of Hippocrates, or Asclepios, were too closely associated with other gods, while the elaborate purification rituals of the Jews represented the "law" that Jesus's teaching had superseded. The Christians lived in a world entirely dominated by their god's immanence; disease and health, if they had any importance at all, acquired such importance as manifestations of God's power and will.

Further, demons populated the world. "Disease" to the early Christians (and to some other segments of Roman popular culture as well) meant above all possession by demons, whether that possession took the form of physical illness or not. For the early Christian, then, "healing" most often meant the exorcism of demons, an exorcism that might take dramatic physical form, as the sufferer (actually the demon who possessed him) roared and shook as the demon was expelled. What resulted was—to the early Christian, if not to the puzzled pagan onlooker—"health." The Christians and the pagans therefore employed different definitions of disease and health, and a visit to a Christian service might be a far different experience from a visit to an Asclepian temple or a Greco-Roman physician. So when we say that the Christianity of the third century (for example) appealed to the Roman population as a "healing" religion, we must be careful about what we mean by "healing."

Yet some correspondences surely existed. Before the Passion, Jesus had appeared to his followers perhaps most dramatically as a healer who could make the lame walk, the blind see, and raise Lazarus from death itself. Such healing powers, Christians believed, were transferred to Jesus's apostles and then to the disciples. Early Christian communities took on the nursing of the sick as an important obligation. Some of the early growth of Christianity coincided with periods of serious epidemic disease in the Roman world, notably the "plague of Cyprian" in the mid-third century; the chronic pressure of malaria, tuberculosis, and a variety of other ailments had long weakened the Roman physical fabric as well. In such times the Christians both promised the power of a healing god and practiced diligent care of their ailing colleagues. Did some Romans look to Christianity as a source of solace for the body? Although one could not become a Christian casually (at least before the fourth century), perhaps Christianity gained followers in epidemic times as a healing religion.

In fact the relation of Christianity to classical culture was not simply one of rejection. By the third and fourth centuries a number of Christian thinkers, especially such Greek Fathers as Origen and Basil, advocated a synthesis of classical and Christian learning. Specifically they urged Christians to accept the medical knowledge of the Greco-Roman world as one of God's gifts. Those who practiced Galenic medicine might be reviled, but they might also be praised for carrying on a profession that illustrated the supreme Christian virtue of charity. The Christian *anargyroi*, the healing saints, inspired cults whose practices resembled those followed by Asclepios' devotees. Their shrines and their relics, Timothy Miller says, presented "more than the god Asklepios in Christian dress," but the therapeutics of each overlapped the other.[12]

Romans and Greeks alike had long offered sacrifices to the gods, and Christians made offerings to the saints. Some of the *anargyroi* were historical persons of early Christianity; others were clearly mythical figures, and some of those were related to analogous Greek and Roman gods. Some saints, like the localized gods of polytheistic paganism, specialized in particular ailments or body organs; St. Lawrence, for example, martyred by roasting, had special care of the back. The Asclepian tradition's emphasis on the role of dreams in both prognosis and therapy was mirrored in the appearance, to Christians, of the healing saints Cosmos and Damian in dreams. The bathing rituals of Asclepian medicine found an analogue in Christian baptism and sprinkling with holy water. The dietetic approach of humoral medicine could be given a moral interpretation, and could thus be brought into harmony with a view of disease as a consequence of misbehavior. At least some Christian holy men cooperated with physicians, using profane remedies as well as performing exorcisms and miracles.

By the fourth century, especially in the eastern part of the Roman Empire, healing in Christian communities bridged the medical and ecclesiastical worlds. Priests and physicians alike might be found at the shrines of the *anargyroi*. The first true hospitals—meaning places that provided beds, food, nursing care, and medical therapy to all classes of the population, with the intention of restoring the sick to health—emerged (according to Miller) from this combination of Christian charity with the classical-Christian synthesis urged by the Greek Fathers. When Christianity suddenly gained favor at the imperial court (under Constantine, 313–337) and then became the official religion of the Roman Empire (under Theodosius, 379–395), the cult of Asclepios was perceived as a dangerous rival that worshipped a competing healer-savior, and the destruction of some Asclepian temples followed. But if Miller is correct, pagan followers of Asclepios may have felt some of the same ambivalence toward the "rational" world of Galenic medicine that bothered their Christian successors. The early hospitals apparently drew on some of the traditions of the *anargyroi* cults (of Cosmos and Damian, for example), but those in turn had borrowed from Asclepios, and all had overlapped with Galenism. Thus Theodore of Sykeon, a Byzantine holy man who died in 613, prescribed folk medicines, applied salves, and massaged limbs. According to Peregrine Horden, stories of Theodore's career contain "descriptions of acts of healing which seem to efface whatever imprecise boundaries we might care to draw between the medical and the miraculous."[13] Aline Rousselle has found a similar mixture of classical-Galenic, folkloric, and Christian healing practices in fourth-century Gaul.[14]

The old Greco-Roman medical orthodoxy felt pressures other than the obvious political ones that stemmed from the empire's conversion to Christianity. In the western part of the empire, where more drastic social and economic change occurred, threads between Christianity and classical culture snapped more decisively. Peter Brown, contrasting the healing of the Christian Martin of Tours and the pagan Marcellus of Bordeaux in the fourth century, notes that Marcellus lived in a society that had lost touch with learning, cities, and professional physicians; what Marcellus could offer was a manual of traditional folk remedies that might enable an individual to enter into a wide world of magical sympathies and forces.[15] Brown's Marcellus and Horden's later Theodore may be seen as occupying different points along a continuum of approaches to healing. Marcellus purveyed folk medicine in which elements of magic punctuated natural explanations and empirically derived procedures. Theodore, a Christian, performed miracles and exorcised demons, yet he applied natural remedies himself and referred some sufferers to others who specialized in them.

The empirical and philosophical approaches that emphasized a "naturalistic" conception of disease never had a firm and unambiguous hold on the Greco-Roman mind. That hold became much weaker by the fourth century, in part because of the pressure of successful Christian competition and in part because the social conditions for the maintenance of a specialized urban healing culture had changed. By the sixth century direct acquaintance with the texts of Hippocrates, Aristotle, the Alexandrian anatomists Herophilos and Erasistratos, and Galen had virtually disappeared from the western part of the old Roman Empire. The eastern half retained some hold on such texts. The Arabs who swept over Egypt, North Africa, Spain, Palestine, and Syria in the seventh century reestablished the Galenic traditions, but in the Christian West the ancient Greek ideas of naturalism did not resurface until after 1000.

Two

Medieval Diseases and Responses

Most historians now accept the idea that "Western" civilization emerged sometime between 300 and 800 C.E., a fusion of elements of Greco-Roman civilization (including the Christian religion or at least its Latin branch) and the Germanic, Slavic, and Celtic peoples of northern and eastern Europe. The "Middle Ages" conventionally begin in that period and extend down to some time between about 1350 and 1550, when they were succeeded by what is called the "early modern" period. The "Middle Ages"—to which the term "medieval" is applied— should therefore more properly be called the "Early Ages" of Western history.

Until about 1000, Western life was overwhelmingly agricultural, long-distance or specialized trades were few, town life almost nonexistent, political authority highly fragmented, literacy rare. Some important discontinuities therefore existed between the early Middle Ages and the ancient Mediterranean, discontinuities that affected the disease environment. The early West, profoundly rural, lacked the urban concentrations that encouraged such airborne or "crowd" diseases as tuberculosis, influenza, and diphtheria. Diseases of the digestive tract may not have spread as rapidly either, although sanitation was, if anything, less effective.

One catastrophic plague pandemic did strike late antiquity between 541 and about 750, and its effects on mortalities, societies, and economies may have contributed to the transition from "ancient" to "medieval" civilizations in both East and West. After that visitation abated, major epidemics were largely (and perhaps fortuitously) absent from the West until plague returned in the fourteenth century. But early medieval people also lived in very close proximity to their animals, so zoonoses (diseases that moved from animals to humans) persisted. So too did dietary deficiencies (of protein, iron, vitamins), spoiled foods, and their

19

resultant diseases: rickets, scurvy, ergotism. Greater continuity existed in the realm of attitudes toward disease and health, where the gradual transition begun in late antiquity from pagan to Christian views and from responses based on literate traditions to those rooted in oral folklore continued in the early West.

Between about 1000 and 1300 cities grew up, the local self-sufficiency of economic life broke down as trade and specialized crafts increased, political complexity and authority grew, and a rich and sophisticated culture emerged. The disease context changed accordingly. Those remarkable developments in Western history that began accelerating around 1000 were accompanied by, perhaps preceded by, and in some senses caused by a rapid increase in population. At the root of that population increase may have lain some combination of improved agricultural techniques (hence more and better nutrition), benign climate, and the relative absence of serious epidemic diseases. On the base of a rising population could be built more varied economic opportunities, improved political security, and a refined religion and ethos that inspired greater respect for human life, all of which in turn magnified the population increase. The population as a whole was almost certainly "healthier" in 1150 than it had been in 900, for some combination of the above reasons. But as will be shown later in this chapter, conditions for a revival of serious epidemics had also been created.

In the years after 1000, and especially after about 1100, Western thinkers began rediscovering the works of the ancient Greeks and Romans. In many cases these discoveries occurred through the intermediary work of Muslims, so that such Arabic authors as al-Rhazes and Avicenna deeply influenced Western medieval thought. But however they reached Western thinkers, the "new" ideas made a staggering impression. By the thirteenth century Aristotle was simply the Philosopher, the master of all who knew. As we have seen in Chapter One, the early Western Christians had often scorned the classical explanations of the natural world, explanations that seemed of little importance when set beside knowledge of God and a spiritual or supernatural eternity. But for whatever reason, twelfth-century European intellectuals became enormously excited by the astronomical ideas of Ptolemy and by the anatomical and etiological theories of Galen. In the course of the twelfth and thirteenth centuries schools in European towns evolved into "universities," in which the new ideas of classical antiquity were taught in harmony (or so it was hoped) with Christian doctrines. Among the disciplines that emerged in those years was formal medicine, and physicians began to assume separate professional status, dependent on postgraduate university training and qualifications.

The effects of these new ideas and this new profession on disease and health remained slight, however. Better health, or an increased life span, or a lower rate of mortality did not result from an actively more successful "medicine." The medical profession and the theory of disease underwent important changes in the medieval period, but those changes had relatively little effect on mortality or health. The ideas of Galen often meant little change in practices, and in any case the formally trained physician who employed them might be found only in larger towns. Although some people from all social classes consulted such physicians, the upper classes most often enjoyed their benefits (if benefits they were). For most of the medieval population, healing remained intimately associated with religion, especially with its popular manifestations, which included an ambivalent mixture of prayers to saints both recognized and not, charms, and a variety of traditional "medical" responses, particularly herbal. Examples of some of these different responses, both Galenic and traditional, emerge from a closer examination of two diseases that attracted particular attention in the central Middle Ages: leprosy, about which the ideas of the official religion strongly affected medieval responses, and scrofula, around which a variety of political and magical ideas clustered. More such examples will follow in Chapter Three, which concerns the great medieval plague epidemic, and in Chapter Five, which will explore more systematically the relations between magic, religion, science, medicine, and popular healing practices.

Leprosy

In the centuries before the fourteenth Europeans experienced many diseases, but one—leprosy—attracted the most attention. Historical writing about medieval leprosy has been dogged by problems of identification and even etymology, and some discussion of what leprosy was and is will clarify both medieval responses and historical views of them.

Leprosy is now most often called Hansen's disease, taking its name from the nineteenth-century investigator who discovered the bacterium responsible for it. That bacillus, *Mycobacterium leprae*, may be responsible for a number of different manifestations or types of disease. It may or may not be very communicable, depending on the individual case; in most cases it can be communicated only after a prolonged and close exposure, and even then hereditary powers of resistance may intervene. Its incubation period is quite long; that is, a prolonged period of years separates infection and visible symptoms. The last fact especially complicates the epidemiology of the disease.

Hansen's disease, especially in the form called lepromatous leprosy, eventually manifests itself in dramatic symptoms. Lesions toughen the skin of the face; the lesions worsen and destroy nerves and tissues. Serious deformities may result, as facial bones are damaged or destroyed and the extremities become misshapen or "fall off" entirely. Such symptoms are repellant, to be sure, and so sufferers of the disease attract attention by their mere appearance. But some of the symptoms, especially if they are imprecisely described, are not unique to Hansen's disease; advanced stages of syphilis and yaws may produce some of the same effects, for example, and the number of diseases that result in skin lesions is legion. Some historians have questioned whether medieval "leprosy" was really Hansen's disease at all. Did medieval diagnosticians loosely group a panoply of ailments under the blanket—and condemnatory—word "leprosy"? A second historical question enters into that problem: what connection exists between medieval leprosy and the disease stigmatized in the Old Testament book of Leviticus as a mark of impurity? Leviticus provided an important source for medieval responses to "leprosy"; were those responses consistent with the ancient Hebrew traditions?

It now seems that what medieval people called "leprosy" really was Hansen's disease, lepromatous leprosy. Although there undoubtedly occurred many misdiagnoses, medieval definitions turn out to have been remarkably good. The most convincing evidence comes from paleopathology. Cemeteries known to have been set aside for "lepers" have been exhumed, notably in Denmark, and the skeletons (or a high percentage of them) show damage of the kind caused exclusively by lepromatous leprosy; the same damage is not found in the bones from other, more "general," burial grounds.[1] Modern students of medieval leprosy have also argued that medieval descriptions of leprosy are consistent with a diagnosis of Hansen's disease; Luke Demaitre, who concurs with their views on the accuracy of medieval diagnosis, adds arguments against the likelihood of a confusion with syphilis, a subject to which we shall return.[2]

Medieval Europeans mistakenly thought the leprosy suffered by their contemporaries was the same disease referred to in Leviticus 13 and 14, a connection that made the lot of the medieval leper even more miserable than it might have been. This mistake emerged from a historical and etymological tangle. Leprosy— Hansen's disease, lepromatous leprosy—may or may not have been known in the ancient Near East. In Leviticus, the Hebrew word *tsara'ath*, roughly meaning (according, to E. V. Hulse) "repulsive scaly skin-disease," is very thoroughly discussed as a serious matter offensive in the sight of God.[3] The chapters describe careful examinations to be undertaken by priests, who decide if the sufferer has *tsara'ath*; if the answer is yes, the sufferer is pronounced unclean, and Leviticus 14 specifies elaborate sacrifices and rituals that when performed atone for the uncleanliness and thus appease the angry god. Leviticus further insists that the sufferer be isolated from the community until he is clean.

The Greek language rendered the Hebrew *tsara'ath* as *lepra*, but the Greeks were also familiar with Hansen's disease, for which good descriptions may be traced to the Hellenistic period. The Greeks called that disease *elefantiasis*, and it was under that term that Hansen's disease (medieval leprosy) existed in the Greco-Roman civilization. In modern terms elephantiasis is yet another disease, a chronic lymphatic complaint found most often in the tropics. This latter disease—modern elephantiasis—was known to the Muslims, who used a term equivalent to the Greek *elefantiasis* (by which the Greeks meant Hansen's disease) to describe it. A different Arabic word was found for Hansen's disease *(juzam)*. When the revival of learning associated with Arabic authors began in Europe, a fatal etymological misunderstanding arose. The Arabic *juzam*—Hansen's disease— should have been equated with the Greek *elefantiasis*, which had no particular ritual or religious significance. But because Arabic had already used a similar word for what we now call elephantiasis, Latin scholars equated *juzam* with the Greek *lepra* and hence with the Hebrew *tsara'ath*.

Hence the "scaly skin disease" of the Hebrews, the mark of a ritual uncleanliness, was equated by medieval Christians with leprosy, a disease that in ancient Greece and Rome (and in the world of medieval Islam) was known and had no such ritual associations. In addition, medieval Christianity placed different emphases, or perhaps even different meanings, on the concept of uncleanliness. How much was uncleanliness brought on by the sufferer's wrongdoing, or by his *sin*? According to Saul Brody, the most thorough modern student of medieval literary responses to leprosy, the original Hebrew intent divorced "ritual uncleanliness" from "moral guilt."[4] Later medieval Christian writers erased such distinctions, perhaps with some Old Testament support, for it is certainly true that the God of the Old Testament frequently punished wrongdoing with disease.

Leprosy was found in the early centuries of Western history, for skeletons from the fourth and fifth centuries show leprous damage and laws commenting on leprosy date from the early Carolingian period of the Franks, in the eighth century. But comment about leprosy, consciousness of it, and vigorous response to it all peaked in the years between about 1000 and about 1250, coinciding with the period of rapid European population growth. In those years leprosaria, or other forms of leprosy "institutions" or communities, were founded in considerable numbers, and the Church formalized its rituals in response to an evidently widespread disease. Reports of leprosy began declining between 1250 and 1350, so that when the great plague epidemic began in the late 1340s many leprosaria had already been gradually depopulated. Leprosy became rarer yet on the heels of the plague epidemic, and by 1500 it was unusual, except apparently in Scandinavia, where it persisted through the early modern period and even revived in intensity in the early nineteenth century.

In the years between 1000 and 1250 leprosy was the subject of heavy ecclesiastical and legal intervention. Sufferers became the objects of harsh laws that might sever them from society. Although the laws varied from one community to the next, and may not always have been enforced, the leper might find himself (or herself) ostracized by legal pronouncement. The process might begin with a public accusation made by neighbors. An examination followed, often conducted by a priest (as specified by Leviticus 13), but committees of magistrates and physicians (especially later in the Middle Ages) might be involved as well. Clearly a real possibility of misdiagnosis existed. In 1179 the Third Lateran Council formalized the leper's separation from the community into an awful ritual. The leper knelt before the church altar under a black cloth, with a black veil over his face. An office for the dead was pronounced over him, and the priest threw spadefuls of earth from the cemetery on him. The priest then read a series of prohibitions:

> I forbid you to ever enter the church or monastery, fair, mill, marketplace, or company of persons. I forbid you to ever leave your house without your leper's costume, in order that one recognize you and that you never go barefoot. I forbid you to ever wash your hands or anything about you in the stream or in the fountain. . . . I forbid you to touch anything you bargain for or buy, until it is yours. I forbid you to enter a tavern. . . . I forbid you to live with any woman other than your own. I forbid you, if you go on the road and you meet some person who speaks to you, to fail to put yourself downwind before you answer. I forbid you to go in a narrow lane, so that should you meet any person, he should not be able to catch the affliction from you. I forbid you, if you go along any thoroughfare, to ever touch a well or the cord unless you have put on your gloves. I forbid you to ever touch children or give them anything. I forbid you to eat or drink from any dishes other than your own. I forbid you drinking or eating in company, unless with lepers.[5]

After this pronouncement the leper donned his distinctive costume and was led outside the town walls to the leprosarium that would henceforth be home. The priest offered consoling words, urging patience and trust in God's mercy.

The priest's prohibitions suggest that several different but complementary views existed about leprosy. On one level the leper presented a religious, ritual danger to the community, in line with the text of sacred scripture. That view was especially important in the early years of concern about leprosy, when it led to isolation that had many overtones of religious penance.[6] Life in some leprosaria included some of the features of monastic devotional obligations, and the pre-scribed dress was clerical in style. Belief that the disease was a heaven-sent pun-ishment for sin was widespread. According to Brody (and to Richard Palmer), the sin most often held responsible was lechery; lepers were schemers and deceivers who cuckolded the faithful, and they burned with overpowering sexual urges.[7] Whether as a ritual defilement or as a punishment for grave misconduct, leprosy was a fit subject of clerical intervention. And as Palmer points out, the medieval church placed great weight on the importance of formal confession as a therapeu-tic tool. A series of papal bulls and pronouncements between the thirteenth and sixteenth century obligated physicians to call in priests for their patients, because at least in some cases the disease might be cured by confession.

From the twelfth century on, physicians in the "new" Galenic tradition began adding other emphases, more focused on the body than on the soul. Galenic humoral medicine offered more detailed rationalizations about symptoms, and especially believed leprosy to arise as a disorder of one humor: black bile. Black bile, overcooked and "burnt," affected blood in turn, and that accounted for such symptoms as "hideous" lips and fetid breath.

Physicians (and others) particularly associated the disease with fornication, an act that actively disturbed two of the humoral "non-naturals" (exercise and excretion). Maintaining a proper balance of such non-naturals was essential for health, and the sex act might threaten that balance. Intercourse with a leprous woman was a "particularly predictable cause," a belief that neatly joined humoral explanations, fears of contagion, and gynephobia.[8] Some opinion, following the most direct humoral route, saw leprosy as dietetic, the product of bad meat and wine. And it is worth noting that physicians rarely referred to the biblical texts of Leviticus when they wrote about the disease.

Ancient authorities also contributed two other causal concepts about leprosy: that it was hereditary, and that it was contagious. Hippocratic texts generally endorsed hereditarian notions; sanguine parents or bilious parents produced sanguine or bilious children. Conception by a leprous mother, or being nursed by a leprous mother or wet-nurse (an idea that combined hereditarian and contagionist strands), might cause leprosy.

Concepts of contagion were also applied. Arataeus of Cappodocia (a contemporary of Galen) had discussed flight from leprosy, and Muslim authorities were drawn to that concept, although with reservations owing to their faith's overriding conviction that all diseases were heaven-sent.[9] A contagionist idea entered the 1179 prohibition cited above: "I forbid you to go in a narrow lane, so that should you meet any person, he should not be able to catch the affliction from you." By the later Middle Ages the doctrine of contagion was more and more frequently applied to leprosy, perhaps because contagionism seemed to explain other diseases (especially plague), perhaps because physicians came to have more influence in the diagnosis and proclamation of lepers. In the case of leprosy the contagionist argument also gained strength from the Levitical horror the disease inspired and the isolation insisted upon by the scriptures. Physicians in the fourteenth and fifteenth centuries who decided that leprosy was contagious had to reach that conclusion in the face of powerful contrary evidence, particularly the frequent cases of lepers who did not pass on the disease to their spouses. Despite that evidence, by the fifteenth century lepers were being compelled to enter hospitals or leprosaria, and—more telling—expulsion from leprosaria for misconduct no longer occurred, as it had when the leprosarium was a place of devotional isolation; the leprosarium had become an isolation ward for contagion.[10]

Was there any hope of cure? Perhaps not much, but physicians certainly prescribed regimens that they hoped would attack leprosy's causes and palliate its symptoms. Diets should avoid acidic or salty foods, sex should be shunned (in fact some authorities urged castration), and the burnt humors (black bile and blood) should be purged. Folk remedies ("Take a bushel of good barley in the month of March, add half a bushel of toads") abounded. The leper might hope for miraculous intervention for a cure, but even that might be suspect. Both the Church and physicians looked askance on the claims of irregular or folk healers to cure leprosy, and such claims might be taken as prima facie evidence of witchcraft.

Without such a miracle, lepers faced a lifetime of isolation in the leprosaria. These institutions varied widely. Surviving regulations of the larger leper houses of the thirteenth and early fourteenth centuries suggest that some enjoyed good supplies of drink, food, and fuel. In some cases the property of the lepers was left untouched, so that their wealth accumulated in the leprosaria. But such cases were probably unusual. Even if the upper orders suffered disproportionately high rates of leprosy, the majority of medieval lepers were poor; while some rich lepers took advantage of high admission fees to use a leprosarium as a posh nursing home, lepers and leprosaria were too often the objects of charity, and that charity always depended shakily on the general level of prosperity. Lepers paid admission fees to the administration of the leprosarium, and brought their movable possessions; a particularly poignant detail was the requirement that lepers supply the wood and nails for their own coffins when they entered the leprosarium.[11] Most frequently small and poor leprosaria survived on the fees squeezed from their occupants and on uncertain local charity, customary dues, and payments in kind. Even when the leprosarium had some potential assets, the lepers did not control them: alms were collected by a "proctor," or administrative official; and, as some English law cases of the 1290s illustrate, those enjoying guardianship of a leper hospital might abuse their position and enrich themselves.[12]

Originally the leprosaria developed under Church control, but as the medieval centuries advanced lay political authorities assumed power over many of them. In some cases these institutions could be prisons for people declared legally dead. Lepers might lose ownership of their property as well as their rights to make contracts or to inherit, although such restrictions varied with time and place. Their property might in some cases devolve upon a seigneur. The position of spouses presented a legal and theological tangle; in some cases the spouse of a leper might be regarded as a widow and allowed to remarry, while in some leprosaria husbands and wives might both live, but often in quarters segregated by sex.[13]

The isolation of lepers in separate institutions might mean danger for them, for leprosaria collected an identifiable minority in one place.[14] On at least one disastrous occasion—in France in 1321—society turned on the lepers with fierce royal proscriptions and murderous local assaults. Wide-spread rumors, amounting to mass delusion, claimed that lepers, together with Jews and Muslims, were engaged in a plot to poison true Christians everywhere. The "plot" had the characteristic features of an imagined conspiracy by heretic outsiders: oaths, secret meetings, and significant blasphemous gestures such as spitting on the crucifix.

Jews and Muslims were traditional victims of the persecutions that followed such delusions, but Malcolm Barber also argues that the strains on medieval society in the early fourteenth century (to be discussed more thoroughly in Chapter Three), such as increasing famine and the growth of vagabondage, created a climate for "conspiracy" theories directed against a variety of outsiders or "closed" groups. The religious order of the Templars came under such an attack in France between 1307 and 1312, for example. The lepers, who lived in distinctive communities, whose physical repulsiveness was associated with moral failure, and who had already been the subjects of an accusatory process at the beginning of their isolation, were almost logical victims of such an outburst. People whose humors were so badly out of balance surely were capable of concocting magic poisons from the feet of toads. Lepers might also be involved in a more local social conflict. In the 1290s the lepers of West Somerton violently resisted the Prior of Butley who claimed that leprosarium property was his, not theirs; the lepers seized some goods and smashed some others, in a case that illustrated that the unclear legal position of lepers could lead to violence.[15]

But, as Brody suggests, the leprosaria could also serve as refuges from a hostile world. Some people actually asked to be adjudged lepers, perhaps to gain admission to such a haven, perhaps to gain what amounted to a license to beg. And the "hostility" of the world was in fact inconsistent, both in practice and in theory. The laws restraining lepers often simply didn't work, or were not enforced. Perhaps that was so, as both Brody and Palmer argue, because of ambivalent medieval religious attitudes toward leprosy. On the one hand the lepers were outcasts from society, morally corrupt, stigmatized by God because of their sins. Their appearance inspired repugnance.

But at the same time it was also widely believed that lepers had in some way been singled out for divine grace, the symbols of suffering for us all, the suffering that would lead sinners to repentance. Jesus had suffered too. Perhaps the idea that lepers were the chosen of God was simply offered as consolation, but many people believed it. Certainly pious people, from kings down, gave alms to lepers. This ambivalence may explain why so many lepers escaped confinement in their leprosaria and why so many medieval street scenes involve lepers freely wandering, begging, and wielding their sad clappers to warn the clean of their approach.

Estimates of morbidity or mortality from medieval leprosy are extremely problematic, as indeed are attempts to specify medieval populations as a whole. One source claims that some 19,000 leprosaria were founded in Europe in the Middle Ages.[16] Rotha Mary Clay, in her careful survey of English medieval hospitals, identified 222 hospitals for lepers, or leprosaria, founded in that country between the eleventh and the fourteenth centuries, but even that seemingly precise number tells us little about the total population affected.[17] Most of those foundations must have been very small; whatever the numbers affected by leprosy, no modern authorities have suggested that morbidity or mortality remotely approached that of plague in the mid-fourteenth century, and it is probable that other diseases such as tuberculosis took a greater toll on populations even at the height of the leprosy scares in the twelfth and thirteenth centuries.

Leprosy disappeared from Europe relatively suddenly (outside Scandinavia); its disappearance remains an enigma for historians of disease. It is tempting, for instance, to see a connection between the sudden appearance of plague in 1347–1350 and the rapid decline in leprosy coincident with it. Plague may have played a role in leprosy's decline, but that role was social and intellectual, not biological. Stephen Ell has shown that plague's biological effects on lepers cannot have been great, for leprosy apparently confers some immunity from plague.[18] But leprosaria were heavily dependent on the charity of others, charity both of gifts and of services. The short-term economic and social disruption caused by plague in 1347–1350 meant terrible hardship for lepers in their communities, and probably meant the failure of leprosaria as well as the scattering of their inhabitants and their subsequent physical weakening as a result of neglect and hunger. Plague, therefore, contributed to decreasing the incidence of leprosy by weakening the social network of care and thus increasing the mortality of lepers.

Changing intellectual conceptions of disease also influenced the perceived incidence of leprosy. As Demaitre argues, physicians came to have an increasing role in the diagnosis of leprosy. We may be persuaded by Danish bones that medieval leprosy really was leprosy, but some doubt remains that twelfth- and thirteenth-century village clerics always made an accurate diagnosis before they packed off a manor's nuisance to a leper "hospital." If Demaitre and others are right that by the fourteenth century physicians were both better at diagnosis and more involved in it, the number of "lepers" in the society might well have declined as a result of changing diagnostic procedures. Plague's appearance may have contributed to etiological thinking as well. As we shall see in Chapter Three, the universality of plague made it more difficult to sustain the notion that an *individual's* sin caused disease. The causal notions about leprosy began a gradual shift in the direction of contagionism, and hence may have passed out of the fevered comment of Church authorities.

William McNeill, in *Plagues and Peoples*, advanced the ingenious idea that the decline in leprosy was related both to plague and to syphilis.[19] His theory depends on a belief that "leprosy" was often misdiagnosed in medieval times, and that one of the diseases from which some "lepers" suffered was actually yaws, a relative of syphilis (see Chapter Four). Yaws, according to McNeill, may have been commonly spread in medieval Europe by skin contact, but the depopulation of the fourteenth century caused by plague resulted in a higher per capita income and a greater availability of clothing and bedding, which in turn decreased skin contacts in situations such as sleeping. Yaws eventually reemerged as a "new" disease, syphilis, in the late fifteenth century, having found a new skin-to-skin contact route, namely the venereal one. Some parts of this theory are more probable than others. Although plague did result in higher per capita income, and probably a greater availability of bedding, the theory depends on assuming a widespread medieval misdiagnosis; the paleopathological evidence for either yaws or syphilis in pre-fifteenth-century Europe is thin; and discussions of the cuddling habits of cold medieval Europeans remain very hypothetical.

A much stronger epidemiological case relates leprosy and tuberculosis. Those diseases are close bacteriological relatives, both the products of mycobacteria. At different points in history, both have created major social problems as chronic, debilitating diseases; the victims of both have been rejected or stigmatized by societies whose members have been unwilling or unable to care for the chronically ill and weak. The diseases apparently share some cross-immunity, more clearly from leprosy as a result of tuberculosis infection than the other way. Tuberculosis spreads much more rapidly and readily; it is far more contagious than leprosy. Tuberculosis is often contracted in childhood or infancy, and a person so infected would be an unlikely later victim of leprosy. Tuberculosis is also a disease that flourishes in dense human populations, so it has been argued that as Europe became more urban in the years between 1000 and 1300, it gradually provided more favorable conditions for the spread of tuberculosis. Indeed Keith Manchester has suggested that oscillations of tuberculosis and leprosy may follow levels of urban concentration: leprosy gradually displaced tuberculosis as the more urban civilization of Rome gave way to the profoundly rural early western Middle Ages, then gradually surrendered as urban life in the West emerged, bringing a revival of tuberculosis that intensified down into the nineteenth century.[20]

The part of the theory that relates a decline in leprosy to the growth of towns is attractive, but it cannot be a complete explanation for leprosy's disappearance, if only because medieval Europe always remained predominantly rural; the rise of its cities certainly had important historical effects, but their populations remained a minority on the Continent as a whole. It is interesting, however, that the lingering strongholds of leprosy in Europe were in thinly populated Scandinavia, Greece, and Portugal.

Leprosy serves as a touchstone for examining many medieval conceptions of disease. God, and God's anger at individual sin, was an important cause. Disease therefore stood as an important moral lesson. The Church claimed—and was granted by opinion—considerable authority, both in diagnosis and in therapeutics, for divine causes demanded sacred remedies. The ideas of the ancient Greeks, mediated by Arabic writings, formed another set of responses, some of which overlapped with the moral and divine interpretations of Christian belief and provided rationalization for it. Etiological ideas coexisted somewhat uncomfortably: disease might be attributed to contagion, heredity, individual responsibility, and divine whim; and those explanations have remained in uneasy yoke in the Western world since medieval times. Finally, disease—including both its causes and its cures—interacted with cultural beliefs and expectations. "Cures" may have "worked" because they were expected to work. Because leprosy was so closely related to sin and divine wrath, its "cures" remained largely in supernatural hands.

The Royal Touch

Very old connections exist between kingship and magic powers over nature; some of the earliest "kings" of ancient Near Eastern city-states may have achieved their political positions as a result of their exercise of magical healing powers. In the early centuries of Western history Roman, Germanic, and Christian sources all contributed to the notion of magical kingship: the Romans had founded cults that elevated emperors to divinity, even in their lifetimes; Germanic tribal rulers (or so it was believed) possessed powers over the crops and the weather; and when Germanic kings converted to Christianity they began associating themselves with the magical powers of that religion.

Early medieval kings could not rely on strong governmental institutions and hereditary traditions to compel obedience from their subjects. They might only enjoy success if they displayed "charismatic" powers, which they could if monarchy assumed a "sacral" character.[21] Thus the kings of the Franks began anointing themselves with holy oil in the seventh century; that custom was revived and strengthened in the ninth and tenth centuries in part because (according to Michel Rouche) the Church, faced with widespread social disintegration in an especially chaotic age, attempted to "stem the tide of anarchy by enhancing the concept of kingship."[22] In those centuries the line between secular and religious powers claimed by kings became blurred. Kings were regularly consecrated as a part of the ceremonies surrounding their coronations. Were kings endowed with priestly powers? Medieval kings certainly impressed their people with such powers: they took communion in both kinds (wine was ordinarily reserved for the ordained clergy), and they gave their armies signs of benediction. The pious Emperor Henry III (1039–1056) refused to laugh at jests, because canon law denied such pleasures to ecclesiastics.[23]

And aside from the confusions that might have arisen from theological practice, legends and popular beliefs surrounded monarchs and associated them with magic power. Upon the death of Halfdan the Black of Norway, his body was divided into four pieces and buried in different parts of the kingdom to ensure good harvests.[24] Emperor Otto I (936–975) rarely slept, or so a chronicler impressed by his watchful care of his realm believed.[25] True kings could always be determined by an identifying royal birthmark, or by the fact that lions respect royal blood; when in doubt about the true king, put the claimants in the lion's den and acclaim the survivor. Old children's stories such as "The Princess and the Pea" make the same point: royal blood is qualitatively different.

All Western medieval kings were surrounded by some measure of these concepts and powers. All pious kings also had a religious duty to be charitable to the sick, and that obligation strengthened in the eleventh, twelfth, and thirteenth centuries, as the ideals of the revived Western Church gained force. But some particularly saintly kings acquired reputations as healers, and their powers confirmed their sanctity. Two early such examples were Robert II ("the Pious") of France (996–1031) and, Edward ("the Confessor") of England (1042–1066); at such courts there existed "a narrow line between ministering to the sick and healing them."[26]

By the thirteenth century medieval kings—or at least some of them—had acquired other bases of authority in addition to the charismatic. Their powers might now be buttressed by judicial and financial bureaucracy; with such institutional authority, kings might be revered because of their secular abilities as governors. And institutional authority meant that a king's powers might be less dependent on his personal charismatic aura; just being the king was enough. Thus the mystique of kingship may have been transmuted, but it persisted. In two thirteenth-century courts it took quite specific thaumaturgic form: French and English kings asserted their particular power over the disease called scrofula, which was said to submit to the royal touch. This specific conviction grew out of both political factors and a persistent belief in supernatural powers that people—and especially kings—might manipulate. Scrofula is a disfiguring but rarely fatal ailment that manifests itself as putrid blotches on the skin of the face and neck. It is in fact a form of nonpulmonary tuberculosis that affects the lymph nodes, especially those in the neck. We now understand that scrofula is subject to frequent remissions, a fact that helps us understand the apparent success of the royal cures of the later Middle Ages.

As we have seen, all medieval kings surrounded themselves with some measure of supernatural power, and as Western civilization became more settled (in the period 1000–1200) kings deliberately associated themselves with ritual and practice that separated them from their subjects and thus magnified their authority. At the same time, however, the Western Church, and especially the papacy, embarked on a major assertive program of its own, denying sacramental and supernatural powers to lay authority and asserting that only the Church could intervene with divine will. In part the claims of the French and English kings to cure scrofula were political responses to papal "aggression," but the boundary between two other motives—a genuine belief in godlike powers and a cynical manipulation of credulous subjects—was not a clear one.

Marc Bloch, the French medieval historian, claimed (in *Le roi thaumaturge*, originally published in 1924) that the specific royal touch for scrofula began with Philip I of France (1060–1108) and Henry I of England (1100–1135), and he advanced plausible political reasons why that may have been so.[27] More recently, however, Frank Barlow has argued that available sources support such a specific association of royal powers and scrofula only in the late thirteenth century; before that time "royal sickness" expressed a broad category of disease identified not so much by symptoms as by a king's power over them.[28] It is possible that the specific claims about scrofula emerged from a process of trial and error with such maladies, as scrofula's self-remitting character seemed to confirm royal powers. Barlow believes that Louis IX of France (1226–1270), a particularly saintly monarch, may have initiated the touch for scrofula, and that the first clear French documents about the practice come from the reign of Philip IV (1285–1314). In England Henry III (1216–1272) probably started the touch, in imitation of Louis IX, and again clear documentation comes from his successor, Edward I (1272–1307). Although Barlow has convincingly revised Bloch's chronology, something of Bloch's original political argument stands, or at least may be applied to Barlow's thirteenth-century situation. Bloch noted that both Philip I and Henry I represented dynasties that might have been seen as usurpers, and the possession of supernatural powers of healing would obviously bolster their claims to legitimacy. God had sanctioned their rule. In the thirteenth century Henry III of England may have undertaken the practice of healing and thus "reconfirmed the monarchy after the disasters it had suffered since 1215," which included King John's surrender to his aristocracy in the Magna Carta.[29] Philip IV of France became embroiled in a tremendous struggle against the assertions of the papacy, a struggle that culminated in Philip's inspiration of a physical assault on Pope Boniface VIII; his use of the royal touch for scrofula may clearly have had a political purpose, for his political theorists argued vigorously against the upholders of the papal doctrine that royal miracles were invalid.

Touching for scrofula quickly became a ritual in both courts. The king laid his hands on the sufferer's afflicted parts, signed with the cross, and washed his hands in water that was then thought to have some healing power of its own. A coin was sometimes presented to the sufferer; the coin too might confer continuing therapeutic power, and receipt of it certainly helps explain the popularity of the rite. In the fourteenth century the English kings touched upward of five hundred of the afflicted per year: in France people came from all over that extensive realm to be touched. Sufferers from other parts of Europe journeyed to England or France to benefit from the touch. Further, both the French and the English monarchies experienced political crises in the fourteenth and fifteenth centuries, and times of dynastic instability or royal weakness brought more insistence on the power of the thaumaturgic king. One of the most vigorous proponents of the royal touch was Edward II of England (1307–1327), a generally unsuccessful king who was eventually murdered by his aristocracy. In order to shore up his crumbling power and prestige Edward II invented a legend of holy oil, and not only touched for scrofula but distributed rings that protected their wearers from epilepsy. Edward claimed that the miraculous powers inhered in his person, not in God's presence at the altar where the rites were performed.

So the healing touch was a product of political motives, at least in part. But it coincided with a widespread belief in kings as magicians, endowed with near-divine powers, and that in turn formed part of a more general belief in what Bloch called "a whole magical outlook on the universe." Magic played a large role in Europe in the Middle Ages, and not just then. We shall see repeated examples of its role in healing, especially in Chapter Five. Faith in supernatural powers persisted for centuries, and for some it persists still. But the royal touch for scrofula fell into discredit in part because many people stopped believing in what Bloch terms "the supernatural and the arbitrary." When the supernatural and the arbitrary came under heavy theoretical fire in the seventeenth and eighteenth centuries, the royal touch simultaneously lost credit.

Just as political factors partly accounted for the rise of the royal touch, so too did they figure in its demise. The division of Western Christianity that followed the Reformation had some political effect, for Catholics came to doubt the healing powers of the Protestant English kings and Protestants similarly doubted the Catholic French rulers. Internal religious divisions in both kingdoms led partisans to question the touch. Nevertheless Charles II of England (1660–1685) touched thousands; so too did James II (1685–1688), but in his reign the rite lost credibility because he blatantly associated it with his unpopular Catholicism. His successor William III (1688–1702) did not believe in the touch, and in any case was not a proper king by inheritance. The Hanoverian dynasty that succeeded after 1714 likewise had slim hereditary claims to such powers, and—unlike earlier monarchs who used the ritual to bolster their legitimacy—drew its support from parliamentary advisors determined to downplay such associations with a sacerdotal monarchy. The exiled Stuart pretenders kept touching their followers in the eighteenth century, to be satirized by both rationalist thinkers and the political followers of their Hanoverian rivals. Meanwhile in France Louis XIV (1643–1715) was a master of such rituals, but his successor Louis XV (1715–1774) was not. Increasingly criticized by the thinkers of the Enlightenment, the custom apparently died out under an Enlightenment king, Louis XVI (1774–1792), only to be reborn, fittingly, in the reign of the self-consciously medieval king Charles X (1824–1830), the last monarch in Western history to touch for scrofula.

The Medieval Disease Environment

By 1300 medieval Western civilization had changed almost beyond recognition from the poor, rural society that it had been four or five hundred years earlier. Cities had grown both in size and importance. Locally based political power, often of a very rough-and-ready sort, had given way to much more elaborate and centralized authority, with relatively sophisticated bureaucratic, taxing, and judicial machinery. An increasingly specialized economy of both rural raw materials and urban crafts, traded across impressive distances, had replaced local self-sufficiency. Arts and letters flourished in a culture that both recalled the triumphs of ancient civilization and embroidered a rich religious tradition.

This advancing civilization certainly assisted the health of its population in several generally important ways. Gradual agricultural change contributed to important nutritional shifts. At the beginning of the common era northern and western Europe was heavily forested and boggy, and some sections remained so for centuries. The Germanic and Slavic peoples who settled those lands slowly cleared and drained them, and gradually developed agricultural technology that took advantage of the northern soil and climate. From the sixth century the heavier plow, pulled by a larger team of animals (eventually including the powerful horse) exploited the rich soils of the north, while the "three-field" system provided for two growing seasons per year in the wetter climate. The Western civilization that emerged thus had the capability to grow more grain per acre than its Greco-Roman predecessor, and could ultimately sustain a larger population.

By the eleventh century the agriculture of the West could supply more calories to its people, although in other respects nutrition may have suffered. The northern diet that emerged in the years after the sixth century included more meat and dairy products, so it may have been richer in calcium and protein. But animal fats, especially butter, tended to replace vegetable oils, to the likely detriment of European cardiovascular systems. Fruits in the north played a smaller role than they did in the Mediterranean, and green vegetables were still few, despite the cultivation of peas and beans. Vitamin-deficiency diseases remained rampant: scurvy, rickets, beriberi, stunted growth, and eye trouble from lack of vitamin A. Maldistribution of wealth put too much food—especially meat—in the hands (and constipated digestions) of a few, and left the great majority heavily dependent on grain. Dependence on grain meant dependence on the weather; and although the period between about 700 and about 1200 was one of generally favorable climate, without variety of crops the failure of one crop in one season, whether from not enough rain or too much rain at the wrong time, meant physical hardship and hunger.

But despite these qualifications, improved agricultural technology and better security for both farmers and trade routes sustained a growing population with better nutrition—certainly more calories, and perhaps a greater variety of nutrients—at least until the middle of the thirteenth century, and in some places well into the fourteenth. The smoothly functioning Italian city-state of Siena still ate well into the 1340s. The stronger and surer hands of central political authority meant more than simply safer trade routes. The security of life in general was improved between the tenth century and the thirteenth, perhaps most notably for women. Our knowledge of medieval demographics is hampered by large lacunae in the evidence, but some data suggest that men may have considerably outnumbered women in early medieval centuries, perhaps because female infanticide was practiced and perhaps because conditions of life—including the hazards of childbirth, random violence, and a lesser share of scarce calories—bore more heavily on women.

In fact the centuries between roughly 400 and 1100 were unusually violent ones, and the character of violence in them differed from that of succeeding periods. Local political authorities, whose power seldom extended beyond a day's ride, dominated life. With a settlement of relatively thin density, and relatively little movement across distances, massive chains of infection were less likely; the infrequency of movement, whether stimulated by violence or trade, meant relatively little biological exchange. Too often, however, conditions approached political anarchy. Where order was maintained at all, it was enforced by bands of armed men who swore personal allegiance to the leader who promised to support and protect them. The lower orders remained almost entirely at the mercy of these rapacious gangs; brute force maintained the peasantry in poverty, a poverty whose inadequate nutrition opened the door for secondary infections and whose daily realities meant living quarters shared with animals and hence with microorganisms and disease vectors.

But in the "high Middle Ages," between about 1100 and about 1300, political power began to concentrate in fewer territorial hands, especially in western Europe. Kings and other rulers of substantial territories began bringing the local lords and their violent henchmen under control. A knight with his own landed estate might be beholden to no one, but an armored soldier equipped and paid by royal coin had less independence. To the extent that some twelfth- and thirteenth-century kings were thus able to impose some form of "law" on their armed retainers, those centuries were more peaceful ones.

Reinforcing royal efforts in those centuries were both a growing commercial population that desired protection from piracy and brigandage and a powerful institutional church that wished to rein in the casual violence. The Western Church, from an increasingly strong political position, gradually persuaded brutal lords and their followers that gentleness, especially with the relatively helpless, might be a more effective key to the kingdom of heaven than violence. Women were beginning to live longer than men, and their proportion of the population increased. The Church suggested another key as well: charity. An outpouring of philanthropy occurred in the high Middle Ages, a movement that founded a vast number of institutions for the care of the sick and the poor. However ineffective or corrupt such institutions might have been, their sheer number is striking, as the figure of 19,000 leprosaria testifies.

A more formal medicine emerged in those centuries as well. Physicians received a "professional" education in the universities, and this training brought them into contact with (above all) the traditions of Galenic medicine, anatomy, and physiology, often as mediated by Arabic authors. Physicians thus joined the clerics and those learned in the law as the educated professionals, whose learning carried certification. And their formal medical practice was at least partially based on tenets of human reason; supernatural explanations may have still predominated, but they might now be employed to explain final or ultimate causes, not proximate ones.

Formal medicine's impact was mixed, however. The numbers of practitioners remained small; although modern scholars have identified a surprising number of such physicians, I will argue in Chapter Five that for most medieval people physicians were only a small part of a wide spectrum of healing alternatives. Although Galenic medicine had many impressive features, it still lacked satisfactory principles of either etiology or therapeutics; leprosy illustrated its fundamental impotence, and plague, as we shall see in Chapter Three, would overwhelm it. At the same time formal medicine began its long attack on other, competing, forms of health care, attempting to drive out traditional folk healers whose trial-and-error remedies might have had some validity.

The growth of cities and of trade was not an unmixed blessing for health, either. Medieval cities became intensely crowded and intensely dirty. Medieval people bathed because it gave them sensual pleasure, not because it made them "clean."[30] Provisions for fresh water and sewage removal fell considerably short of those of the Romans. Vermin infested the population. And regardless of sanitation, or lack of it, the mere crowding of the population in cities presented opportunities for some diseases to spread. If the lack of sanitation meant high levels of intestinal infections—diarrhea, dysentery, typhoid fever—the crowds meant tuberculosis, influenza, smallpox, measles, and (dramatically in 1347–1350) plague. Another measure of "progress" intervened as well: the frequency and complexity of trade and travel. By the late medieval and early modern centuries, as will be apparent in Chapters Three and Four, Western civilization took part in what William McNeill calls the sharing of disease pools. Plague spread rapidly through fourteenth-century Europe; typhus and syphilis did the same in the sixteenth century, although they might have already had an earlier foothold; smallpox rapidly moved from Europe to the Americas. The European population grew prodigiously between 1000 and 1250 in part because it could shelter within a still-isolated biological environment; its growth, and that of its "civilization," ended that isolation.

Leprosy made clear some of medieval civilization's limitations in the face of disease, particularly its inadequate etiology and therapeutics, its association of disease with the divine will, and its association of disease with the sins of individuals and groups. The arrival of plague in the fourteenth century further illustrated those weaknesses, which were then paradoxically magnified by the greater complexity and sophistication of an increasingly urban world.

Three

The Great Plague Pandemic

1347-1353 *30-60% of Europe died*

The most serious epidemic outbreak in Western history began in Sicily in October 1347. Between that date and the end of 1353 most of Europe was affected. The disease most likely responsible was the plague, apparently in both its bubonic and its pneumonic forms. In the course of this massive epidemic between 30 and 60 percent of Europe's population died, a nearly inconceivable human disaster. The event—much later and for unclear reasons called the Black Death— had a profound impact on the imagination of the time, and has attracted considerable historical attention in recent decades. What caused the epidemic? Where did it come from? Where it go, and how did it spread? Was the Western society of the 1340s ripe for such a catastrophe? What did medieval people make of the epidemic? What did they do about it? What were its consequences? And finally, why and when did plague cease its hold on the West? All these questions have generated historical controversy and will repay careful review.

Plague

Plague is caused by a microorganism, *Yersinia pestis* (or as it was formerly known, *Pasteurella pestis*), parasitic in various burrowing rodents. The microorganism is carried from rodent to rodent most frequently by fleas, which bite infected rodents and then carry the bacteria to other rodents. Many rodents may carry plague, including marmots, ground squirrels, and prairie dogs, but the rodent most often involved with human epidemics has been the rat, and especially the so-called black rat *(Rattus rattus)*, an adept climber that is particularly at home in human dwellings. Plague may remain enzootic (that is, endemic among animals) in a population of rodents for a long time. If it reaches epizootic intensity (that is, becomes epidemic) the larger number of animal deaths will

37

increase the number of their accompanying fleas who will seek new hosts. Those fleas may become vectors—carriers that convey an infectious agent from one host to another. In the case of the black rat, the rat flea *(Xenopsylla cheopis)* is a frequent vector, but other flea species may play a role, including (although this is controversial) the human flea *(Pulex irritans)*. The new host may—perhaps only by chance—be a human.

When a flea transmits the microorganism to a human, the form of plague called "bubonic" results, a disease that apparently depends on a continuing epizootic of infected rodents during which humans inadvertently get in the path of a rodent-flea-rodent transmission. Plague may, however, pass from one human to another. Some authorities believe that the human flea, *Pulex irritans*, sometimes carries *Yersinia pestis* bacilli between people, making the spread of bubonic plague possible without the constant necessity of an epizootic rodent reservoir. And all agree that the pneumonic form of plague requires no vector. Pneumonic plague occurs when *Yersinia pestis* settles in the lungs, and from there spreads by drops of saliva into the respiratory tracts of others. Pneumonic plague was almost certainly an important element in the great epidemic that began in 1347, but the fact that it is almost invariably and rapidly fatal limits its power of diffusion, for its victims perish before they travel far or contact many others.

Many questions persist about the identification of the microbe responsible for the great "plague" of 1347–1353. Some of those questions focus on its apparent epidemiology. How could an epidemic on the scale of the 1347–1353 events be generated by accidental encounters with fleas that generally have little interest in human hosts? How could the epidemic spread so rapidly across a subcontinent when it depended on populations of infected rodents that move from place to place only very slowly? To drive so many fleas to seek human hosts, rats must have died in immense numbers; why didn't contemporaries notice an unusual pile of dead rats? On the basis of such questions some biologists, epidemiologists, and historians have argued either that the disease of those years cannot have been plague, or that (if it was plague) the generally accepted mortality figures must be highly exaggerated.[1]

Such arguments, however persuasive, fly in the face of considerable historical documentation of both the extent of the disaster and the symptoms of the disease. Bubonic plague manifests itself most dramatically in "buboes," the large, hard, painful swellings in the groin, armpit, or neck that form when the infection reaches the lymphatic system. Devastating symptoms rapidly ensue: a rapid rise of body temperature, delirium for some and stupor for others, and progressive failure of vital organs as the microbe reaches them. Death follows in three to five days for about 60 percent of those infected. Death from pneumonic plague is even more swift and certain, occurring in less than three days. Many contemporary accounts of the Black Death and from subsequent later visitations of the disease vividly describe these symptoms.[2] While the meaning of fourteenth-century testimony about disease (from authors whose mind-sets were quite different from ours) is always open to interpretation, much contemporary evidence supports a diagnosis of *Yersinia pestis* infection; the repeated references to buboes are particularly persuasive.

Some of the epidemiological improbabilities posed by *Yersinia pestis* may be overcome if: (1) we grant the importance of pneumonic plague as a massive killer in some populous localities; (2) we consider the possible role of the human flea (*Pulex irritans*) as a human-to-human vector; (3) we remember that while rats may not move very far or very fast on their own, they frequently ride with human travelers both by land and sea; (4) we similarly realize that fleas can carry plague microbes for considerable times and distances, while living in grain, textiles, and other goods; (5) and we argue that fourteenth-century witnesses didn't record the deaths of rats because they had no reason to think that fact important.

In addition, alternative explanations—anthrax, typhus, an unknown "hemorrhagic virus" or some other now unknown infection—have their own weaknesses. Difficulties have been raised with each; for instance, the patchy distribution of the victims of the Black Death seems more consistent with an insect-borne disease than with a airborne virus, and anthrax simply doesn't pass from person to person in any way.[3] It may be that (as Ann Carmichael has argued) the vast mortalities of 1347–1353 (and later) resulted from a number of diseases acting in tandem, with plague their greatest but not sole killer.[4]

Could the causative organism of the Black Death be identified by molecular biology? Procedures now allow the accurate sequencing of DNA from small quantities of surviving soft tissue, and some such tissue has been recovered from dental pulp. Results have to date been inconclusive, and hotly debated. At least some samples from, for example, 1348 Montpellier seem to reveal the presence of *Yersinia pestis*. But even if so, that would at most prove that *some* fourteenth-century deaths were due to plague, not that millions were. On balance, it seems that *Yersinia pestis*, for all its epidemiological uncertainty, remains the "least lousiest" solution to the puzzle of the Black Death. It may not be conclusive, but it is better than the alternatives.[5]

If *Yersinia pestis* was the chief culprit in the Black Death, then the ecologies of rodents and fleas form important parts of the history of the pandemic. Fleas are sensitive to climatic variations and flourish only within certain ranges of temperature and humidity. Generally they find those conditions in summer months, which may account for the particular severity of bubonic plague in the summers of 1348 and 1349. But fleas may also find ideal conditions both within rodent burrows and in human clothing and bedding, so that epizootics may persist year-round in rodent colonies and risks may persist for humans in all seasons. In the fourteenth century the dominant rat of Europe was *Rattus rattus*, or the black rat, exceptionally companionable with humans and their dwellings; the characteristic European materials of domestic construction—wood, wattle-and-daub, and thatch—made comfortable homes for rats and fleas alike. And while fourteenth-century Europe had some densely populated cities, where large numbers of people constituted a critical mass for infections, we should remember that the great majority of the population was rural. For that reason an important epidemiological consideration was the density of rat and flea populations, greater (especially in proportion to the human population) in rural settlements. Rats especially gathered around grain stocks and grain mills, whence human traffic also moved. Plague therefore posed many dangers to rural communities, which may have suffered as much or more than cities.[6]

The Path of the Black Death

The course of the 1347–1353 epidemic has been well authenticated, although its point of origin remains uncertain. Various areas in central or western Asia have been proposed, without any conclusive evidence. In any case, the disease spread across the Asian steppes in the 1330s and was then carried by ship from the Crimea to Sicily in 1347. Alexandria and Constantinople also faced the disease that autumn, and before the year's end plague had gained footholds in Italian ports (notably Pisa, Venice, and Genoa) as well as southern France (Marseilles) and the coast of Dalmatia. After the end of 1347, plague spread across Europe by both land and sea; thus it reached Florence (by land) and the Aragon coast (by sea) in early 1348, much of the rest of Italy by that spring, and southern France in the spring and summer. Northern Spain was also infected, in part from Bordeaux by way of the sea. By late in the summer of 1348, plague had come by sea to England's south coast, Ireland's east coast, and northern France, while it gradually spread overland from Italy into southern Germany in the same year. In the course of 1349, plague's spread continued from the south and west into central Germany and the Danube valley; into northern England and the rest of Ireland; and by sea to western Scandinavia and some points on the Baltic coast. By 1350 Scotland, Sweden, Denmark, and northern Germany had plague; in 1351, eastern Baltic lands; and in 1352 and 1353 plague reached first western Russia and Ukraine, and then Muscovy. The epidemic had therefore completed a clockwise circuit through Europe, from the Black Sea into the Mediterranean, then from southern and western Europe into northern and eastern parts. The regions first affected (the Crimea) and last affected (Muscovy) were not that far apart.

A few anomalous pockets of land remained relatively free of plague: the largest of these was Bohemia and part of Poland, and some cities elsewhere escaped with lower mortality, notably Milan, Nuremberg, Liège, and some towns of Flanders and Brabant. Many different factors may have lain behind their comparative immunity. Plague spread in its bubonic form in the summer months, when fleas flourished in the air as well as in burrows and bedding; if bubonic plague appeared in a town in the spring or early summer, its epizootic reservoir in the local rodent community might be exhausted in a few months and the rate of infection of humans might then rapidly decline. Such a pattern repeated itself in many European towns, which suffered three months of devastating bubonic plague and then relief. But if bubonic plague only began in the late summer, a town might then face the horror of pneumonic plague in the fall and winter, as plague intersected with pneumonia and other respiratory ailments that flourished in cold, damp climates and spread through populations confined indoors. So differential mortalities may have depended on the timing of the plague's arrival. And—as we shall see—human actions may have moderated the plague's impact on some towns.

Europe before the Black Death

This great epidemic made its way across a Europe whose social and economic stability, and the very health of its inhabitants, had been weakening in the earlier years of the fourteenth century. When we consider plague as an agent of social change, that weakness must be kept in mind. Not all the disasters of the fourteenth century can be ascribed to the epidemic, and the preplague condition of the society helps explain the epidemic's course.

Europe's population perhaps doubled between 1000 and 1300, driven in part by the agricultural technology discussed in Chapter Two. But by the end of that time, and perhaps even before 1300, the society's ability to produce food may have reached an upper limit for the available technology. Growing cities, for example, had become increasingly dependent on food supplies imported from greater and greater distances; their vulnerability to famine increased accordingly, for too many fragile links existed in the medieval transportation chains that brought food to cities. New lands pressed into cultivation in the thirteenth century were often marginal ones, whose productivity—never good—could fall quickly. Soil erosion became more and more serious. David Herlihy's studies of the Italian town of Pistoia between 1240 and 1350 illustrate that by the beginning of that period the area was already badly overcrowded, and that during the subsequent century the population declined, as social and economic factors that discouraged population growth accumulated in Pistoia.[7] Certainly Pistoia was not alone in suffering repeated bad crops and famines in the years before 1348. The years from 1315 to 1317 were perhaps the most serious famine time in European medieval history, begun by two seasons of heavy rainfall and cold temperatures in 1314–15; by 1316 grain stocks in many places were exhausted. In five months in 1316 the Flemish town of Ypres lost 10 percent of its population.

How important was lack of adequate calories for the spread of an epidemic such as plague? In some broad sense it can be argued—as Robert Malthus did and as more recently Thomas McKeown has done—that inadequate food supply has worked together with unrestrained human fertility to hold human populations in a grip of scarcity, one that has only relented in the last two hundred years in the West.[8] In this view inadequate nutrition causes high levels of mortality, above all because the poorly nourished more easily fall prey to infections. Against this attractive hypothesis some difficulties have, however, been raised. It is not clear that infections *do* prey more easily on the poorly nourished. Microorganisms need a certain level of nourishment too, and the cells and tissues of the starving may not provide it. Infections may develop more successfully in hosts who are only slightly malnourished, not severely so.[9] Some infectious epidemics illustrate that victims may be the healthy and well-fed; the great influenza pandemic of 1918–19 resulted in particularly high mortalities for healthy young adults. Plague's incidence may have had little relation to the nutritional health of its victims. What may have been more important, Ann Carmichael argues, is that "secondary infections"—pneumonia piling on top of a primary infection such as plague or influenza—struck poorly nourished people who were more quickly weakened by the simultaneous assault of several microbes.

But other consequences followed such episodes as the 1315–1317 famines. Extended periods of malnutrition weakened the population, perhaps had a depressing effect on the birth rate (if only for psychological reasons), and certainly increased infant mortality, which in turn changed the later age structure of the population in a way that adversely affected productivity. Witnesses testified to increased geographical mobility, as the hungry repaired to cities and monasteries that might have grain stocks. Their departure removed field hands and thus further weakened agricultural output. Such rural migration also broke down the isolation of villages, promoting the possible spread of contagious disease. The preplague world in Europe was one in which food was scarce and hence expensive, land was in short supply and hence also expensive, and labor, being plentiful, was cheap. But the evidence (from Pistoia, for example) suggests that the overpopulated world of 1300 was already losing people before the great epidemic, so that while the plague may have exaggerated changes, it did not initiate them.

Medieval Opinions

What did medieval people make of this epidemic? In their view, what caused it? For most of those who thought about that question, divine wrath provided the most satisfactory general answer. Other causes were often cited, but for most writers such other reasons were "secondary," explaining how plague came in a particular time or place. Only God's wrath could explain such a comprehensive disaster. Furthermore, God's anger did not in this case fall on particular sinners, as was the case with leprosy. The scale of the plague suggested rather that the whole civilization, or the whole human race, was being punished.

The general social and economic hardships of the previous hundred years gave such arguments credence: man had sinned, the judgment of God was at hand. Millenarian expectations were close to the surface already; they had emerged in Italy around 1260, and the great epidemic would call them forth again.

Within the general framework of a heaven-sent scourge, medieval thinkers offered a number of more immediate causes, and on the basis of those causes proposed (or put into effect) some remedies. At the head of the list of such immediate causes was "bad air," the official doctrine of the medical faculties of some universities, where it was integrated with Galenic theory. Hot, moist air, putrified (ultimately by God's action, to be sure), entered the lungs and caused a blood disorder. Plague resulted. But if widespread agreement existed on the role of bad air, great disagreement ensued about the source of that air. Some found its origins in the heavens; thus the Sorbonne cited an unfortunate conjunction of the planets that engendered bad air. Eclipses, always regarded as grave astronomical events, were another possibility. Comets—sublunary phenomena in the dominant Ptolemaic astronomy—were likely disturbers of sublunary air. For some the moon influenced the stages of the plague, as it seemed to affect other periodic human physical events such as menstruation. Others maintained that "plutonic," not astronomical, forces produced bad air: corruption poured from openings in the earth such as volcanoes. Sicily, with both Mount Etna and early cases of plague, was especially suspect. Or perhaps the bad air merely accompanied a variety of natural cataclysms; the Sorbonne instanced earthquakes as "provoking an unaccountable abundance of frogs and reptiles."[10] Bad air as well as frogs might result from such disturbances.

But for many medieval people such causal explanations were too "natural"; they preferred to see supernatural beings: angels or demons, the small blue flame in the sky seen in Düsseldorf in 1348, the witchlike apparition called "la Mère Peste" or "l'Ulcéreuse."[11] With explanations such as these we enter a murky area between environmental and contagionist explanations of disease. Does God send the small blue flame to pass plague from one individual to another (contagion), or to infect the entire atmosphere (environmental)? When individuals ("l'Ulcéreuse") were specified in the transmission process, contagion was close at hand, despite the universities and their bad air. Certainly European cities and people reacted almost instinctively as though they accepted contagionism. In 1347 Catanians attempted, without success, to keep those fleeing Messina out of Catania, and in 1348–1350 their efforts at quarantine were many times repeated all over Europe. In fact European thinking about the plague did not fall into clear categories of "contagionism" or "environmental cause." Europeans accepted God's power as the primary cause and saw that power working in many ways. Bedeviled by guilt, they saw humankind as a whole as provoking divine wrath; perhaps reacting in fear and denying their individual guilt, they blamed other individuals, either because those people had sinned or because they maliciously and deliberately spread disease. Lepers and Jews, both groups outside the framework of Christian society, were likely candidates for such accusations. So too were domestic animals.

Part of the pattern of causal explanation involved not just God's mechanism (bad air, bad individuals, bad animals), but also the victim's propensity for the disease. It was perhaps not satisfying enough to say simply that God was scourging the human race; had some individuals made themselves susceptible by their actions or their temperaments? Galenic theory generally viewed plague as a blood disorder, and some physical types seemed prone to diseases related to that humor: fat, florid people, and the sensually hot-blooded, especially women. As in the case of leprosy, the fornicator was a likely victim, perhaps as a sinner who displeased God, perhaps as a fool who sapped his strength; for men especially, sex was thought to weaken the constitution. Some thought revolved around questions of age, social class, or profession. The rich—especially the very rich and powerful—seemed less susceptible; physicians, surgeons, apothecaries, and members of religious orders were thought vulnerable. Others believed in a "natural predisposition," or a hereditary propensity for the disease, consistent with some Hippocratic traditions.

Out of these varying theories of cause—operating within the grand general cause of God's wrath—came medieval responses and remedies. The scale of the disaster was quickly appreciated and gave rise to widespread panic and flight, the latter of course easier for the rich than for the poor. Omens were consulted. Belief in God's anger led to numerous local attempts to propitiate the divine rage. Town after town held religious ceremonies and processions. Cities resolved to build new churches. Legislation attempted to enforce a purer morality on the populace, as in Siena where the city government outlawed gambling in an attempt to win divine favor, or in Tournai where swearing was forbidden and cohabiting couples were ordered to marry. In some dramatic cases groups of individuals took on themselves the sins of society and hoped by their suffering to assuage God's anger. That response was most vivid in the processions of the Flagellants that moved through the towns of Germany and the Netherlands. The Flagellants were among the most striking manifestations of medieval millenarianism; they came to see themselves as armies of saints whose very blood had redemptive power, as they not only assumed the burden of humanity's sins, but through their suffering (in their self-flagellation) assumed Jesus' role as redeemer.

But the plague came anyway. Probably the gathering of city populations in processions and religious ceremonies offered more opportunities for contagion, as would the enthusiastic war bond rallies in the midst of the World War I influenza epidemic. Many responses were based on a more "natural" explanation of the disease's cause. Many people believed in some type of contagion, regardless of official "bad air" environmentalist doctrine. Port cities refused to allow ships with plague victims to land. Pistoia imposed quarantines on the movement of people and goods. Bodies of the victims were shunned, thrown over town walls, hastily buried in mass graves while their clothes were burnt. Dogs and cats, possible bearers of contagion, were massacred, allowing the rats more license. Belief in bad air led some to flee to the pure mountains; an extreme (and well-known) example of a search for good air was afforded by Pope Clement VI, who barricaded himself, surrounded by fires, in his palace in Avignon. He survived. Measures of public health—quarantines, burning the clothes of the sick, disposing of bodies outside town walls—might also be the outcome of a "bad air" theory, if clothes or bodies were thought to produce the corruption.

Immediate Effects

The immediate effects of the plague on communities varied, although mortality was high in most places affected by the disease. Studies of particular places in the midst of the epidemic leave different impressions. In some places the fabric of the social order seems to have been surprisingly resilient; after a few months' interruption, city government resumed its functions, men of the professions went about their business, and social order was consistently maintained. In other cases communities embarked on frenzied searches for scapegoats, and grave social revolution threatened. Almost all communities apparently ground to a halt for a few months. Thus Siena's economic and political activity largely ceased in June, July, and August 1348: the woolen cloth industry stopped working, olive oil imports ceased, and the city's courts recessed, while the government ordered religious processions and ended legalized gambling. Fields in the surrounding countryside were neglected, animals wandered uncared-for, and mills closed. From Perpignan in April, May, and June 1348 the only legal documents that survive are wills; other legal or political business apparently simply stopped.

Modern historical studies of Siena, Perpignan, Pistoia, and Orvieto all suggest that after a few months political and legal machinery once again functioned, and that at least in some cases city governments tried to assist their populations in coping with the disaster. In Perpignan the persistence of will-making even at the height of the epidemic was impressive; a will written by professionals, with witnesses, was a "fairly sophisticated document, representing a rather high level of social organization" that did not break down in panic.[12] When the worst months passed, legal documents reappeared in full flower, and their character reveals a community rebuilding itself: there were again estate settlements, disputes among heirs, restorations of dowries, and apprenticeship contracts as new workers were recruited to fill gaps in trades. The finances of the city government of Siena recovered rapidly, as the governing council successfully raised taxes and imposed forced loans, all of which met the higher demands of the city's mercenary army. Individuals who had fled the city began returning, and the city government attempted to assist the reconstruction of the rural hinterland of Siena: taxation of hard-hit villages was remitted and rent payments were canceled. A city government that could actually boast of a budget in balance, as Siena could do in 1353, was hardly a demoralized or disorganized community; a balanced government budget in Siena, according to William Bowsky, rarely happened even in prosperous times.[13] The government of Orvieto was perhaps less effective than that of Siena, but there too the council resumed its regular meetings and appointed new city employees.[14]

Similarly mixed evidence comes from rural communities in England, where several locales have been studied. In some respects agricultural activity, like its urban counterpart, came to a near halt during the three or four months in which plague peaked. Many landholdings were vacated by either the death or the flight of the tenants; mills fell into disuse, buildings deteriorated, and livestock wandered unsupervised. Rural societies might depend heavily on the management skills of a bailiff or other agent; a very high turnover of management positions occurred in the manors of Cuxham, near Oxford, between 1349 and 1359.[15] A cleric's death might also unhinge a village, and many English studies document the high mortality of the clergy.[16] Yet in Midlands manorial society, legal procedures and their routines were maintained (as they were in Perpignan), even though those procedures for a time concentrated almost wholly on the registration of deaths, conveyances of vacant holdings, and wardships arising from the great epidemic.[17]

But while communities showed considerable resilience in the face of human calamity, social and political systems did suffer shocks that manifested themselves in later years. Siena provides a good illustration. The epidemic apparently furthered a considerable social and economic upheaval there, involving newly emerging rich and newly created poor. The new rich showed their political power by ending monopolies enjoyed over tax-farming by a narrow circle of bankers. The city government, alarmed by the new rich and their ways, passed sumptuary legislation to limit their fancy-dress display. While new wealth vied with an established oligarchy, new citizens flocked into the city, encouraged by the government's immigration policies. Political tensions between these groups intensified, and the existing government (the Council of the IX) was unable to defuse them. In 1355 a revolution overthrew the IX, thus ending seventy years of continuous oligarchic domination. In Bowsky's view the great epidemic served not so much as the immediate disrupter of society as the catalyst that set in train or accelerated larger social and economic effects.

Long-Term Effects

When we extend the question of effects over the balance of the fourteenth century and into the fifteenth, more complications arise. How rapidly did the population of Europe recover its pre-1300 level? Did the depression in population have major effects on wages, prices, land tenures? Did productive processes or land uses change? Were authorities—ecclesiastical, political, intellectual—called into question? Clear answers to all those questions are difficult, but the great epidemic certainly had some weight in all such issues.

First, the Black Death of 1347–1353 seriously reduced the population of Europe. Mortality may have ranged from 30 to 60 percent, in some places higher, in some places lower. But the plague's impact on the European population did not end in 1353. Although controversy continues about just when the population began to grow again, much local evidence suggests that repeated visitations of plague in the years after 1353 contributed to holding populations down. The population of Cuxham in 1377 had reached only one-third of its 1348 level.[18] Many writers, in fact, see no real recovery of growth in the European population until the end of the fifteenth century. For this remarkable period of declining or stagnant populations the plague bears at least some responsibility. Once plague established itself in the 1340s it remained an almost constant menace for over three hundred years, in what may be properly called a prolonged plague pandemic. Jean-Noël Biraben has compiled tables which claim that plague was present somewhere in Europe every year between 1347 and 1670.[19] The most serious and widespread episodes followed on the heels of the great Black Death; thus the epidemics of the early 1360s and middle 1370s, though overshadowed by the 1347–1353 catastrophe, rank as demographic disasters in their own right. Such massive after-shocks hampered the recovery of population levels late in the fourteenth century; and although the intervals between major plague waves seemed to have lengthened in the fifteenth and sixteenth centuries, the disease could still be a powerful brake on growth in some localities.

The social and economic consequences of the great decline in population between the mid-fourteenth and the late fifteenth centuries have been much discussed, and some points remain controversial. As we have seen, Europe in the early 1300s manifested many signs of a society with cheap labor and expensive land. To some extent the Black Death reversed that picture; Europe, now population-short, experienced rising labor costs and falling land costs. Especially in western Europe, the drastic depopulation forced landlords to lower rents, to replace fixed-term rents with share-cropping arrangements, to offer higher wages for agricultural labor, and to commute the traditional labor services demanded of peasants by lords. Considerable regional variation in such effects could be found; in some cases, for example, deaths among the tenantry enabled landlords to let out lands on new terms that freed them from long-term customary arrangements favorable to a tenant family.[20] But in many places in western Europe the lives of peasants improved as the obligations of manorialism fell away. Emmanuel LeRoy Ladurie's classic study of the peasants of Languedoc shows them enjoying the results of abundant and cheap land and high wages in the second half of the fourteenth century and the fifteeenth century.[21]

For many European landowners the serious depopulation of 1347–1353 created problems: lower rent receipts, a shortage of tenants, perhaps higher wages to pay, perhaps lower prices for the produce of their lands as demand for those products fell. Landlords had several options. They could join employers everywhere in attempts to hold wages down by statutes that could be enforced with state power, or to use other legislative or judicial means to control labor (such as restricting the laborers' geographical mobility). Several European states adopted such measures in the years after 1348—for example, the English Statute of Labourers of 1349—and serious social and political grievances often resulted.

Another possibility for the landowner was greater efficiency. Labor apparently became more productive, if only because (in agriculture) it was possible to abandon the cultivation of marginal lands and concentrate on richer soils. Still other landlords converted their fields from arable to pasture and thus reduced their labor costs. That point relates to a subtle but significant shift: that in the years after the great epidemic, what we may loosely call "luxury" products and crops prospered, at least in relation to more "staple" items.[22] Several likely factors combined to cause this trend. Survivors of the Black Death possessed greater per capita wealth than they enjoyed before 1348, for such sources of wealth as land, tools, or plate did not vanish in the same proportion as the people who shared them. Survivors also perhaps enjoyed marginally higher incomes, if land costs fell while wages rose. With both greater wealth and greater income came marginally higher disposable income, and items that had been unimaginable luxuries might become desirable possibilities.

Producers—large and small—might respond to this new situation. The demand for grain products fell with the fall in population; half the population will not eat twice the bread it had eaten even if the price falls in half (that is, the demand for such "necessities" as bread is relatively inelastic, or constant regardless of price). The years after 1348 were therefore difficult for producers of grain, caught between higher labor costs and declining absolute demand for their products. For some, the answer lay in the production of goods for which demand might be more elastic, goods that appealed to the new wealth and higher level of disposable income. And so in Spain and England the importance of pasture for wool increased. More land, proportionally, was also given over to crops from which drink could be made: barley for beer in England and Germany, grapes for wine in France, northern Italy, and southern Germany. More varied fruits and vegetables appeared, especially in France and Spain, while the demand grew for exotic substances such as sugar. Crops from which industrial materials came prospered: dyestuffs, flax and hemp, mulberry trees (for silkworms). Meanwhile, areas that had lived by the export of grain, such as Sicily and southern Italy, suffered hard times. Finally, the position of smallholding peasants in this changed market might be mixed; as subsistence farmers they benefited from lower land costs, but as producers for a market they might lose.

The Black Death and subsequent plague assaults may have eased the lives of surviving peasants in western Europe, making their land cheaper, increasing their wages, and decreasing the traditional labor services expected of them. But the general experience of the peasantry of eastern Europe should make us wary of the power of the plague as an overwhelming historical cause. At least in theory the same change in the positions of laborers and landlords occurred there, although it is possible that the plague's incidence and hence mortality was lower in eastern Europe. Perhaps more eastern peasants survived, but that point remains speculative; certainly the position of the eastern landlords strengthened. They seized opportunities that made the east increasingly the supplier of large-scale agricultural products to the more developed western European economies. A different political milieu made it possible for landowners to tighten the bonds of serfdom on the large estates on which they pursued those profitable activities. Disease and its resulting depopulation is clearly not the single determinant of social, economic, and political change.

The industries of towns likewise found a different climate in the post-plague era. Without doubt the great epidemic caused tremendous short-run disruption, as the social mechanisms of markets, transportation, money institutions, and production collapsed in varying degree; a sudden dearth of artisans, or merchants, or seamen might each bring their trade to a standstill, with effects that rippled through an entire local economy. In the somewhat longer term, urban industries shared some—but not all—of the circumstances that affected the rural economy. A peasant in the countryside could benefit immediately from more or better land after 1348; an urban artisan did not have those advantages. Productivity of urban crafts may have declined per capita, at least temporarily, owing to the loss of hard-to-replace skills. But some evidence suggests that such a decline was very temporary, and that both productivity and prices rose in the years after 1350. For that prosperity both demand for manufactured goods and greater efficiency of production may have been responsible. The same factors that promoted the sale of "luxury" agricultural products also applied to manufactures; with more disposable income, consumers demanded more clothing (or fancier clothing, involving silks and dyestuffs) and the products of skilled artisans. Not all manufacturers profited; wool cloth made in Florence declined relative to the luxurious silk, and hard times for some artisans (also facing competition from wool producers elsewhere) resulted. Certainly contemporary observers noticed that conspicuous consumption was a common reaction among survivors of the Black Death.

In the century after the great epidemic, Europe embarked on one of its seminal periods of technological innovation. The sternpost rudder and the ship outfitted

with both square-rigged and lateen sails expanded the possibilities of ocean navigation, and Europeans simultaneously adopted compasses from Asian civilizations. By about 1450 the various technologies involved in printing by movable
type had been brought together. In the 1400s the use of firearms made headway;
what in the 1300s had been a battlefield curiosity became before the end of the
1400s a decisive weapon of war. These technological changes are dramatic and
well known, but others of great importance also appeared in the late 1300s and
the 1400s. Especially significant were the spinning wheel and the rapid spread of
such instruments of power as water- and windmills (especially the latter) in
industrial processes. In some manner we may see all of these technological
changes as "labor saving," whether printing presses that save the labor of copy-
ists, mills that save the labor of fullers, or cannon that save the labor of battering-
ram carriers. Is it too much to wonder whether the scarcity of labor in the century
after 1350 encouraged such innovations?

Plague and the European Spirit

The great epidemic had serious consequences for "authority" in several
respects. The landed class had dominated European social, economic, and political life for centuries. On balance in western Europe, the Black Death damaged
its economic position, especially in respect to the peasantry which it had
exploited for so long. Its power over the peasantry did not end in 1350, but in the
later medieval centuries its authority did gradually weaken. Many factors contributed to that immense change in social relationships, including the changing
power of towns and trading wealth, the growing authority of central political leaders such as kings, and the development of military technology that supplanted
the armored horseman. Although it would be foolish to claim that the Black
Death ended the power of the western European landed class, it would also be
foolish to assert the epidemic's irrelevance.

The institutional authority of the Church received several blows. To the extent
that it depended on learned and administrative talents, it suffered. Such talents
and learning could not be quickly replaced, and the death of a parish priest, for
example, sometimes resulted in the rapid ordination of a replacement with little
training or vocation. Such a circumstance might worsen an already bad situation
if the deceased priest had shirked his pastoral duties while the plague raged.
Many did (as many did not), and contemporaries held the secular clergy up to
unfavorable comparison with the mendicants; some members of the clergy had
abandoned their flocks, and others had enriched themselves in the crisis. And
even if a clergyman remained devoted to his parish in its travail, his powerless-
ness was manifest; the extent to which members of the clergy commanded
respect because of their "superhuman" qualities was weakened by their inability
to stem the disease, and by their own vulnerability to it.

The epidemic touched off long-simmering resentments against the Church as well as against other symbols of authority. The direction taken by the Flagellant movement in Germany provides an illustration. Flagellant processions, especially in Germany, quickly passed out of clerical hands and control. The Flagellants were often highly organized groups, under the direction of a master—a layperson—who heard confessions and imposed penances, thus seemingly poaching on the preserves of the clergy. A millennium was thought to be at hand, in which Christ (perhaps accompanied by the Emperor Frederick Barbarossa, awakened from his mountain tomb) would come again, slay the priests who oppressed the people, and take from the rich to give to the poor. Flagellants saw themselves as armies of saints. In some horrific cases the coming of such an army ignited savage massacres of the Jews, the most obvious outsiders who might serve as scapegoats for the tragedy of the epidemic; thus the Jewish populations of Frankfurt, Mainz, Cologne, and Brussels were put to the sword as a part of the mass hysteria. As Norman Cohn describes the episodes, their revolutionary potential was very real, not only against the authority of the Church but also against the wealthy and the entitled.[23]

These plague-inspired popular movements fed other, later fourteenth-century currents. For while the epidemic may have weakened the institutional authority of the Church, it did not diminish the piety of the population. Although "piety" is hard to measure (as is "authority"), the same civilization that denounced the laxity of the clergy left bequests to churches for prayers and buildings, went on pilgrimages, and manifested signs of intense personal piety that found an outlet in such movements of the laity as confraternities. By the late fourteenth and early fifteenth centuries such expressions of lay piety boiled over in what the Church judged to be heresy, as with the Lollards in England and the Hussites in Bohemia.

Did public morality decline during and after the epidemic? Some witnesses claimed that the horror of the plague loosened the bonds of behavior. Boccaccio reported: "Others . . . maintained that an infallible way of warding off this appalling evil was to drink heavily, enjoy life to the full, go round singing and merry-making, gratify all one's cravings whenever the opportunity offered, and shrug the whole thing off as one enormous joke. Moreover, they practiced what they preached to the best of their ability."[24] But the same author also told of those who lived abstemiously in the hope of avoiding plague, and it is possible as well that the plague overstimulated moralists to find "sin" everywhere to explain the catastrophe. The drastic mortality laid the basis for conspicuous consumption by the survivors, nevertheless, and there were those who adopted a tonight-we-drink-for-tomorrow-we-die attitude. And as we have seen, in some cases the social fabric was badly torn by revolutionary movements and hysterical massacres of innocents.

As hard to measure as "piety," "authority," and "morality" is the notion of a civilization obsessed with death and its images. Johan Huizinga, in a famous book

written in 1924, drew a memorable picture of a post-plague world of extreme contrasts, of silences and noises, a highly strung civilization quick to violence and
outward displays of emotion, one in which the smell of blood mixed with that of
roses.[25] Millard Meiss, who studied Florentine and Sienese art in the wake of the
plague, showed that art grew more "religious" and "conservative," perhaps from
a general desire for intense personal religious expression in painting, but perhaps a reflection of the typical *arriviste* tastes of those enriched by the changed
circumstances.[26]

Certainly much evidence says that Europeans reacted to the Black Death with
mingled guilt and fear: convinced that their sins had brought on God's wrath,
fleeing in terror when and where they could, and savagely turning on scapegoats.
To many Europeans the Apocalypse seemed at hand. Michael Dols's study of the
same epidemic's effects on another civilization both offers interesting contrasts
and reinforces the view of European guilt and fear.[27] Dols found that Mamluk
Egypt, where the mortality in 1348 rivaled that experienced in Europe, was
generally free of most of the hysterical reactions found in Europe. According to
Dols, differences in religious background and ideas account for the different
reactions. A plague epidemic (part of the first great plague pandemic, mentioned
in Chapter Two) had ravaged the Middle East in the earliest years of Islam,
so that the faith's original writings discuss the plague specifically and with (for
Muslims) enormous authority.

Muslims regarded the plague as God's gift, not his scourge—"a mercy and a
martyrdom" for the faithful. Flight was therefore wrong, for it was flight from
God and God's will (although there was some theological disagreement about
that point, Dols admits). Because plague came directly from God, Muslim
thinkers more consistently held to a heaven-sent miasma as the immediate
cause; doctrines of "bad air" did not slide into ideas of contagion, as they did in
the Christian world. Hence Muslims did not turn on alien minorities who might
be blamed for contagion. More generally, the Muslim tradition lacked the
Christian emphasis on original sin, which lay behind both the guilt felt by
Christians and the punishment which Christians believed that someone deserved.
Mamluk Egypt, Dols argues, reacted with reverent resignation to the disaster of
the Black Death.

But Dols's contrasts may be too sharp. Did Westerners characteristically react
with flight, guilt, and a search for scapegoats? Remember the speed with which
communities rebounded from the social and economic blows of the epidemic;
remember not just the wild Flagellant hysteria, but the legal routines of
Perpignan, the effective governments of Siena and Cornwall, the rising prices
and productivity of craftspeople, and the prosperity of surviving peasants.
Furthermore, millenarian traditions did not necessarily involve Flagellant
excesses and threats to the social fabric; on the contrary, Robert Lerner

observes, the traditions of chiliastic prophecy in the West provided a framework of belief that enabled some men and women of 1348 to find comfort when faced with the awful event of the Black Death.[28] Nancy Siraisi reminds us of another truth: that medieval Western civilization constantly lived with hardships and its people were inured to disaster; Christian traditions of the transitory character of earthly life gave them resiliency or at least some comfort.[29]

The Continuing Pandemic

The Black Death of 1347–1353 was the first and gravest episode of what became a pandemic lasting over three centuries. In the succeeding centuries plague both persistently disrupted Western civilization and stimulated responses from people whose concepts of plague gradually shifted from the environmental to the contagionist. These two subjects were in fact interrelated, for the accumulated experience with the plague contributed to the shifts in etiological perceptions, and it is at least possible that human agency ultimately diverted plague.

The particular effects of the long-term pandemic still need much study. Some large-scale generalizations have been made (of the sort discussed earlier in this chapter) about the social and economic effects of the prolonged demographic downturn between the fourteenth and late fifteenth centuries, in which the plague is at least heavily implicated. Certain specific places and times have been subjected to close study, but satisfactory generalizations may be difficult, especially because most such studies concern only parts of England, France, and Italy. The subject remains a fruitful field for hypotheses. Such giant periods of Western history as the Renaissance, the Protestant Reformation, and the "general crisis" of the seventeenth century were all played out on a plague-infected stage. And what may be an important point about the stage: even in the comprehensive disaster of 1347–1353, and much more thereafter, the visitations of plague had wide local variations. Some regions and cities felt its effects more than did others, or felt those effects at different times. Did Bohemia's escape from the worst of 1347–1353 lay the basis for the remarkable period of Hussite political power in the early 1400s, when the Bohemians repeatedly defied German imperial authority and laid waste sections of Germany itself? Did the plague epidemics that swept Italian cities in the late sixteenth and early seventeenth centuries disrupt their economies and thus contribute to the end of their centuries-old European economic dominance? Did Milan's comparatively light brush with plague in 1347–1353 aid its relative rise among Italian cities? Was Antwerp similarly favored in the sixteenth century with respect to other towns in the Low Countries? A large number of such attractive speculations suggest themselves.

It is possible to be more concrete about changes in European beliefs about disease. Scholarly concentration on Italy in the years after 1350 has introduced us to the changing conceptions of the plague and to changing responses of political authority. Between 1348 and the 1500s—at least in northern Italian cities—the idea of plague as a contagion gained great force, and if governments were not yet ready to deny that plague was God's visitation, in practice they took more and more measures designed to combat the spread of infections. Remarkable and intrusive systems of public health developed, which in turn gave rise to basic questions about the limits of state authority exercised in the name of the public good. In early modern Italian cities the power of public health machinery clearly interfered with both the freedoms of individuals and the traditions of social groups.

As we have already seen, the great 1347–1353 epidemic prompted some reactions that seemed based on the idea of contagion. But most of the official medical (and theological) opinion spoke of "bad air," or "miasma," as the immediate cause of the disease and based most preventive measures on that assumption. Even if the cause were universally bad air, perhaps it might be escaped through vigorous actions. Sometimes—because there might be "secondary" causes of a local origin to explain the bad air—a general cleansing of the environment might be undertaken. Thus Venice, for example, appointed an ad hoc committee of influential citizens to "preserve public health and avoid the corruption of the environment." In the course of repeated plague visitations in the fifteenth century, such ad hoc committees multiplied and in some cases became standing boards. From 1486 on in Venice, three noblemen were annually elected to a Commission of Public Health, which in turn supervised the activities of subordinate local boards in towns in Venetian territory. Florence adopted a similar course in 1527. Milan, governed more despotically than either the Venetian or the Florentine republics, followed stronger measures in the 1348 epidemic, and as early as 1437 the reigning duke appointed a standing "health commissioner." A five-member board replaced this officer in 1534, after which date all three of the large northern Italian city-states had standing commissions. These boards were primarily administrative, not medical, in both their duties and their composition, although the Milanese board was to include two physicians among its members.[30]

Initially the chief task of these boards was the elimination of possible sources of corruption of the air, a charge reflecting the general miasmatic theory prevalent in 1347–1353. In fact the early boards, whether ad hoc or permanent, undertook actions on a diffuse front, for (as we have seen) the number and variety of possible "secondary" causes of plague was very large. So in their pursuit of corruption-free air, commissioners inspected wine, fish, meat, and water supplies; they worried about sewage; they regulated burials, and decreed the destruction of the clothing of the deceased.

But by the fifteenth century the members of health boards gradually began acting on more clearly contagionist assumptions. Those assumptions led to more direct interference with both individuals and groups. Occasions that brought crowds together became suspect, and were thus objects of regulation: schools, church services, and—especially—the very religious processions that so many towns had sponsored to propitiate God's wrath. The movements of the suspiciously transitory classes—especially beggars, soldiers, and prostitutes—came under scrutiny. Boards of health also, in their attempt to stay informed, began recording the causes of death in their cities. These early censuses of death themselves contributed to changing conceptions of cause.

Doctrines of contagion led to two particularly important forms of public health control, both clearly articulated and practiced in the fifteenth-century Italian city-states: municipal quarantine and isolation of the victims. A health commission's declaration that plague was present in a city set in chain a complex series of administrative and political measures whose goals were quarantine and isolation. By the end of the fifteenth century the cities had introduced the "health pass" as part of the quarantine process. Other cities would erect a *cordon sanitaire* around themselves, stopping traffic on roads and demanding health passes from travelers, or perhaps halting all people and goods at their borders entirely. As Giulia Calvi's microstudy of Florence in 1630 has illustrated, travelers could be the subjects of zealous monitorial interest.[31] (Of course such a *cordon*'s effectiveness was limited, for the early modern state lacked the rapid transportation, communication, and electrical detection gadgetry that a modern state could employ; seventeenth-century Florence could not erect a Berlin Wall.)

Within the affected town, families of plague victims would be confined to their houses, with the doors locked and barred from the outside; supplies were passed in through windows, preferably above ground level. Objects used by the sick and the deceased were seized and burnt; houses were disinfected, painted with vinegar and fumigated with sulphur. A pesthouse might be established wherein sufferers would be immured. Ideally a city would have not only a pesthouse but a convalescent house as well, for those recovering from their brush with plague. All these measures could entail considerable civic expense. Extra staff had to be paid: physicians, surgeons, inspectors, guards for the *cordon*, grave-diggers. Food had to be provided for the isolated, and items destroyed might have to be replaced.

The sweeping powers assumed by the boards of health, and the measures that they enacted, led to conflict with both vested interests and the traditional cultures of the society. The clergy took offense at the suspension of divine services and processions in the name of public health. The business community soon found that a quarantine could cripple a city's trade and industry. Isolating a single victim's house, especially in those times of essentially home-centered crafts and industry, could cause loss that rippled through the city as raw or finished materials were destroyed. Urban artisans, who might live close to the margin of survival anyway, could face ruin if health officers proclaimed plague in the town: trade would stop, workers might be confined to their homes, stocks of material might be seized and burnt. And as Calvi has made clear, more than economic

loss loomed for the common people of a city. Accumulated belongings had important cultural value as symbols of family continuity, and their destruction by the
all-powerful health bureaucracy stirred deep resentment.

Finding a suitable pesthouse could present a difficult political problem, for no
one wished his property to be so used. "Hospitals" in these centuries did not exist
as institutions specifically for the sick, and when plague was accepted as a contagion, separate isolation houses were required. For that purpose the states seized
private property and thus alienated property owners. And for the designated victims and their families, forcible removal to the pesthouse was a horror that broke
the family's cohesion and was often perceived—with reason—as a death sentence.

Small wonder then that the boards of health could be unpopular. Sometimes
this unpopularity boiled over into disorder, such as the Milanese board confronted in 1630 when "[t]hey were execrated by the ignorant populace which lis-
tened to a few physicians who, caring little for the public health, kept saying that
there was no question of plague . . . Fed and imbued with such delusion, the populace began to slander Tadino and Settala [members of the health board] and
when by accident they moved through the narrow streets of the popular quarters
they were vilified with foul and unseemly words, and they were even pelted with
stones."[32] Giulia Calvi found no riot in Florence in the same year, but she turned
up even more suggestive—and probably more common—popular reactions to
public health regulations. Many possibilities existed for corruption: surgeons
could be bribed to report plague as something else, grave-diggers could be
swayed to bury a body in the church rather than in the mass shallow plots set
aside for plague victims outside the walls, confiscators of condemned material
could overlook prized possessions, officials commissioned to lock up a house or
shop could forget to do so. These acts might be seen as corruption, but they
might also be acts of mediation between the bureaucracy and the traditional community whose property and values were under assault.[33] In those ways the populace cushioned the blows directed at them. The health bureaucracy was clearly
and deeply unpopular, in part because its rules broke families and rode
roughshod over important customary beliefs (such as veneration of corpses),
but also in part because some bureaucrats seemed to take their powers as license
to loot for their own gain. Health officers not only took bribes but extorted them,
sometimes in property, sometimes in sexual favors. They accordingly met the
sullen resistance of deception and evasion.

Perhaps in the face of such resistance, whether overt as in 1630 Milan, or
more subtle and pervasive as in Calvi's Florence, city governments gave the
health bureaucracy broad powers and made attacks on its officers a major crime.
As early as 1504 Venetian health officers were empowered to arrest people and
inflict torture on them, and Florence in 1630 resorted to torture almost routinely
to enforce its health ordinances. It was, in addition, important that the health

boards consist of, or at least include, men of wealth and rank in the community, who might be able to overcome resistance to unpopular seizures of property by a status to which others (especially lesser property owners) might defer.

The contagionist measures of governments, then, stimulated various levels of political opposition. But in addition the health measures themselves were sometimes the products of political forces, and we should not understand them solely as reactions to the pressure of epidemic disease. Measures of isolation and quarantine included an element of social control, and the actions of a state against disease might occur in the larger context of a period of greater state economic and social manipulation, as early modern governments assumed some paternalist characteristics. And the actions of the states themselves sometimes contributed to changing etiological views.

The last point emerges clearly from Ann Carmichael's study of Florence in the fourteenth and fifteenth centuries.[34] As the Florentine government amassed facts about the incidence of plague (both in time and particular place), it became convinced by the disease's patterns that it spread by contagion. But the government also concluded that the poor (and especially their children) were the most likely carriers and hence in most need of control—not an unwelcome message to the property owners of the city, frightened as they were by such disorders as the Ciompi uprising of 1378. In Carmichael's perhaps-extreme view, the plague may have been little more than a convenient excuse for the dominant classes of Florence to exert social control. Her argument gives short shrift to the divisions within the propertied classes themselves, but it also makes the interesting case that while plague undoubtedly occurred in post-1348 epidemics, the death toll in those episodes was swollen by other illnesses that *were* likely contagions in the congested, poorer, quarters of the city.

Paul Slack's study of the plague in Tudor and Stuart England provides some support for Carmichael's view, but Slack is more cautious.[35] English governments remained well behind the Italian cities and their aggressive policies. In part the English reflected continuing doubts about the contagion theory of plague; even in seventeenth-century Florence, etiological doctrines contained elements of "bad air" or "universal corruption," and the persistence of the custom of giving grave-diggers the clothes of the deceased testifies to the popular weakness of contagion concepts. Slack also explores the nuances of religious views, in which tensions persisted between "providential" and "natural" explanations of plague, and shows how those theological perspectives—somewhat curiously—reinforced some social policies by the seventeenth century. For churchmen who emphasized the power of divine providence, the tensions proved especially strong; on the one hand, resistance to God's will was futile, but on the other, the clergy of the state (Anglican) church were obligated to support government measures, including those meant to counter plague. Perhaps for such churchmen the answer lay in

viewing individual sin as at least a "secondary" cause of plague, a view that might
license state action against sinners. And English "natural" interpretations became
congruent with such a view; although the English lagged behind Carmichael's
Florentines in reaching this conclusion, by the seventeenth century English opinion saw plague as a disease of the poorer urban districts, a social problem associated with poverty and disorder. Religious and secular opinion thus agreed with
government attempts to (at first) strictly isolate plague victims, and then (slightly
later) quarantine borders and establish pesthouses. Etiological theory, morality,
and the desire for order thus neatly coincided.

Slack would also agree with Carmichael's view that governments took contagionist actions against plague for their own reasons, not necessarily connected
with plague itself. English royal government, he found, was more apt to take vigorous measures in periods of aggressive paternalism (or maternalism, in the
reign of Elizabeth I). And Slack usefully explores the differences between the
regulations and intentions of the central government, and the actual government
practice at the local level. In 1578 Elizabeth I's government ordered the isolation
of plague victims in their households and provided for a system of *local* taxation
to fund measures against contagious disease. These orders received the support
of parliamentary statute in 1604, but when royal policy moved to favor the construction of pesthouses, such expenditure remained a matter of local discretion,
as indeed the tax rate was levied locally. The orders of the town of Bridport
(Dorset), in 1638, clearly illustrate both the local direction plague policy might
take and the way in which fear of plague overlapped other worries: "to use all
good and lawful means to prevent the same Contagion & other mischiefs and
inconveniences that may ensue unto this town for want of constant warding," the
town council ordered the provision of a night watch by six householders.[36] What
the good householders were to do if they saw plague is not specified, but they
clearly might prevent the disorder of "other mischiefs and inconveniences."

Government did not have an enviable task. To what extent did it respond to
the demands of the propertied for order? Carmichael and Calvi—and to a lesser
extent Slack—would say that in the face of plague, order was a great priority. By
the eighteenth and nineteenth centuries quarantines and isolations sparked
more disorder from the same lower ranks whom governments wished to control;
government public health policies in the time of cholera precipitated major riots
in some European cities, as we shall see in Chapter Seven. But Carlo Cipolla sees
a different problem for Renaissance and early modern Italian city-states, for the
interests of the propertied might conflict with antiplague measures. As Cipolla
puts it, health boards often faced painful conflicts between their "moral obligation to mankind" and "unspeakable economic losses" if they suspected or discovered plague in their cities.[37] Should they publicize the presence of plague, or
attempt to hush it up and thus preserve the commerce of the city? Cipolla
believes that "moral obligation" most often won out, if only because an outbreak

of plague was impossible to hide. Other cities and their health boards received reports from ambassadors, after all. Were health officers urged on by "moral obligation," behind which lay fear of discovery, or by a desire to discipline the turbulent lower orders?

The growing conviction of the contagious character of plague certainly led governments to remarkably active public health policies. Did those policies have an impact on the course of the great pandemic? For it was true that plague lost something of its tremendous grip between 1347 and 1670, and after the latter date it became infrequent in the West. By the sixteenth and seventeenth centuries plague had ceased to be the "major demographic regulator" that it had been in the fourteenth and fifteenth centuries in England, although the magnitude of its periodic assaults was still considerable.[38] Plague carried off as many as 100,000 Londoners in 1665, out of a total estimated population of 459,000. Such an experience makes it clear that the bacillus had remained lethal over the centuries; the plague evidently did not gradually fade away. Rather, it simply disappeared. According to Biraben 1671 was the first year since 1346 when northern and western parts of Europe were free of plague.[39] Further outbreaks of the disease occurred in Spain and Germany between 1678 and 1682; in Poland between 1708 and 1710; in southern France, notably Marseilles, in 1720–21. Thereafter plague in the Western world was confined to the Balkans and Russia, with occasional minor outbreaks in southern Europe, until the next great pandemic began in the late nineteenth century.

The disappearance of plague remains one of the interesting unresolved questions of Western history. After seemingly recovering demographic momentum in the sixteenth century, Western civilization's population stagnated through much of the seventeenth. It then began to rise—rather dramatically—sometime in the first half of the eighteenth, and that population growth was sustained over most of the Continent until the early twentieth. This population surge coincided with the rise of Europe to world domination. Many factors (some to be considered in Chapters Six and Eleven) contributed to that rise, and many factors lay behind Europe's demographic burst. But certainly the disappearance of the disease that had been the chief epidemic killer for over three centuries must have helped.

Many theories have been advanced to account for plague's retreat, and no one theory is totally convincing. The number of possible variables is large, since the disease involves humans, rodents, insects, and microorganisms and their possible shifts in behavior or even genetic makeup. Perhaps the climate provided discouraging conditions for fleas, for the period between about 1590 and about 1850 has been called the "Little Ice Age," when European mean temperatures probably reached their lowest points since the true Ice Age. But the first great epidemic of 1347–1353 occurred during a similar, if less severe, climatic downturn. Andrew Appleby has argued that rats developed greater immunity; plague-carrying fleas are less likely to abandon living rats and thus accidentally light on a human.[40] Robert Sallares speculates that the periodicity of plague epidemics during the three centuries of the pandemic may have reflected population cycles among rodent reservoirs, and he concludes that changing rodent immunities may be the best answer to why the pandemic eventually disappeared.[41] But as Slack has noticed, the disappearance of plague was extremely patchy geographically.[42] The last cases in Italy occurred in the 1650s, while neighboring southern France was affected in the 1720s; plague struck Moscow in the 1770s and persisted in the Balkans until the 1840s. Could rat immunity have been so unevenly distributed?

Another opinion, given particularly wide currency by Karl Helleiner in the *Cambridge Economic History*, credits a shift in the dominant rat species, as the larger *Rattus norvegicus* ousted *Rattus rattus*.[43] The theory notes that the former species is less companionable with humans and lacks *Rattus rattus's* skill as a climber, so that it maintains a greater distance from human habitations and especially human roofs; thus the chain of rat-flea-human might be broken. But the chronology of plague epidemics almost completely disproves this theory of a shifting balance of rat power. *Rattus norvegicus* did not arrive in England (where the plague last visited in 1665) until 1727, while it had been long established in Moscow at the time of that city's 1771 plague.[44]

Hardest of all to prove are possible changes in *Yersinia pestis* itself. It is now believed that that bacillus is a member of a genus that includes other pathogens "genetically almost identical" but with very different clinical effects.[45] Further, *Yersinia pestis* has apparently manifested itself in three different strains, or "biovars." Have some shifts occurred in the makeup of the organism that would explain the pandemic's disappearance? Aside from the molecular possibilities of such a shift, historical circumstances cast doubt on it. London suffered a major plague epidemic in 1665 and never saw plague again, yet when *Yersinia pestis* resurfaced again in Asia in the late nineteenth century (see Chapter Nine) it was still very virulent.

Did human actions inadvertently interfere with plague? If housing construction methods and materials changed, perhaps the result distanced humans from rats and fleas. London suffered not only a serious plague epidemic in 1665 but a major fire in 1666. After the fire much of the city was rebuilt with brick and tile, which may have provided less happy homes for rodents than the previous wood and thatched roofs. But how general was London's experience? All across the European world, plague disappeared more quickly than old housing materials. Similarly, the general possibility of improved sanitation, on the surface an attractive hypothesis, falters from lack of clear correlations between sanitary changes and the plague's disappearance. Plague last visited Naples in 1656, yet Naples became notorious as a supremely unsanitary city. Did European nutrition improve in the late seventeenth and early eighteenth centuries? Perhaps for some, but most likely for a wealthy minority by then not much affected by plague. Longer-term nutritional improvements for many may have occurred, as European diets were supplemented by new crops such as the potato and by legumes in new crop rotations, but significant improvement for the masses was surely very slow.

Conscious human action against plague presents another possibility, one that Slack has argued strongly. Quarantines especially, he says, may have decisively interfered with the intercity movement of plague.[46] Cipolla cautiously concurs, arguing that on balance the public health bureaucracies of the sixteenth and seventeenth centuries did a good job.[47] Both Slack and Cipolla admit that many of the public health measures had little effect, and some were positively harmful. The killing of dogs and cats, undertaken because of their supposed role as contagious agents, continued into the seventeenth century and clearly allowed rats to run riot. Household isolation of victims most often harmed their families, and had little to do with the rat-dependent transmission of plague from house to house. It may, as Cipolla notes, have slowed the frightening spread of the pneumonic plague that made the 1347–1350 epidemic so horrific. Although the value of quarantines almost certainly was real, questions remain about their practical efficiency. Appleby, noting that plague disappeared from Italy but flourished in the Near East, doubts the effectiveness of Mediterranean quarantines as an explanation of the contrasts.[48]

Many mysteries still surround the end of the great pandemic that stretched from the fourteenth century into the eighteenth. Human agency may have assisted, but the case remains far from proved. The vigorous measures of public health were of course undertaken without any clear knowledge of the etiology of plague, or indeed of any other disease. But they were undertaken out of a growing conviction that plague was "contagious," and that a cause such as contagion could be subject to human intervention. The Italian health commissioners were surely pious Christians, but their actions anticipated Alexander Pope's advice:

> Know then thyself, presume not God to scan,
> The proper study of mankind is man.

The health boards created precedents for an active role of the state in the name of public health, and in doing so they raised questions about the state's regulatory powers that remain meaningful today. Their activity may reasonably be seen as an aspect of the scientific revolution of the sixteenth and seventeenth centuries (see Chapter Five), when a conviction in human powers over nature took root. And when another great plague pandemic got under way late in the nineteenth century, Western public health machinery began to employ a powerful new etiological concept against it, thus strengthening the hand of regulation over individual lives.

Four

New Diseases and
Transatlantic Exchanges

In its long history the human species has been both extremely mobile and extremely isolated. This paradox has had several different consequences for humanity's relations with disease. Prehistoric humans fanned out widely from their original central African homeland, across Europe and Asia; they apparently reached the Americas and Australia over land bridges (or at least narrow, shallow sea passages) at times of significantly lower ocean levels. These vast movements diffused the human genetic pool over the globe and may also have diffused a common pool of parasitic microorganisms as well. But in subsequent millennia geological changes separated different groups of people as the land bridges that connected Asia with the Americas and Australia were re-submerged. Humans on different continents, and their accompanying parasites, had a period of separate evolution.

At least in the great Eurasian land mass (including Africa), however, isolation was never total. Human movement resulted in some interchange of the vast number of other organisms that accompanied it, some of those organisms more obvious (because visible) than others. Perhaps assisted by human traffic, diseases endemic to one area of the land mass might make their way to other regions, as did plague in the fourteenth century. To at least some extent Eurasians shared McNeill's "disease pool" of common vectors, microorganisms, antigens, and antibodies. The inhabitants of the Americas and Australia, as well as of a variety of oceanic islands, did not share some of the elements of that pool. For several millennia they had been out of contact with Eurasia, with the occasional exception illustrated by the voyages of the Scandinavians to North America in the eleventh century.

That isolation came to an abrupt end in the late fifteenth and sixteenth centuries with the voyages of Columbus and his successors. Those voyages not only initiated the movement of a wide assortment of animals, insects, and parasitic microorganisms; such transfer was solidified by the establishment of an imperial hegemony over much American territory, in which European domination ensured the uninterrupted movement of both people and their accompanying flora and fauna. What those movements have meant for the history of disease has generated considerable historical speculation, both about the export of disease to America from the Old World and about America's returning the favor. And while each of the several migrating diseases has inspired different historical questions, the overall experience with diseases such as syphilis, typhus, and smallpox strengthened the Western belief in the importance of contagion. Because this book emphasizes Western civilization's disease experiences, this chapter will devote more attention to Europe. But the American civilizations now came into contact with the Euro-African world, and disastrous disease consequences for them ensued that deserve some discussion as well.

Newly Recognized Diseases in Europe

Late in the fifteenth century several diseases appeared in Europe that (at least apparently) had not previously affected Western peoples. The most prominent of these ailments were what later scholars have called syphilis and typhus; the mysterious disease called "English sweats" appeared at that time as well, and Europeans also became conscious of a great variety of "fevers." Syphilis and typhus both had considerable effects on the society of early modern Europe, and syphilis especially stimulated interesting medical and social responses in the sixteenth and seventeenth centuries. But the "newness" of each of these diseases remains in doubt, and hence their relationship—so attractive at first glance because of coincident chronology—to the great age of exploration also may not be a simple one.

Syphilis

Syphilis apparently first appeared in Italy in the middle 1490s, in the wake of warfare; contemporary accounts associated it with the invasion of Italy by the armies of Charles VIII of France in 1494–95. Armies of that era were almost ideal disseminators of disease: dirty, ill-disciplined, drawn from the far corners of the Continent, disbanded at the end of each campaign to scatter back into the far corners. After its first appearance in 1494–95 syphilis spread swiftly, to be reported all over Europe by 1499. By that date it had also reached the Middle East and North Africa; China experienced it within the next decade.

Where had it originated? A few years later—and just when is open to different interpretations—it came to be believed that Columbus' men had brought it back from America, and this "Columbian" theory of syphilis commanded scholarly support for a very long time. Some contemporary Europeans, convinced of its novelty, blamed it on someone else: "Naples disease," "French pox," "German pox," "Polish pox," for instance. But clinical descriptions of disease from before the 1490s, in either Europe or Asia, remain subjects of scholarly controversy. Nor is there consensus about the evidence of syphilitic bone damage (or lack of it) in Old World skeletal remains.

But not all observers of the early sixteenth century were convinced either that the disease was American, or that it was new. There were, to be sure, some contemporaries of Columbus, themselves witnesses—Oviedo, Diaz de Islas, Las Casas—who later said that they associated the disease with people returning from America in the 1490s, but their writings were retrospective, with Oviedo apparently the earliest in 1526. Other contemporaries, however, spoke more generally (and traditionally) about the causes of the disease as the wrath of God and/or unfortunate conjunctions of the heavenly bodies. The common sixteenth-century terms for the disease—Naples disease, French pox—reflect a view that the horror came from sinful neighbors, not necessarily American Indians. Finally, early in the sixteenth century some scholars found biblical or classical texts that seemed to describe some similar ailment; certainly Europeans (and Muslims as well) had long been bedeviled by diseases that caused appalling skin lesions, with leprosy only the most famous.

Was this disease simply some new (or perhaps old) variant on such familiar visitations? That old question, debated over the centuries first by reference to the medical texts of antiquity and then (since the nineteenth century) by paleo-pathology, has gained new complications from modern bacteriology and molecular biology. Venereal syphilis results from an invasion of the body by a bacterium of the genus *Treponema*; this genus is part of a group of bacteria called, from their shape, spirochetes. Several species of *Treponema* exist, whose genetic relation-ships (according to recent molecular analysis) form a "tangled skein."[1] They are responsible for several distinct diseases (distinct in the sense of clearly different symptoms), including, in addition to venereal syphilis, yaws and pinta (tropical diseases most common in, respectively, Africa and Central America), and "endemic" syphilis (called bejel in the Middle East), a relatively benign complaint.

This complex bacteriology has provided fodder for considerable historical speculation. Some have maintained an extreme "unitary" position, arguing that only one treponematosis exists, that it has existed in the human population as a whole for millennia, and that it has taken different forms depending in part on its transmission route into the body.[2] Yaws and bejel flourished as endemic childhood diseases in hot climates, among communities of little clothing and (in E. H. Hudson's words) "low levels of personal and community hygiene"; when the organism reached urban populations in temperate climates it found its person-to-person routes (skin contacts) broken by clothing and more regular bathing habits, and so it gradually evolved as an adult infection transmitted venereally.

In this view Columbus (and the American Indians) had nothing to do with its sudden appearance in Europe, which was not so much sudden as a suddenly noticed phenomenon that had been slowly evolving. Some modifications of this basic "unitary" position maintain that different treponematoses are responsible for different diseases, and that they may have evolved differently among different, and geographically isolated, human populations.[3]

Was venereal syphilis new to Europe in the late fifteenth century, and did it reach Europe from the Americas? Paleopathological conclusions are ambiguous, although treponematoses were both "present and variable" in America before European and African contacts,[4] and more American skeletons have treponemal bone lesions than are found in those of the Old World. At least some contemporary Europeans were convinced that they confronted a new disease (wherever it originated), and their writings provide some clinical evidence for that belief.[5] The virulence of the disease in the early sixteenth-century European population was characteristic of an epidemic striking new ground. Strengthening the "new disease" case is a weakness in one of the countering possibilities: for medieval leprosy seems to have been just that, not syphilis. But it is also very likely that some form of treponemal disease existed in Europe centuries before Columbus's voyages. Perhaps bejel had made its way to Europe from the Near East; perhaps yaws had migrated from Africa. Certainly both were long established on the Eurasian/African landmass, so the possibility remains that the apparent Columbian explosion of a new disease really started within Europe itself as a mutation of one of those other treponematoses.

Wherever it came from, the disease made a great impression on European observers in the early sixteenth century. Its dramatic symptoms gave rise to expressions of horror, as writers described the initial genital chancres and then the succeeding skin lesions and skeletal aches that accompanied the several years of the disease's secondary phase. No estimates have been made of its mortality or morbidity in the early decades of the sixteenth century, but contemporaries leave little doubt of its wide extent. The symptoms, especially the initial genital sores, led most (though not all) to associate the disease with sex. Fear of such a contagion fed already-existing suspicion of indigent transients; in sixteenth-century France statutory attempts were made to isolate such dangerous characters, or to lock them up. "Pox" victims were an especially obvious and inviting target for such regulation, although its implementation remained ineffective. Syphilis and its association with sex conferred on prostitutes a particular air of danger, and demands grew that they be regulated, confined, or outlawed. Sixteenth-century attempts to do so did not work, but in subsequent centuries—especially the nineteenth and twentieth, when the regulatory efficiency of the state vastly strengthened—prostitution and syphilis assumed the central roles in important social morality plays, the subjects of further discussion in Chapters

Eleven and Twelve. And certainly the sixteenth century conviction of the contagiousness of the "Great Pox," as it was known, also strengthened a growing general predisposition to see diseases in a contagious light.

This terrible "pox" showed some signs of abating (in both incidence and virulence) as the sixteenth century advanced. Perhaps more people now survived its
earlier stages, so that tertiary stages could become clearer. Descriptions of it
came to focus on the persistent lesions and frightening disfigurements that
marked its later stages, and writers paid more attention to the symptoms of those
who had clearly had the disease for a long time, rather than noticing a continuing
increase in new cases. (The different stages of syphilis, interrupted by periods of
latency, undoubtedly complicated and confused descriptions and diagnoses;
"pox" remained a broad brush for what may have been a variety of diseases.) If
contemporaries were right, and the disease receded from its savage first attacks,
such a recession would be consistent with a "Columbian," or at least a "new,"
view of the disease, as after several generations people and microorganisms may
have been reaching a balanced relationship.

Galenic theory generally held that the pox was a disorder related to humoral
imbalances, and that theory underlay most sixteenth-century therapy. While different authorities cited different humors as the offenders, phlegm emerged as the
favorite. So while bleeding was sometimes urged, the usual treatment involved the
expulsion of phlegm by the promotion of spitting and sweating. Two substances in
particular came to be employed for that purpose: guaiacum and mercury.

Guaiacum, one of the hardest woods known, is found in the West Indies and
Central and South America. Its European use as a cure for syphilis began sometime after 1510 under unclear circumstances; its popularity owed much to an
influential book by the German humanist Ulrich von Hutten (1488–1523), *De
guaiaci medicina et morbo gallico*, published in 1519.[6] Von Hutten's tract carried
the authenticity of a sufferer from syphilis as well as the vigor of a controversialist active in the defense of Martin Luther. The Augsburg banking and merchant
house of the Fugger established control of the marketing of guaiacum and heavily promoted its sale, an example of the antiquity of enthusiastic peddling of
remedies. Its virtues were hailed, its prices soared, and pieces of the wood were
hung in churches as objects of veneration. It received names consistent with
such faith: *lignum vitae*, or even *lignum sanctum*. Some of the belief in its efficacy arose from its American origin. If the disease was American, the widely
accepted "doctrine of specifics" argued that since God always paired diseases and
remedies, an American disease must have an American remedy. (Later opponents
of the Columbian theory wondered whether the argument did not run the other
way: since this American wood was a cure, the disease must be American. A precise dating of the first use of guaiacum, and of the first belief in the Columbian
theory, would be revealing.)

According to von Hutten, the guaiac medicine was prepared by grinding the wood to a powder and then boiling the powder in water for a specified time. The resulting liquid was the medicine, drunk as a potion. While he administered this medicine, the physician confined the patient to a heated, sealed room, wherein—drinking much liquid potion—the patient perspired profusely, thus expelling the offending phlegm. Different sixteenth-century authorities prescribed variations on this therapy, but they generally agreed on conditions that promoted sweating.

Not all physicians concurred with the guaiac treatment. Many combined it with mercuric compounds, or used those compounds exclusively. Mercuric ores, and substances prepared from them, had long been favored (especially by Arab physicians) in the treatment of skin disorders and sores. "Arabic ointment," most often ore cinnabar (mercuric sulfide), was rubbed on the lesions. This treatment was applied to the earliest "new" cases of the disease in the 1490s, only to be overshadowed for a few decades by the rage for guaiacum.

One of the most influential authorities on syphilis, Girolamo Fracastoro (1483–1553), took a cautious position that advocated both remedies. In 1530 Fracastoro wrote a long poem about the disease, *Syphilis sive morbus gallicus*, notable as the origin of the modern word for the ailment; "Syphilis" was a shepherd who brought the pox on himself by his acts of blasphemy, illustrating that the connection of the pox with sex was still not universally accepted. (The word "syphilis" did not, however, begin to supplant "pox" until the eighteenth century.)

If Fracastoro illustrated ambivalence about the use of guaiacum and mercury, his contemporary Paracelsus had no doubts, and his arguments helped mercuric compounds regain their primacy. Paracelsus stands as one of the major figures in the history of science, medicine, and disease; his philosophy and its implications will be discussed in Chapter Five. For the moment it is sufficient to notice that Paracelsus' general objections to the ideas of Aristotle and Galen led him to oppose many of the plant and herbal remedies associated with the Galenic and Hippocratic traditions, and to urge instead the use of metallic or inorganic chemically prepared substances. For him mercury was a particularly sovereign substance, for he (following some Arab traditions) believed that mercury was one of the fundamental "principles" of nature. By the mid-1500s mercury compounds had resumed their place as the favored treatment for syphilis, a position that they held into the nineteenth century. Their effects pleased not only Paracelsus but the Galenists whom he opposed. Their use produced immense quantities of saliva (the offending phlegm being expelled), which was in fact a classic symptom of mercury poisoning. And while mercury compounds became the favored treatment, guaiacum remained as an alternate (it was, for example, listed in the *British Pharmacopeia* until 1932), although its only possible curative effects were psychological.

The history of syphilis in the sixteenth and later centuries has attracted some historians of medicine in part because of its associations with the ailments of notable persons. Thus the policies, personalities, and careers of such rulers as Francis I of France (1515–1547), Henry VIII of England (1509–1547), and Ivan IV of Russia (1533–1584) have sometimes been interpreted as influenced by their supposed syphilitic afflictions. It is an exciting prospect to explain by a clear simple cause—a disease— Henry's apparent infertility, his increasing ill temper, and, indirecdy his break with the Roman Church, or Ivan's paranoid cruelty that had such a crucial effect on later Russian history. Such arguments make disease (as it has affected individuals in this case) an important causal agent in human history as a whole.

Two substantial difficulties with such easy answers should be remembered, however. First, precise physical diagnoses of individuals, when undertaken across the centuries, are very chancy. Henry VIII may serve as an example of the pitfalls. That monarch threw his life, and nearly his entire kingdom, into a turmoil in his search for an heir who would secure his shaky dynasty. He had at least four children (by four different women) who survived infancy, but none of them had children in turn. Did their failure to conceive stem from an inherited syphilitic infection? Add to that circumstance Henry's headaches and sore throats, ulcerated legs, and changes in his character as he aged, and a case might be made for Henry as a syphilitic.[7]

But close students of Henry VIII, including his modern biographers, have convincingly argued against the diagnosis of syphilis. They have suggested depression (perhaps brought on by his worries about the legitimacy of his first marriage) and the serious effects of the ulcerated legs that developed as he aged. Milo Keynes, in a recent medical analysis of the case, cites the absence of the telltale rash of the "Great Pox" in Henry, as well as the king's continuing mental acuity. And—most convincing—no evidence exists that Henry was ever treated for syphilis, although he lived in a time when the disease attracted great attention and when cures for it were widely prescribed. Francis I of France *was* treated for syphilis. If Henry had syphilis, why didn't his doctors treat it?[8]

There exists a second, substantial objection to the use of royal illness to explain decisive points in history. Simply put, historians are—and should be—suspicious of any simple, unicausal explanation of complex historical phenomena. That the fall of the Napoleonic Empire can be attributed to the great man's ulcers, or to his stomach cancer, is a laughable oversimplification. This is not to deny that individuals and their actions have an important and often crucial role in the pattern of historical change. But a very risky trail leads from want of a nail to the fall of a kingdom. Sensitive and careful studies of the relations of an individual's health and his public policies do exist—for example, Roger Williams's *The Mortal Napoleon III*—but they require thorough biographical and historical understanding of contexts more than a diagnosis that provides a magic key.[9]

English Sweats

Syphilis appeared in Europe simultaneously with two other noteworthy diseases, a fact that has encouraged speculation about the widening of world disease pools. Both these "new" diseases, like syphilis, were first associated with warfare and the movement of troops; they were typhus and the ailment that came to be known as "English sweats." In the former case the military association was probably a sound one, but in the latter it was likely coincidental. The English sweating sickness first appeared in that country in 1485, which later gave rise to the theory that mercenary troops involved in the Wars of the Roses (specifically the invasion of England by Henry Tudor) carried the disease. The sweats reappeared in England four other times—in 1508, 1517, 1528, and 1551—on each occasion remaining in that country only; they made one appearance elsewhere in Europe, in 1529–1530. Contemporary descriptions carefully differentiated this disease from plague, typhus, and malaria; they further noticed that young upperclass males were particularly susceptible to it.

The English sweating sickness made a dramatic impression in part because of the prominence of its victims and in part because of its sudden and lethal character. Accounts from 1517 speak of its victims perishing very quickly: "Some within two houres, some merry at dinner and dedde at supper."[10] But its demographic impact was relatively slight, and it did not establish itself. After 1551 it vanished. John Wylie and Leslie Collier, careful students of the English sweats, have concluded that an arbovirus originating in northern and eastern Europe caused these epidemics. Such arboviruses may be enzootic among small mammals (such as mice) and carried to people by insects. A new virus strain, Wylie and Collier theorize, invaded England and attacked those people in the society who might most frequently encounter insects (active young males) and those who might have constituted an immunologically virgin population, especially young adults.[11] The attack on young adults may also have characterized sixteenth-century syphilis in Europe, and such a pattern might explain the violence of the early epidemics of English sweats. The latter's disappearance from the scene after 1551 may have been the product of changing small-mammal populations and their immunities, or some other interference with the complex virus-reservoir-vector-human route.

Typhus

The English sweats remain a subject of historical conjecture, if only because their disappearance makes certain diagnosis impossible. The third "new" disease in Europe in the age of Columbus, typhus, rapidly established itself as a major problem and remained so for centuries. Typhus first claimed attention as a new disease in 1489–90 in the course of military operations in Spain, where the Moors resisted the attempts of the Spanish Christian kingdoms

to conquer Granada. The victims of the new disease suffered an acute fever, followed by a rash, headaches, delirium, and general debility, followed in turn by
an alarming proportion of deaths; not perhaps as high as that inflicted by plague,
but serious enough, especially among the armies where the disease seemed
most at home. Contemporaries believed that typhus came either from corpses or
from soldiers who had been in the East, perhaps Cyprus where the Venetians
employed an army against the Turks. As with syphilis and plague, conviction
that typhus was contagious dominated sixteenth-century etiological thinking.

In fact these contagion notions, and their associations with armies, were fairly
accurate, although the "newness" of typhus in the late fifteenth century remains in
question. A very small organism, of the family called *Rickettsia*, causes typhus.[12]
Such organisms are smaller than bacteria (though larger than viruses); they are
responsible for a number of diseases, including Rocky Mountain spotted fever and
Tsutsugamushi fever as well as typhus. Different *Rickettsia* species are at home in
populations of small mammals and insects: fleas in the case of typhus, ticks in the
cases of Rocky Mountain spotted fever. Ordinarily the organisms infect only their
rodent and insect hosts, and humans enter the picture accidentally when they interrupt the path of a flea or tick that customarily prefers another host. The *Rickettsia*
diseases therefore share something of plague's epidemiological pattern.

But also like plague, typhus can become epidemic in human populations and
be passed from one human to another. Typhus in its murine form, passed from
rodent to rodent by fleas, probably originated in Asia and most likely reached
Europe long before 1489, infecting the occasional European who got in the way.
Only in 1489 did it reach a serious epidemic stage, when it began to be transmitted directly from one person to another by lice. Human lice (both "body" lice and
"head" lice) make their homes on humans and their clothing, unlike fleas, which
hop on and off. Lice therefore have much more dangerous potential as carriers
of *Rickettsia* organisms. In 1489 an epidemic most likely began when a critical
mass of humans—some infected—gathered, and within that mass a person-to-
person transmission of typhus began via lice.

For that purpose the armies of late medieval and early modern Europe
afforded nearly ideal conditions: they contained large masses of unwashed and
ill-nourished people living an undisciplined life in which they foraged over the
countryside and lived in close proximity to others. And not only did armies prop-
agate typhus; warfare disrupted whatever public health measures might be
attempted. From the standpoint of health, the European armies of the sixteenth
and seventeenth centuries often combined the worst features of their predecessors
and successors: shakily controlled by still-impoverished governments that sometimes could not afford to pay them, yet equipped with the fearsome firepower of
cannons and musketry, the early modern mercenary army was a particular threat
to whomever got in its way, whether friend or foe. Not only did it practice direct

violence, whether under discipline, or told to forage plunder for itself, or given the freedom of a captured city; it remained basically unwashed, itinerant, and promiscuous, a powerful agent for the diffusion of disease. And its enhanced destructive powers made it all the more likely that its incursions could completely break down the fabric of a community it attacked, including whatever provisions for health and sanitation existed.

So while the contagious character of typhus was appreciated early (although the role of the louse—and of course that of *Rickettsia*—was only understood in the twentieth century), early modern states had trouble controlling its spread. They erected barriers to the spread of contagion, as we have seen in the previous chapter. But it is hard to imagine the thousands of members of an armed rabble stopping at a border to show their health passes; and states never considered disbanding their armies in the name of public health.

Once typhus epidemics established themselves in the wake of armies, they both played a major role in the military campaigns per se and eventually (perhaps by the 1560s) built up a pool of infected Europeans that sustained typhus epidemics in Europe continuously from that date until World War I. In that long period typhus hounded every European war and persisted in every poor, overcrowded, unwashed population. Only a few examples are necessary here to make the point.[13] In the prolonged struggles between Hapsburg Spain and Valois France in the sixteenth century, typhus sometimes played a decisive role, as for example in 1528 when it broke up and scattered a French army besieging Naples. Spanish primacy in Italy was thus strengthened, which in turn affected the Hapsburg-Spanish position in Reformation Germany. Hans Zinsser, the author of a classic study of the history of typhus, calls the Thirty Years' War (1618–1648) "the most gigantic natural experiment in epidemiology to which mankind has ever been subjected"; certainly no collection of military campaigns in Western history presents such a grim picture of invading disease accompanied by pillage and rapine.[14] By the eighteenth century some governments placed their armies under more reliable control (which included more reliable pay), so that their menace to health may have declined. But terrible examples persisted: Napoleon's failed Russian campaign of 1812, for the disasters of which winter weather is often blamed, suffered massively from diseases of which typhus was the most notable. Any student of the military history of sixteenth-, seventeenth-, and eighteenth-century Europe must take the ravages of typhus into account. Yet appalling as some of those numbers may be (17,000 Christian soldiers dead of typhus in Granada in 1489, against 3,000 killed by the Muslims), the losses to new diseases in early modern Europe are dwarfed by the contemporary experiences of the Americas. For the natives of America, encounter with European diseases proved disastrous, and their experiences form an important part of the story of the West's disease relations with the rest of the world.

New Diseases in America

The European expeditions across the Atlantic begun by Christopher Columbus in 1492 led to the conquest of a sizable proportion of the Americas within a century and precipitated the greatest demographic disaster in history. Although scholarly debate persists about the numbers, the population of the Americas in 1500 may have been between fifty and one hundred million. By the middle of the seventeenth century that number had almost certainly fallen below ten million, and perhaps below five million.

This horrific depopulation had numerous (and interrelated) causes, among which disease may take pride of place. Much attention has been focused on the sudden appearance of new epidemic diseases in the American population, and those terrible episodes undoubtedly played an important role both socially and demographically.[15] But some of the demographic collapse of the Americas may be explained by less dramatic workings of disease, in which illness worked conjointly with the drastic social effects of an alien conquest.

In the centuries before Columbus American populations had undergone some fluctuations, and some evidence suggests that about 1500 those populations may have reached a high point, near (or at) the upper limit that the existing agricultural technology could support. America's demographic condition in 1500, therefore, may have paralleled that of Europe two hundred years earlier, at the time when an overpopulated continent suffered famines in the decades that preceded the plague epidemic of 1347–1350. The capacity for food production in the Americas may have already been stretched thin before the Europeans arrived. Massive human sacrifices, it has been suggested, may have been "an unconscious mechanism for the control of population expansion."[16] In addition the population density in some parts of America—notably the Valley of Mexico and the *altiplano* of Peru—had become very high. The cities of Cuzco and Tenochtitlan may have been among the largest urban concentrations on earth.

The density of the American populations of Mexico and Peru remains a controversial point, however. If Bernard Ortiz de Montellano is correct, neither high population density nor inadequate nutrition characterized pre-Columbian Mexico.[17] The vulnerability of its population to epidemics therefore may not have paralleled that of Europe in 1347. But social and biological factors certainly did add to the vulnerability of Americans. Although many Americans fled in response to the new epidemics, at least some may have valued ties to kin and to tribe and so dispersed only reluctantly. Without clear theories of contagion, Americans may have regarded disease fatalistically and hence passively. But it is also true that many inter-American trade routes existed (including some by sea) that could contribute to the diffusion of epidemics, as could of course flight.

More important was the biological problem. Beyond doubt, the American population had been biologically isolated from the Old World for many centuries.

That isolation meant epidemiological vulnerability, although disagreement persists about its nature. The causative organisms of some diseases—notably smallpox but also measles, typhus, and plague—were evidently all new to the Americas; when these maladies traveled with Europeans to the Americas they fell on what is sometimes called "virgin soil." Subsequent documented experience with virgin soil epidemics has illustrated the savage character of such outbreaks, which for some reason strike the young adult population with particular severity.[18] That may have occurred in sixteenth-century America, although we have no age-specific statistics of mortality. Certainly the Americans had inherited no immunities to the diseases suddenly loose among them. But were the Americans also genetically predisposed to higher mortalities from diseases such as smallpox? That possibility remains in question. In either case—whether they simply lacked antibodies, or because their genetic makeup led to higher mortality from some diseases—the first American generations to meet the microorganisms suffered very high mortality. Subsequent generations perhaps fared better, either because the survivors acquired antibodies or because natural selection eliminated those with genetic susceptibility to high mortality, or both.

Smallpox was probably the first of the epidemics, and it caused perhaps the greatest single ravages. By 1519 the Caribbean islands of Hispaniola and Puerto Rico had been devastated by smallpox, and in that year the disease moved to Mexico. Its role in the astonishing conquest of the Aztec Empire by Cortez (and his Amerindian allies) was considerable.[19] By 1524 smallpox had spread through the American mainland from Mexico south to the populous Peruvian civilization of the Inca, so that by the time of Pizarro's arrival in 1532 Peru had already been crippled by disease, which the Inca regarded as a terrible omen. Measles arrived in the Caribbean in 1529 and reached Mexico two years later; typhus, perhaps accompanied by influenza, spread from Mexico to Peru between 1545 and 1547. Another outbreak of some form of influenza was at large in the 1550s. Smallpox reached Brazil in 1562, originally from Portugal, but by the seventeenth century Brazilian smallpox epidemics were being fueled by the slave trade from West Africa. The 1570s and 1580s were particularly catastrophic decades for the Americans, as typhus and influenza assailed Mexico in the middle 1570s, smallpox and measles fell on the Venezuelan coast, and smallpox worked its way north from Peru through New Granada (Colombia). This repeated epidemic pressure meant a continuing drop in populations. The pre-1492 population of the Americas may never be known, but it is likely that by the seventeenth century the population had fallen by about 90 percent from its 1500 level.[20]

The sheer number of different diseases, all new, differentiated the sixteenth-century American experience from the fourteenth-century European one. In Europe plague alone was not responsible for the death tolls of the 1340s and later, but it was not simultaneously accompanied by other great *new* killers.

The Americans suffered a succession of different "plagues," in the manner of the ancient Egyptians at the hands of Jehovah, over a prolonged yet overlapping period. Diseases spread, or became more severe, in the wake of one another. Smallpox, measles, typhus, and plague were of course great killers, even of non-virgin populations. And surviving one epidemic might leave an individual help-less to face the next. Influenzas that might simply weaken had lethal results too, for they left the system feebly unable to resist other "opportunistic" infections such as pneumonia, or they weakened the people who provided care for infants. The highest death rates in the Americas in the sixteenth century were consis-tently recorded in the tropical, coastal, and island territories, perhaps because the new diseases there fell on populations already weakened by malaria and other insect-borne fevers.

The new diseases in America also interacted with a social and economic situa-tion that had been radically changed by the abrupt European conquest. Violence had been inflicted on the population, especially on the males; some demographic data suggest that in sixteenth-century Spanish America females came to out-number males significantly, as the latter fell victim to both violence and brutally hard work. The imposition of plantation agriculture on parts of the New World resulted in monoculture, poor diets, and situations in which livestock took over the best arable land and left the natives cultivating soils of marginal productivity. Cultural imperialism also took unexpected tolls on the diet of Americans; well-meaning Christian missionaries insisted that the natives be clothed, arranged for the plantation of cotton to provide cloth, and so removed arable land from food cultivation.

The combination of inexplicable diseases, alien conquest, and brutal rearrangement of social and economic systems contributed to widespread loss of will, which in turn affected demography. Ill parents may simply have given up hope and thus doomed their young children, perhaps through inadequate food, nursing, and shelter from the elements, perhaps—more drastically—through infanticide and suicide. But were native Americans simply helpless? Or did they in fact demonstrate powers of resistance or cultural adaptation? Did they retain some independent agency in their lives?

Unanswered questions about the epidemiology of the terrible sixteenth-century diseases remain, and to consider some of them an introduction to small-pox will help, although the disease receives a more thorough discussion in Chapter Six. Smallpox is the product of infection by a virus, or rather one of a closely related group of viruses. Little doubt exists about its antiquity, and clear descriptions show that it was established in medieval Europe and the Middle East. Smallpox is an acute infection, exposure to which confers a high degree of immunity from further attacks. It passes directly from person to person, usually by way of the respiratory system; only actively sick people can transmit it.

It meets, therefore, many of the requirements of a classic "childhood" infection, since it persists in previously unexposed populations that (especially if it has been long established in a population) it finds in the young.

Moving such an infection across the Atlantic in the early sixteenth century must have involved a certain measure of chance, for the voyage was generally longer than a month, the average length of an active smallpox infection. Unless the passage were unusually fast, more than one previously unexposed person would have to be on board for the disease to be sustained across the Atlantic and thus passed to the Americans. The death of a victim would of course cut short the period of possible infection and thus make transoceanic transmission more difficult.

But deaths of Europeans from smallpox may, in the sixteenth century, have been relatively unusual, so that smallpox's chances of crossing the ocean were thus marginally improved. According to the recent arguments of Ann Carmichael and Arthur Silverstein, smallpox had been a relatively mild childhood disease in Europe for some centuries, down into the sixteenth.[21] Medieval commentators, both Muslim and Christian, regarded smallpox as a benign and perhaps even necessary part of the maturation process. If that was so, smallpox's transmission across the Atlantic may be more easily understood, but another epidemiological problem then arises.

The benignity or malignancy of smallpox may be accounted for by the fact that the viruses are part of a genus whose members are in many ways indistinguishable, but whose effects are drastically different. *Variola major* may kill 25 or 30 percent of its victims; *Variola minor,* 1 percent or less. What happened between Europe and America? Carmichael and Silverstein suggest three possibilities. Perhaps, while most smallpox cases in Europe had been mild (probably *Variola minor*), there had occurred occasional virulent *Variola major* outbreaks in later medieval Europe, and (by terrible chance) one of those was transmitted across the Atlantic to the American population. Alternatively, common *Variola minor* made its way across the ocean, and in America underwent a mutation to *Variola major.* As a third possibility, the American population carried genetic weaknesses that made it susceptible to high mortality from the benign smallpox known to Europeans. In any case, by the end of the century (or by the beginning of the seventeenth) smallpox became a serious disease to Europeans as well, although when its more lethal form spread in the Old World much of the population already enjoyed some immunity from the centuries of experience with the less virulent version.

Did the Europeans, especially the Spanish, deliberately foster disease among the Americans? Did they practice bacteriological warfare and thus achieve a desired genocide? First, we should remember that the great depopulation of the Americas, especially in those zones conquered by the Spanish (the Caribbean,

Mesoamerica, and the Andean regions), occurred by the end of the sixteenth century. In that period simple contact with the Europeans often brought disaster, and in some cases diseases actually ran ahead of the physical arrival of the Europeans themselves, as was true in Peru preceding Pizarro's conquest. The Spanish did not need to deliberately spread disease, but in any case they lacked both a motive to do so and a clearly understood means. Europeans had no precise notion of the causes of smallpox, typhus, and plague. Although by the sixteenth century doctrines of contagion were commonly held, any attempt to create biological weapons out of human bodies or their clothing would have been extremely awkward.[22] In addition, the Spaniards founded colonies whose economic bases were plantation agriculture and mining, both of which led to the enslavement of large populations of workers. The Spaniards' interests surely lay in keeping the work force alive, not in the deliberate massacre of it.

This does not deny an abundance of malice in the European conquerors of America, for they clearly stand responsible for deliberate horrors aplenty. Some of those horrors grew out of the attempts of Europeans to exploit the labor of the Americans, especially in the Spanish colonies. The interests of the later English settlement differed somewhat; at least in some areas the English, settling the land and replicating European society, wished to evict the natives, not put them to work. So the English settlers might have had an interest in disposing of the Americans. But by the seventeenth century, when the English arrived, smallpox had become a lethal disease to Europeans too. Even had they known more of its epidemiology than they did, the English may have been leery of using such an obviously two-edged sword, which might spread from the Americans back to the settler population. But it is also true that by the eighteenth century much clearer notions of smallpox's contagious character had become generally known, for inoculation (see Chapter Six) came to be practiced under a variety of circumstances in many parts of the Western world, some of them on the "frontiers" of America. Malicious English settlers (or their United States successors) who wished to clear the natives away may well have hurled blankets soaked in the "matter" of smallpox, and thus sowed a bitter legacy. But the great damage had been done unconsciously and earlier.

Five

Continuity and Change

*Magic, Religion, Medicine, and Science,
500–1700*

As we have seen, the Western world experienced new diseases in the late medieval and early modern ages. Although in some respects those periods of Western history present remarkable continuities in human responses to disease, some important new thinking about nature and disease also developed. This chapter will first discuss widely shared social and individual responses, and then consider new ideas that undermined many of the premises on which those responses were based

Between the fifth and the eighteenth centuries the people of the West lived predominantly, or even overwhelmingly, in rural surroundings. Human and animal muscle performed most work. Beliefs in supernatural powers explained the workings of the universe, whether those beliefs were simply grounded in traditional folk culture or highly elaborated in Thomistic Aristotelianism. Life expectancy remained low and disease most often inspired fatalism, however much beliefs about diseases and their causes may have changed. To such a sweeping set of generalizations must be added many qualifying caveats. In some areas—northern Italy and the Netherlands, for example—urban life early assumed considerable importance and fundamentally changed economies and societies. The "simple machines" of the science of mechanics, such as wedges and levers, magnified muscle power, while wind and water alike were harnessed in a variety of ways. By the eighteenth century the supernatural powers of the universe retreated (at least for some thinkers) into the distant recesses of a mechanical deity muscle-bound by the laws of human reason.

But the ailments of Western people, and the responses to them, remained on the whole remarkably constant. Those responses included the employment of a few pain-dulling narcotics and appeals to religion, to "magic," to the services of a wide range of empirics, and to the official mercies of professional medicine. Sometimes those responses overlapped; indistinct boundaries divided science, religion, magic, empirical healing, and folk custom. And to some undoubtedly considerable extent, people also responded to their ills by doing nothing, sometimes with iron stoicism, sometimes with vocal complaints of a kind as familiar to the twelfth century as to the twenty-first.

Much of this book concerns the effects of, and response to, more or less violent epidemic visitations: plague, leprosy, smallpox, tuberculosis. But all through the medieval and early modern periods everyday ailments affected the people of the West as well. Many of those troubles stemmed from nutritional deficiencies. Others were not so much chronic as occasional, especially the wide range of gastrointestinal disorders and the even wider variety of viral ailments and "colds." Some natural immunity to those complaints might develop, but the causative viruses themselves underwent frequent variation. A population that worked with the strength of its muscles and the leverage of its bones fell victim to osteoarthritis, bursitis, rheumatism, and other sorts of aches and pains. Diseases of physical degeneracy and aging awaited those who survived epidemic infections; cancerous tumors were well known; and psychiatric illness, called by a wide range of names and treated in an equally wide range of ways over these centuries, added to popular burdens. And of course difficult physical work often meant high rates of accidental injury; the maimed were a common sight in the medieval and early modern centuries, the products of accident, violence, birth defect, or progressive disease.

Modes of Healing

For centuries people of Western civilization found in alcohol (sometimes in combination with opium or mandrake) their first defense against pain, and some evidence suggests that alcoholic drinks became more important and pervasive in the later Middle Ages, perhaps as a consequence of the greater disposable income available in the labor-scarce, land-cheap economy of the years after the onset of plague.[1] But when the consolations of alcohol failed to relieve pain or banish care about illness, sufferers called for the aid of others. Those others might employ religion, magic, empirical remedies, and perhaps "medicine"; and while those categories were partially congruent, a consideration of each of them may clarify attitudes toward disease and practices of healing in the long preindustrial, preurban age of Western history.

Religion

Christian religious practices played a major healing role. For a start, God's will loomed as a major—perhaps *the* major—etiological explanation of disease, a notion that certainly antedated Christianity but that Christians maintained. Particularly important in medieval Christianity were the cults of the saints, for saints might intervene with God on behalf of a sinful (and ailing) suppliant. Saints and their relics emerged as important healing aspects of Christianity for a number of reasons. The competing deities of the old Roman Empire had claimed some healing powers (as did, notably, Asclepios and his votaries), and some of those pagan traditions merged into Christianity (see Chapter One). Some early healing saints were certainly Christian versions of pagan gods. Early Christian missionaries found the performance of miracles (such as healing) a strong card to play when they confronted, and converted, the heathen Germans and Slavs. Furthermore, the relics of the dead (such as bones) both shared a powerful juju with other religious traditions and could be easily carried by itinerant missionaries.

A large number of shrines associated with such holy relics grew up in the Middle Ages. Some shrines became famous all over Western civilization, including those of St. James of Compostela in Spain and St. Thomas à Becket in England. They drew pilgrims from considerable distances, and might therefore be crowded with those with the means to undertake lengthy and expensive journeys. A much larger number of shrines enjoyed a strictly local celebrity. In some cases the hierarchy of the Church recognized these places as associated with "official" saints, but in many others the local population venerated semilegendary figures, those who had not been canonized at all, and subjects of folk legend that perhaps antedated Christianity.

The story of St. Guinefort, unraveled by Jean-Claude Schmitt, illustrates well the tangled relationships of such shrines and popular faith in their healing powers.[2] St. Guinefort was originally associated with Pavia, in Italy, where his relics were venerated for their curative strength. His cult spread to regions of France, and popular belief there conflated the saint and a legendary "Holy Greyhound," a loyal dog slain by its owner in the mistaken belief that the hound had killed the master's child. The master had returned home to discover a blood-spattered dog and house, and had reached his awful conclusion. When the mistake was discovered—the child safe, the blood that of a serpent killed by the dog defending the infant—the repentant master buried the dog with great ceremony and the grave became a site of healing rituals for sick children. In the thirteenth century the Church's Inquisition denounced this story (and its associated practices) as superstition, but, as Schmitt has shown, some version of belief in the holy greyhound's healing powers persisted until the early twentieth century.

The Church made many efforts, especially from the twelfth century on, to bring such beliefs into conformity with orthodox theology. But as Ronald Finucane notes, "public demand for relics was far stronger than public obedience to church regulations," so attempts by the hierarchy to regulate the shrines often had little effect.[3] And in any case, even the most orthodox and approved shrine might be the object of unorthodox beliefs and hopes. Why did a pilgrim travel to a shrine? The answer might lie locked in his or her heart, or even subconscious. R. A. Fletcher, speaking of St. James of Compostela's shrine, puts the matter clearly: "The solemn notes which have been sounded here—contrition, amendment of life, deepening of Christian observance—may not have sounded for him [the individual pilgrim] at all. Most pilgrims (we may suspect) were perfectly ordinary people with only the humdrum problems of daily life to contend with; provided always that we bear in mind that that little word 'only' can mask whole worlds of tempestuous and ghastly experience."[4] Fletcher's study of visitors to St. James's shrine shows people fleeing from plague, barren couples hoping for a child, paralytics and cancer victims seeking cures, and even those theoretically on pilgrimage but in fact engaged in an armed expedition to loot the Mediterranean basin.

Among those drawn to the shrines, regardless of the orthodoxy of the holy places, were the sufferers. Perhaps the shrine's reputation, either in a locality or as specializing in particular ailments, attracted them. Perhaps they came only after other recourses—alcohol, their local priest's prayers, the medications of an empiric—failed them. According to Finucane, who studied the records of English shrines, the most common ailments for which relief was sought varied according to social class.[5] The lower orders, both men and women, brought their crippling illnesses and blindness and troubles brought on by malnutrition, lives of toil, and (in the case of women) complications of childbirth. Men from the upper class, not surprisingly, brought their battlefield wounds. All the suppliants prayed at the shrine, hoping to get as physically close to the relic as they could; they also consumed waters associated with the shrine, if any such existed. Procedures rooted in folk custom might help: for example, measuring the sufferer's height with a string and then using the string as the wick in a votive candle to be burnt at the shrine. Pilgrims waited for some signal turn of events: a dream, or a dramatic moment of crisis in their pain. When they were convinced that a cure had taken hold they departed, first making offerings of coins, candles, or objects associated with their affliction such as crutches or slings.

The Church's position on the validity of these curative shrines was very ambiguous. Although the hierarchy inveighed against superstition and the Church theoretically could not compel natural events, priests regularly blessed everyday activities (such as the planting of crops) and extraordinary ones (armies going into battle), and for many onlookers such blessings implied some power over the course of nature. The sacraments, especially the holy water of baptism and the elements of the Mass, possessed apparent magical powers. As a number of authors have noticed, the popular belief in the powers of the elements led to thefts of the bread and the wine, which led in turn to the Church's attempts to secure them in locked monstrances, which security (and display) simply confirmed popular belief in their magical powers.

In addition, in the early Middle Ages, if any knowledge of Greco-Roman medical traditions and writings survived in the West, it could be found in monastic communities, which meant that monks might offer some medical treatment as well as spiritual help. To those drawn to them the distinctions may not have been clear. As the Church's priests acquired some of the learning of the cathedral schools and universities (after the twelfth century) some of them inherited the earlier position of the monk: the person in the village community who might have some smattering of Galenic ideas as well as the power to perform the miracle of the Mass.

The position of kings offered further examples of the Church's ambiguity about religion's power over nature. Western kings increased their prestige and gained respect by surrounding themselves with pomp and ceremony at their coronations, and the Church cooperated in these rituals, consecrating kings with holy oil. When (in the thirteenth century) the papacy contested the miraculous powers of the French and English kings to cure scrofula, it was belatedly realizing that it had encouraged a view that religious ceremony meant control over nature's course. And in any case the Bible itself seemed to license the idea that the God of the Israelites was a supreme magician, who could part the Red Sea and bring the chariot of the sun to a halt when so requested by Joshua. When Jesus was born magi visited him; when he grew to manhood he caused the lame to walk and the dead to rise up.

Magic

All these factors, and their perception in the ordinary medieval mind, lend support to Richard Kieckhefer's argument that neat divisions of the realms of religion and magic are likely to founder on the complexities of medieval and early modern culture.[6] Kieckhefer argues that medieval thinkers came to see different categories of magic: "natural" magic, which dealt with what all agreed were the hidden, or occult, powers of nature; and "demonic" magic, a perversion of religion.[7] And while before the twelfth century (according to Kieckhefer) Christian thinkers saw all magic as "demonic," in fact many classical, pagan, early Christian, Norse, and Celtic beliefs eroded those Christian denunciations. After the twelfth century, natural magic gained acceptance as a legitimate branch of inquiry.

Natural magic, which attempted to understand the hidden powers of nature, was bolstered by philosophy as well as by religion. These relations were clearest in the late Middle Ages and the period of the Renaissance, when neo-Platonic doctrines gained wider currency among thinkers. Neo-Platonic beliefs insisted on the complete interrelation and mutual responsiveness of the different phenomena of the universe. Events in the "macrocosm"—the greater world of astronomical phenomena—affected or even mirrored events in the "microcosm," the individual. Harmonies vibrated between the heavens and the individual, or between large natural events and human physiological processes. To understand man, the thinker must understand the macrocosm. "Understanding" might entail more than a simple process of rational analysis; the thinker should become attuned to the harmonies of the universe, should be sympathetic to microcosm and macrocosm alike.

Studies of alchemy and astrology therefore loomed large in the neo-Platonic understanding of nature. Astrology clearly rested on the belief that events in the heavens influenced or mirrored the lives of individuals; alchemy pursued chemical changes that would lead to "purified" metals (ultimately gold) and elixirs (which would confer health). Before purifying metals or elixirs, the alchemist had first to purify himself. The distinctions that later thinkers, in the Cartesian tradition, made between "matter" and "spirit" simply had no meaning to the neo-Platonist. Renaissance neo-Platonism, or naturalism, filled the universe with life and volition and so approached pantheism. It believed that powers were at large in the universe, powers that might possess their own will to act, powers that the knowing might harness, perhaps to effect a cure.

For many reasons, therefore, the beliefs both of devoutly Christian priests and monks and of Renaissance court thinkers overlapped the practices of folk empirics who, drawing on some arcane knowledge of nature, called down supernatural powers to aid in their healing arts.

Empirical Healing

Folk medicine involved a varying mix of religion, magic, philosophy, and tradition. Activities might include the bleeding and purging consistent with Galenic theory, attention to diet, the herbal traditions of both the classical authors (such as Dioscorides) and the trial-and-error empirics, the practices of surgery and midwifery, careful attention to routine, the employment of what Keith Thomas has called "technical aids," arcane language, and religious formulas and incantations in which the routinely orthodox Christian prayer existed along a continuum with appeals to the occult powers of nature or even to demons. Scholars who have written about the healing activities of medieval and early modern Europe have found generalization difficult, for the local variations were almost innumerable. Some common elements did exist, however.

Many healers employed some combination of herbal remedies, often together with animal parts. Trial and error produced many of these medications, as it had for centuries in different cultures. Perhaps some of the monks and priests who found themselves in healing roles had some acquaintance with ancient Greek or Roman authorities, but perhaps not. For many healers some element of magic inhered in particular herbal remedies. The preparation and administration of these materials might follow a definite routine, which might be designed to ensure reliability or perhaps to avoid taboos which, if violated, would weaken or destroy the healing power of the herb or indeed of the healer. "Technical aids" might accompany the administration of the remedy: ducks' bills placed in patients' mouths, dipping victims in flowing water, examining the belt of a pregnant woman.[8] Because of their local character the symbolism of these acts was often extremely obscure, although some—opening and closing doors and drawers to assist women in labor—seem obvious.

Words often accompanied such actions: prayers, some of them (Hail Marys, Paternosters) ordinary enough, some of them specific to a particular ailment ("Jesus Christ for mercy's sake/Take away this toothache"), and some of them best described as gibberish, at least to the sufferer.[9] Gestures might attend the words; some curative power might reside in the healer's touch. Some touching powers were thought to be God-given, or the gift of inheritance. For obscure reasons of mystical numerology, seventh sons were widely credited with a healing touch, and seventh sons of seventh sons had extraordinary power. The consoling or comforting touch of a healer might not need any magical explanation at all, but such gestures of kindness surely, if insensibly, shaded into the efficacy of supernatural power.

Notable here were the "strokers" of the sixteenth and seventeenth centuries, whose claims in England and France ran the risk of poaching on royal healing preserves. Where the rulers had asserted a specific healing power in their touch (see Chapter Two), they might be jealous of infringements. Thus Jacques-Philippe Boisgaudre, a reputed seventh son, found himself prosecuted in England in 1632, and James Leverett was imprisoned and whipped in 1637, for offering healing competition to Charles I. The most famous seventeenth-century stroker, Valentine Greatrakes, attracted a large following in the 1660s, which included such eminent men of science as Robert Boyle and John Flamsteed. Greatrakes retired from the healing field rather than contest it with Charles II, but although his contemporaries disagreed about whether his powers were "natural" or "magical," they united in respecting them.[10]

Materials had real importance as well. Symbolic considerations entered into the selection of both medications and talismans.[11] Yellow materials might be prescribed for jaundice; amulets offered protection from illness, perhaps because of their inherent virtue, perhaps (if they carried words or letters) because of the talismanic power of the inscriptions.

Women carried on a considerable proportion of empirical practice, especially— but not exclusively—that which applied to women's health in general and to births in particular. Some women could be found at all levels of medieval and early modern healing, including physicians, although few of the latter have been identified. Monica Green suggests that the position of women healers evolved in a way that reflected the increasing complexities of "professionalization" in the early modern period. As surgeons and physicians alike maneuvered for advantage (see Chapters Six and Ten), women practitioners found themselves "gradually restricted to a role as subordinate and controlled assistants in matters where, because of socially constructed notions of propriety, men could not practice alone."[12] Within those roles, however, some women could gain or retain considerable authority, as the career of Angélique Marguerite Le Boursier du Coudray, the eighteenth-century French "King's Midwife," illustrates.[13] But much empirical practice remained outside the scope of the established professions; at the end of the eighteenth century the midwife Martha Ballard still performed a variety of healing services in Maine, despite the growing power of organized (and male) professions.[14]

Physicians and Surgeons

By the late thirteenth century—earlier in some places—many medical practitioners had established their formal qualifications as physicians. Those qualifications might derive from possession of a university medical education (which itself emerged with the general medieval university movement of the twelfth century), from privileges granted by a public authority (lay or religious), or from membership in a guild or "college" that had legal power to grant such privileges to protect the standards of the healing trade. Some practitioners might possess all three: the claims of others might be less clear.

Theoretically these "recognized" physicians practiced healing in accord with their education, one dominated by Galen, Hippocrates, and a number of Arabic texts based on classical authors. Physicians therefore believed that an imbalance of humors resulted in sickness, for such imbalance led to an imbalance of the qualities (hotness, dryness, and the like) that constituted each individual's "complexion." Humors could be returned to balance by bleeding, scarifying, purging, attention to diet that would restore the proper qualities, and medications that might have the same effect. The physician's armory included all those approaches and remedies. In fact most physicians—most of whose patients appeared with self-limiting or non-life-threatening conditions—usually offered relatively gentle dietetic remedies that did not differ appreciably from those of folk healers.[15] That was equally true of medications, which for physician and empiric alike might be drawn from a rich complex of local favorites, well-established traditional herbals, and those derived from written classical sources. "Magic" played some role in those medications, even for physicians.

From the late twelfth century on, surgery developed as a separate healing skill, like medicine rooted in the written texts of antiquity. But while different professional paths of physicians and surgeons developed, those lines were often unclear, especially in Italy and southern Europe. While surgeons often did not have the qualification of university education, both they and the physicians "shared a common tradition of knowledge drawn from the same sources."[16]

On the other side of the profession, surgery was also practiced by a continuum of empirics, such as bonesetters, as well as by members of other guilds such as barber-surgeons. Guilds of surgeons therefore sometimes found themselves in conflict with rivals from both directions. But most agreed that the dressing of wounds, the setting of broken bones, and such serious occasions as amputations and lithotomies (to remove bladder stones) required a surgeon's skills.

Success

A large question remains: in this plethora of techniques and materials, what was believed central to the cure? Did a herbal remedy, by itself, receive credit for a physical effect on the body or on the disease? Were the words that accompanied the remedy's administration decisive? If so, did it matter who uttered the words? Did the words have power apart from the speaker? Or was the cure found in the person of the healer? How important was the preservation of some symbol— a cross, an amulet, words written on a cloth and worn around the neck—by the sufferer? The possibilities of belief, shading across a spectrum involving more or less emphasis on some or all of the above answers, encompassed the worlds of physicians, surgeons, apothecaries, traditional folk healers, priests, midwives, barbers, charlatans, magicians, and villagers with the "gift."

If cures were "successful," on what grounds do we explain the success? The wide range of popular medicine certainly attracted masses of people throughout the medieval and early modern periods. Far more sufferers repaired to popular and folk healers—"wise women," "cunning men"—than to orthodox physicians who worked in the Galenic tradition. Some explanation of that relative popularity lies in social and economic circumstances. Physicians—and to a lesser extent surgeons and official apothecaries—were expensive, and village cunning men and wise women were not. Outrageous charlatans who charged high fees did exist, but they were relatively rare.

More important even than cost, however, was accessibility, both geographical and social. Physicians were rare and overwhelmingly urban, in what remained (in most of the Western world) a predominantly rural society. Village healers were convenient. They also represented a familiar world, one of villagers from the same social stratum, who shared common experiences and trials of life. However much some folk healers wrapped themselves in arcane language and mystery, they remained more familiar to most patients than the university-educated, urban, pretentious physician. And village healers also offered, most frequently, gentle healing arts: herbal remedies and baths (even if they insisted that the bath must be taken in a stream flowing in a particular direction, or during a certain phase of the moon). Contrast such therapy with the violent bleedings and purgings sometimes undertaken by the Galenic physician, or—worse yet—the ministrations of the surgeon, offered with no anesthetic except alcohol or opium.

The activities of popular healers may also have appealed because they corresponded to contemporary perceptions of illness and hence of cure. Such perceptions were, as Finucane puts it, often a "consensus of opinion," as indeed they are in all times and places.[17] Medieval understanding of human anatomy and physiology lacked much of the precision that it acquired in the centuries after the sixteenth. "Causes" of disease bore no clear relation to cellular biology or microorganisms; pathology related largely to externally observed symptoms. Changes in condition, seen externally, might well be considered a "cure," even though they might (by modern lights) be temporary or partial or even a new and more alarming stage of a disease. At the extreme limit of this "consensus of opinion" lay contemporary views of death itself. Modern definitions of death have become increasingly confused, as technology replaces failing organs; how many contemporary laypeople still think (in good Aristotelian terms) that death occurs when the heart stops beating? Well into the eighteenth century considerable popular doubt persisted about when death occurred, dramatically illustrated by the numerous cases of people hanged but later revived by their friends and relations.[18] Some medieval "miracles," in which saints and their relics brought the dead to life, might be explained by different definitions of death in the twelfth and twenty-first centuries.

Many cures, of course, "worked" by any standard. The trial and error of centuries of folk tradition had winnowed the vast field of herbal remedies. Still other cures succeeded at least temporarily (or could be perceived as successful), especially with the large variety of diseases that had remissive traits or that we would, today, call "self-limiting." The myriad viruses that produce colds and influenzas usually run a limited course. We have already seen (in Chapter Two) that scrofula's remissive stages conferred on the kings of France and England apparent power over that ailment.

And, perhaps most important of all, many popular cures "worked" because the sufferers believed that they would. Disease ultimately is self-defined; psychosomatic symptoms are "real." At least by the seventeenth century (and probably much earlier) some healers knew the reality of the mind's power over "disease." Keith Thomas quotes a fascinating example of such seventeenth-century knowledge:

[A] French doctor had a patient who was convinced that he was possessed by the Devil. The doctor called in a priest and a surgeon, meanwhile equipping himself with a bag containing a live bat. The patient was told that it would take a small operation to cure him. The priest offered up prayer, and the surgeon made a small incision in the man's side. Just as the cut was given, the doctor let the bat fly into the room, crying, "Behold, there the devil is gone!" The man believed it and was cured.[19]

Diverging Categories

In important and fundamental ways the responses of religion, medicine, and folklore remained in a close and mutually supporting relationship over the medieval and early modern centuries, and that relationship only began to founder in the seventeenth century.[20] Even then, the symbiosis did not rapidly dissolve; rather it broke apart gradually and partially, in different times and places.

Religion's connections with magic were considerable, but also always fraught with tension. If in the high Middle Ages the Church brought "natural magic" within its fold, in the same period it undertook a prolonged effort to regularize popular religion and bring it under central control. The denunciation of numerous local magical powers, cures, and shrines followed, as of course did more general attacks on movements judged heretical. In addition, the elaborated theology of the medieval Church attempted to clarify the limits of human powers to compel nature to obedience. Cunning men and wise women might not clearly understand those limits, and so could claim no theoretical support from organized religion.

The Protestant Reformation of the sixteenth century significantly widened the gaps between religion and magic. Protestants simply dismissed the cults of the saints as accretions that lacked scriptural authority. Even more fundamentally, most Protestants refused to grant special powers to the priesthood. Ordination was not a sacrament. And, in any case, for Protestants the sacraments themselves lost their magical powers; for Calvin the Mass ceased to be a literal reenactment of Christ's sacrifice, in which wine was transsubstantially changed to blood, and became instead a simple memorial service. The Christian religion, at least in its Reformed guise, no longer had priests who performed miracles.

If religion was transformed in the early modern centuries, the world of "magic" ultimately suffered particularly heavy blows. Intellectual and social changes alike played roles in diminishing magic's appeal. The Christian religion, especially in its Protestant form, more clearly separated itself from "magic"; in the short run, some historians have argued, magic flourished in sixteenth- and seventeenth-century Protestant Europe precisely because orthodox religion had left a vacuum for it to fill. Without saints' shrines to repair to, sufferers turned all the more readily to the "white witches," the wise women and cunning men, the benign faces of the contemporary "witch craze." But in the longer term religion's antipathy turned opinion against the practitioners of magical healing, much as rationalism ultimately dampened the ardor of witch-hunting.

Although religion and magic may have diverged, their difficulties with each other paled before the challenges to both posed by new scientific beliefs. The "scientific revolution" of the sixteenth and seventeenth centuries undercut traditional Christian orthodoxy and demanded new ideas about the relations of God, nature, and humankind. And although the Renaissance naturalism that supported some aspects of magic and empirical healing formed an important component of the scientific revolution, other components that suggested a mechanical philosophy of nature called that spirit-laden naturalism into question as well.

The Scientific Revolution
Cosmology

Medieval cosmology made it easy to believe that God's power and providence totally dominated the universe, and that God had awarded man the special central place in that universe. In fact the entire universe literally revolved around humankind, which inhabited the stationary central sphere of the earth. And while medieval people might regard the earth as a sinkhole into which the universe's corruption fell, the earth and its inhabitants were also clearly unique. They occupied the central and privileged position, the stage on which the great human and divine drama of salvation was played. Humankind capped God's creation; sun, moon, stars all deferred to sinful man. How natural, then, to believe in God's providence, to believe in God's constant intervention in human affairs, to believe that individual sickness and health were the concerns and products of the divine will. Between 1500 and 1700 belief in the salient features of that cosmology collapsed, to be replaced by quite different conceptions of the relationship of God and man, and quite different explanations of the causes of natural phenomena, including, ultimately, the causes of disease and health.

This story conventionally, and properly, begins with Copernicus (1473–1543), who proposed, in effect, that the earth and the sun switch places, with the sun taking the earth's central place in the universe and the earth joining the other planets and the stars in their revolution about it. The theory faced massive difficulties before it could win general acceptance, for it removed the earth from its privileged central position in the universe and hence posed grave psychological barriers; even in the present century, people must be educated out of their instinctive sense that the earth is central and motionless. It seemed to contradict Scripture, inasmuch as Joshua had commanded the sun to stand still, which implied that ordinarily it moved. And a moving earth demanded an entirely new view of the motion of bodies, perhaps even a completely different mind-set. Copernicus himself hardly addressed such issues at all.

Little wonder, then, that Copernicus' ideas made few converts in the balance of the sixteenth century. But in the hundred years after his book appeared, the notion of heliocentricity both gained important adherents and underwent interesting modifications. One was the gradual association of Copernicanism with the radically new idea of an infinitely extended universe. Although this conception was not found in Copernicus himself, he opened the door for it by his belief that the universe was much larger than the prevailing cosmology maintained. By the end of the century Giordano Bruno had advocated an infinite universe, without any notion of a central place. Another interesting modification of Copernicus came from Johannes Kepler (1572–1630), a German astronomer who argued that the planets moved not in perfect unchanging circles—as both the Aristotelian tradition and Copernicus had agreed—but instead followed elliptical paths around the sun (for Kepler was in that sense a strong Copernican).

Kepler's work led to precise laws of planetary motion, laws that made the case for Copernicus more convincing from the standpoint of the connections between astronomical theory and observation. And on a broader front the ideas of Galileo Galilei (1564–1642) established the feasibility of Copernicanism as a physical explanation; perhaps the earth really moved. Galileo began the construction of a new science of motion that would explain the apparent anomalies that followed a belief in the rotation of the earth. What caused the motions of the heavenly bodies, and what caused the motions of bodies on earth? What kept the planets in their courses around the sun, especially since—if Kepler was right—those courses did not follow an unchanging circle? How to account for the heavy body dropped from the tower, when the tower itself—if Copernicus was right—moved in the "circle" characteristic of heavenly motions? Some seventeenth-century thinkers believed that the causal question was secondary; better to ask how the motion might be described mathematically? than to ask why the motion occurred. Galileo and Kepler, for instance, both believed that the universe could best be understood in mathematical terms. But questions of cause did not go away easily, even for Galileo, Kepler, and others with their mathematical vision of nature. Two broad physical interpretations of motion emerged in the course of the seventeenth century. For some—most notably the great French philosopher René Descartes (1596–1650) — motion arose from the mechanical interactions of matter. An object moved because some other object pushed it. Others saw motion caused by some natural "force" that could act at a distance, without objects being in direct physical contact with one another. In this view natural objects had powers which extended outwards. Thus while for Descartes the motions of the planets resulted from the whirlpoollike pressure on them of a medium that filled all space, for Kepler the planets were swept along by a force emanating from the sun.

Anatomy and Physiology

Regardless of the explanation of motion, these two schools of thought, one mechanical and the other finding a perhaps-"vital" force in natural bodies, had great influence in fields beyond cosmology and mechanics. Their impact may be seen in both the chemical and the anatomical traditions of the scientific revolution, two fields that ultimately bore on concepts of health and disease. Challenges in those fields were associated with two contemporaries of Copernicus: Paracelsus and Vesalius. Paracelsus certainly mounted the noisiest and most immediately effective attack of the three; Vesalius was more deferential, but eventually similarly subversive of old ideas.

Galen's authority in the fields of anatomy and physiology bolstered his authority as a physician, and his physiological and anatomical ideas went largely unchallenged until the sixteenth century. Although Andreas Vesalius (1514–1564) was, like Copernicus, a reluctant revolutionary, he was a pivotal figure in a revolution in thought nevertheless: a revolution that ultimately overthrew Galenic anatomy and physiology.

Some groundwork for a challenge had been laid in the medieval period. For one thing, thirteenth-century physicians and surgeons (in the universities of Italy and southern France) resumed the practice of human dissection, a practice that had been abandoned before Galen's own time. In 1316, on the basis of this limited experience with the human frame, the leading medieval anatomy text was composed: that of Mondino de Luzzi. Mondino's text was copied and recopied many times in the next two centuries, and for that period became the authority through which an understanding of Galen was transmitted to students. Mondino and others may have had direct experience of human anatomy, but Galen's authority led them to see the body through Galen's eyes. If Galen said that the stomach was a sphere, so did Mondino; if Galen said the liver had five lobes, so did Mondino; if Galen said the heart had three ventricles, so did Mondino.

Before we condemn Mondino and his successors for slavish obedience to an authority contradicted by their own eyes, we should remember the practical constraints on the practice of anatomy. One constraint was social: dissections performed for the benefit of students were done not by physicians but by surgeons or their assistants. The physician-professor sat at a high desk and read Mondino's text, while below in the pit the surgeon and his assistant worked away on the cadaver. No necessary correspondence existed between what the professor read and what the surgeon exposed. Another constraint was more difficult to avoid. Dissection, though a regular practice, remained an infrequent one; the corpse was often that of an executed criminal, for Christian resistance to such treatment of the dead ran deep. Christians, after all, believed in the literal resurrection of the body. Since corpses for dissection were therefore rare, each was precious for anatomical instruction; the demonstrator used it all, as rapidly as he could, for there were no effective means of preserving its organs. A demonstrative dissection might therefore be conducted hastily and carelessly.

Two other large barriers interfered with anatomical understanding. One was the lack of agreed-upon terminology, and the other was the lack of accurate reproductions of illustrations. Those difficulties began to be overcome in the fifteenth century, owing to changes in the worlds of scholarship and of art. The humanism of the Renaissance was a complex phenomenon beyond our scope here, but the humanists' demands for pure Greek or Latin texts are relevant. A "pure" text of Galen, for instance, would be "freed" of the Arabic and Christian medieval barbarisms and word usages that interfered with understanding the master's meaning. Such arguments cleared the way for agreed-upon anatomical terminology. Modern medical students may find committing anatomical terms to memory an albatross, but imagine their distress if different professors had different terms for identical organs. Even more important, the rise of more naturalistic artistic representation, when concentrated on anatomical detail, led to more accurate illustration. And in the fifteenth century illustrations could be reproduced precisely, which for the transmission of anatomical knowledge was absolutely crucial. Woodcuts and engravings, which existed by about 1400, came into wide use by about 1450; etchings followed by about 1500. These techniques, linked to the printing press developed by about 1450, made possible what William Ivins called the "exactly repeatable pictorial statement," important in many aspects of modern civilization, of which anatomical illustration is one of the most striking.[21]

By about 1500 some anatomists, notably Berengario, both became more critical of past authority and saw the possibilities of reproduced art for anatomical instruction. Vesalius emphasized these new approaches. Andreas Vesalius, or van Wesele, was born in Brussels, the son of an apothecary in the service of the Hapsburg family. He received a physician's education in the universities of Paris and Padua, the leading centers of Aristotelian and Galenic learning of the age. At Padua he passed quickly from student to master, and while attached to the faculty there he wrote his great textbook of anatomy. *De humani corporis fabrica* (usually just called *De fabrica*) was published in 1543, the same year in which Copernicus' *De revolutionibus* proposed a heliocentric universe. Vesalius' text established for him a European reputation and led to his appointment as physician to the Emperor Charles V and subsequently to his son Philip II of Spain. Vesalius died suddenly while returning from a trip to the Near East in 1564.

De fabrica, unlike *De revolutionibus*, did not set forth a challenging new general hypothesis. In many ways it remained firmly in the Galenic tradition; its novelty lay in its thoroughness, accuracy, and precise anatomical illustrations that approached fine art. Vesalius shared most of Galen's fundamental physiological assumptions (see Chapter One): three different systems of vessels (veins, arteries, nerves) based on three different organs (liver, heart, brain) moved different humors and spirits throughout the body. But a critical spirit pervaded the work, and Vesalius was eager and willing to find Galen's mistakes. He especially delighted in showing how Galen, by relying on dissections of animals other than humans, had been led into anatomical errors in his descriptions of muscles and bones. Galen remained the master, but the disciple proved his mettle by correcting the teacher.

This style of challenge persisted in what became a kind of "Vesalian" school of anatomy in the university at Padua for the remainder of the sixteenth century. Vesalius' contemporaries and successors there continued to find and point out Galenic errors of detail: Eustachi, Fallopio (both of them immortalized by the

names of body parts), Colombo, Fabrizio. And—crucial for the ultimate fate of
Galen's system—some of the details became linchpins in a more general challenge to Galen's authority. One of these details concerned Galen's description of
the heart. Galen believed that the septum, the thick tissue that divides the heart
into right and left sides, was perforated by tiny pores that allowed some "venous"
blood to seep through from one side to the other. Vesalius could not detect those
pores, but—unwilling to challenge Galenic physiology—concluded: "Thus we
are compelled to astonishment at the industry of the Creator who causes the
blood to sweat through from the right ventricle into the left through passages
which escape our sight."[22] One of Vesalius' successors, Colombo, proposed a
solution that would preserve the fundamental Galenic physiology. He traced
what is sometimes called the "lesser circulation" of the blood, in which the blood
passes from right ventricle to left auricle not through pores in the septum—
which are not there—but through the pulmonary artery, the lungs, and the pulmonary vein. This transfer from one side of the heart to the other was very
important in Galen's physiology, because arterial blood, which for Galen was
rooted in the heart, received much of its material (though not its essence) from
venous blood. By moving some venous blood to the left side of the heart,
Colombo "saved" the system, which otherwise would have been imperiled by
Vesalius' failure to clearly confirm Galen's necessary pores.

But the notion of a circulation, in which blood looped through the body from
one side of the heart to the other, proved a dangerous ally. Another Paduan
anatomist, Fabrizio of Aquapendente (or Fabricius), puzzled over another
anatomical detail: the so-called valves in the veins and their function. In Galen's
physiology the flow of arterial blood, venous blood, and the fluid of the nerves
was in each case two-way; in the case of the veins, for example, venous blood
moved back and forth through them from the liver to the rest of the body, carrying a fresh load of humors and spirits to all other organs, then returning to the
liver to be recharged. Fabrizio's "valves" perhaps regulated the flow of venous
blood in some way. The door now opened for an inquiry that would be fatal to
Galenic physiology. One of Fabrizio's students, the Englishman William Harvey
(1578–1657), used such details as the valves of the veins to propose an entirely
new system of human physiology in a book published in 1628: *De motu cordis*, a
masterpiece of experimental evidence, the use of dissection, quantification, and
analogical reasoning. Harvey put forward the general circulation of the blood, in
which blood moved from the heart through the arteries to the extremities of the
body, then returned to the heart through the veins. Fabrizio's valves regulated
not volume of flow, but its direction; blood moved around the body in a grand
circuit, and not in an ebb and flow through three separate systems.

Harvey found at least some of his inspiration in Aristotle, for the Paduan
school that he represented had long been imbued with a careful Aristotelian

experimentalism. More than that, Harvey saw the human heart in fervent, near-mystical terms, as the center of heat and life of the body; Aristotle had seen the heart as the primary organ, a judgment that Galen's tripartite systems had weakened in favor of the brain and the liver, and that Harvey now restored. The blood carried a vital principle of life around the body, one that regenerated the body and gave it spirit. Thus although Harvey himself did not simply consider the heart as a machine, a pump at the center of a hydraulic system, his doctrine of circulation nevertheless invited such a mechanical idea. Seventeenth-century thinkers were to find mechanical explanations of nature particularly convincing.

Paracelsus

Paracelsus (1493–1541) is a major figure in the histories of both medicine and chemistry, and his importance stems both from what he did and what he was later thought to have done. Paracelsus, whose original name was Theophrastus Bombastus von Hohenheim, was born in Einsiedeln, Switzerland, the son of a man who practiced as a physician. When he was a boy his family moved to Carinthia, where his father practiced medicine among the miners of that province. The young Paracelsus' education in medicine was apparently irregular; one writer calls it "inconsecutive," meaning that it probably consisted partly of apprenticeship and trial-and-error practice and partly of peripatetic attendance at different universities. His enemies—and he accumulated a lot of them—questioned his right to call himself a physician. He may for a time have practiced as an army surgeon. By the mid-1520s he had developed a reputation as a healer. Successful cures at Basel resulted in his appointment as official physician to that Swiss city, where he made a great stir and after about a year had to flee the place. On taking office in Basel he delivered an intemperate oration, often quoted since:

> I am Theophrastus, and greater than those to whom you liken me; I am Theophrastus, and in addition I am *monarcha medicorum* and I can prove to you what you cannot prove. I will let Luther defend his cause and I will defend my cause and I will defeat those of my colleagues who turn against me; and this I shall do with the help of *arcana*. . . . It was not the constellations that made me a physician; God made me. . . . I need not don a coat of mail or a buckler against you, for you are not learned or experienced enough to refute even one word of mine. I wish I could protect my bald head against the flies as effectively as I can defend my monarchy. . . . I will not defend my monarchy with empty talk, but with *arcana*. And I do not take my medicines from the apothecaries; their shops are but foul sculleries, from which comes nothing but foul broths. As for you, you defend your kingdom with belly-crawling and flattery. How long do you think this will last? . . . Let me tell you this: every little hair on my neck knows more than you and all your scribes, and my shoe buckles are

more learned than your Galen and Avicenna, and my beard has more experience than all your high colleges.[23]

Clearly a violent and radical character. After fleeing Basel, he wandered from town to town in central Europe, in constant contention with medical establishments. He wrote a great deal, but little of it was published before his death in 1541. He did, however, gain followers, who in the century after his death gave his ideas—or what were said to be his ideas—greater and greater currency. His writings were massively printed and reprinted between 1565 and 1620.

The varied history of Paracelsus and his work has meant that interpretations of him have not been easy, and in any case Paracelsus' thought is forbidding to modern understanding. Some points are nevertheless clear. He systematically (though not always consistently) denied the authority of the scholastics of the Middle Ages, of Aristotle, and of Galen. He also proposed alternatives to those authorities, but those proposals may be clearer if we first examine his criticisms of established views. Just as Galen's humoral medicine (and ultimately the Hippocratic humoral medicine from which it came) was based on the theory of the four elements, so too Paracelsus' rejection of humoral medicine included a rejection of those four elements, especially as they had been expounded by Aristotle. Paracelsus was not entirely consistent about this, but in general he argued for the primacy of what he called the "Three Principles" in place of the Aristotelian quartet of earth, air, fire, and water. The three principles were sulfur, mercury, and salt; as with the Aristotelian four elements, the principles were associated with certain physical qualities. Sulfur conferred on substances that contained it the quality of combustibility; mercury conferred fluidity; salt conferred solidity and color. Although some aspects of these ideas were not new— Arabic thinkers had, for instance, emphasized the primacy of mercury and sulfur—for Paracelsus they formed part of a sweeping attack on scholastic authority, one with a true religious component and at least implied overtones of social radicalism.

Part of Paracelsus' denial of scholastic authority included a vigorous defense of both "experiment" and "experience," not necessarily the same thing although some of their features overlapped. When Paracelsus asserted that "my beard has more experience than all your high colleges," the voice may have been that of the practical man who had labored among the miners and soldiers, the man whose dirty hands scorned mere book learning. But "experience" might also mean that he had *experienced* something akin to revelation of divine mysteries, and so had an arcane (remember *arcana*) understanding of, and perhaps even control over, the forces of nature. Paracelsus, like many of the figures discussed earlier in this chapter, certainly believed in nature's occult powers. He was in fact a leading exponent of that philosophy which imbued all nature with spirits and souls, which made different natural phenomena the products of their own self-willed principles of activity. "Experience" might mean the ability to penetrate (or to have revealed) the secrets of that self-willed principle, to understand its motives.

Paracelsus applied this notion of a self-willed nature to his thoughts about disease. He strongly disagreed with the Hippocratic-Galenic belief that disease was a systemic malfunction. No, said Paracelsus, disease was local, not systemic; it was the product of a disorder of a particular organ. Such disorders, it should be noted, were chemical in character, and they illustrated that each organ had in some manner its own will. Thus:

> A person eating meat, wherein both poison and nourishment are contained, deems everything good while he eats. For the poison lies hidden among the good and there is nothing good among the poison. When thus the food, that is to say the meat, reaches the stomach, the alchemist is ready and eliminates that which is not conducive to the well-being of the body. This the alchemist conveys to a special place, and the good where it belongs. This is as the Creator ordained it. In this manner the body is taken care of so that no harm will befall it from the poison which it takes in by eating, the poison being eliminated from the body by the alchemist without man's cooperation. Of such a nature are thus virtue and power of the alchemist in man.[24]

When this "alchemist" (or as Paracelsus sometimes called it, this *archaeus*), an independent self-willed spirit of a body organ, became incapacitated, disease resulted. The physician should then become the substitute alchemist, correcting the malfunctions by the administration of chemically prepared remedies.

Paracelsus also believed—as did many Renaissance thinkers, especially those influenced by neo-Platonism—in the correspondences of the macrocosm and the microcosm. The human body was a microcosmic representation of the macrocosmic universe; events in one paralleled events in the other. Astral emanations connected the two. The signs of one might be seen in the signs of the other. Hence the importance of observation, not just of the body but of all nature, for healing. Astronomical events were portentious for health, and so astrology had a role; and the body was above all a microcosm of chemical processes, which could be observed in the alchemist's laboratory and then replicated in the body. Book learning—or at least some sorts of book learning—was at a discount, and the physician should gain experience with nature by working with it and observing it. And since the body's actions (or more properly the actions of the "alchemists" of the body) mirrored alchemical procedures, the physician must be adept at such procedures, for they were the keys to maintaining health. Paracelsus therefore emphasized the importance of medications prepared in the laboratory, in addition to the herbals found in nature. We have already (in Chapter Four) seen his advocacy of mercury compounds in the treatment of syphilis, and we may now more clearly understand the philosophy that lay behind that preference.

Paracelsus and his followers were largely responsible for a growing connection between medicine and chemistry in the period between roughly 1550 and 1700. In those years *iatrochemistry*, chemistry in the service of medicine, became both a prominent medical philosophy and the great goal of practical alchemy; the search for the transmutation of metals continued, but was often overshadowed by the practical composition of remedies used by physicians and by the ancient search for the principles that would prolong life. Within the medical profession struggles went on between long-entrenched Galenists and the new Paracelsians, or "iatrochemical" physicians. The struggle was especially bitter and important in Paris, where the Galenists remained in control of the medical faculty of the university but the Paracelsians enjoyed periods of favor at court. These struggles had both religious and political overtones, for sixteenth-century Paracelsians were apt to be associated with other "rebel" ideologies. Sometimes the connections were more temperamental than ideological, but Paracelsianism's most basic beliefs had many conscious affiliations with Protestantism. Paracelsus had founded a new science, purely "Christian" as opposed to scholastic, in which truth was sought first in the Scriptures and then in God's book of nature. Thus in France, Paracelsian power at court coincided with the rise to power of the ex-Huguenot Henry IV (1589–1610). In the late sixteenth century Paracelsians often supported the new astronomy of Copernicus, not because they were persuaded by the astronomical evidence, but because here was another disagreement with established scholastic authority, a disagreement that furthermore had some of its roots in neo-Platonic philosophy.

From about 1600, neo-Paracelsian writings circulated more and more widely, combining iatrochemistry with Paracelsian ideas about health and disease: anti-Galenic, seeing disease as local, pro-"experience," and self-consciously "Christian." At least some seventeenth-century healing practices were conducted in such terms, in some cases by physicians thoroughly converted to Paracelsianism and in some cases because aspects of iatrochemistry crept into even the most devout Galenist's armory. Connections grew between chemistry and pharmacology, pushed along by Paracelsian influence. Pharmacopoeias appeared, inspired by Paracelsianism. In the same spirit, a growing number of chemical texts concentrated on the preparation of remedies, emphasizing such procedures as distillation and tests to judge the purity or composition of remedies. The text by Jean Beguin, first published in 1610, went through forty-one editions in the succeeding eighty years; the text by Nicholas Lémery, which first appeared in 1675, was still being reissued as late as 1757. It is a significant fact that in the age of the scientific revolution the best-selling scientific works were not those of Galileo or Newton but the chemical texts of Beguin and Lémery, found in the homes of physicians and the shops of apothecaries all over Europe.

Paracelsianism did not simply mean more attention to chemical remedies, however. In the seventeenth century it continued to embody an alternative and sometimes revolutionary approach to nature. The Paracelsian philosophical tradition was maintained most notably by Jean Baptiste van Helmont (1579–1644), the most important seventeenth-century figure in what Allen Debus calls the "Chemical Philosophy." Van Helmont, like Vesalius a native of Brussels, became a convert to Paracelsianism in the years after 1609 and spent the rest of his life writing and arguing for the cause, as one of the most eminent physicians and intellects of his age. Like Galileo, his ideas led him into difficulty with the Roman Church, and he was placed under house arrest between 1634 and 1636. For van Helmont religion intersected medicine in fundamental ways; the physician, he said, had a "divine office." In the Paracelsian tradition, he maintained that disease had a local, not a systemic, character. Both the organs of the body and the diseases themselves possessed active, vital principles that combated each other. The outcome of their interaction determined health, as the *archaeus* of disease (outside the body) attempted to intrude its alien seed in an organ.

The remarkable controversy over the workings of the "weapon-salve" illustrates aspects of Paracelsianism as they had emerged by van Helmont's time. The controversy arose within the Paracelsian belief that a healing salve could be prepared that included blood from a wound, and that the salve should then be placed on the weapon that had caused the wound. The resulting action-at-a-distance, Paracelsians claimed, had a curative effect on the wound. Perhaps this happened because of a magnetic action between weapon and wound; perhaps, others such as van Helmont maintained, divine powers as well as magnetism were at work. Notice that the efficacy of the cure did not enter the question; at least until mid-century, Paracelsians took that for granted. Magnetism seemed to Paracelsians an excellent example of sympathetic emanations and attractions occurring across an apparently empty space, especially after William Gilbert thoroughly described magnetic effects in his *De magnete* (1600). Examples of such emanations filled nature: did not flowers open and turn toward the sun?

Mechanical and Animate Forces

Thus two explanatory systems gained strength in the seventeenth century, one explaining natural effects mechanically and the other invoking forces acting across distances. While Paracelsians clearly supported the second, the Vesalian tradition could lend aid to either or both. Harvey may not have been a mechanical thinker, but his system of circulation could certainly be seen as mechanical, with the heart a pump that forced fluid through conduits. Descartes, imposing a mechanical interpretation on the heart, believed it the site of a fire: blood, entering the heart, expands with heat and so pushes into the arterial system; the "most agitated and penetrating parts of the blood" proceed to the brain, setting off impulses in the nerves that ultimately cause muscular action.

> This will hardly seem strange to those who know how many motions can be produced in automata or machines which can be made by human industry, although these automata employ very few wheels and other parts in comparison to the large number of bones, muscles, nerves, arteries, veins, and all the other component parts of each animal. Such persons will therefore think of this body as a machine created by the hand of God, and in consequence incomparably better designed than any machine that can be invented by man.[25]

Seventeenth-century mechanical explanations of life found their most thorough exponent in Alphonso Borelli (1608–1679), whose *On the Motions of Animals* appeared in 1680, just after his death. Borelli subjected both body parts and animal functions to a searching mechanical examination; for Borelli the heart was a piston that exerted a calculable force which kept the blood in circulation, and the muscles and bones presented a tremendous complex of machines at work: levers, pulleys, wedges.

But others invoked vital forces to explain life processes. Descartes himself, the arch-mechanist, allowed that the possession of a "soul" differentiated humans from other animals. Aside from the obvious influence and direction of Paracelsianism and van Helmont, vital forces entered explanations of astronomy and mechanics. Isaac Newton (1642–1727), the English thinker whose synthesis dominated cosmology and mechanics throughout the eighteenth and nineteenth centuries, ultimately appealed to "the very first Cause, which certainly is not mechanical";[26] Newton's gravitation could be described mathematically, but he refused to see it as the product of Cartesian pushes and pulls among matter. He argued that bodies could be, and were, moved by "certain active Principles," which caused gravitational, electrical, and magnetic effects and chemical changes such as fermentation. Modern scholarship has now thoroughly explored Newton's alchemical beliefs. And if Newton—whose system suggested to many eighteenth-century thinkers a universe that functioned as a gigantic, perfect machine—saw vital forces in many physical phenomena, how much more likely must those forces be in the biological world?

The Impact of the Scientific Revolution

The scientific revolution was not confined to the dramatic reconceptualizations of Copernicus, Kepler, Galileo, Harvey, and Newton. The authority of the ancients underwent challenge from many quarters, often simply from floods of new information. In the biological sciences especially, travel and discovery presented new facts, as did the microscope, dramatically employed in the second half of the seventeenth century. Anton van Leeuwenhoek began his systematic microscopic investigations in the 1670s, seeing the microorganisms he called "wee beasties"; Jan Swammerdam used the microscope to support mechanistic explanations of life, and described the subunits of blood called corpuscles; Robert Hooke, in 1665, observed the microscopic structures of plants, which he called "cells"; Marcello Malpighi, in 1661, traced the final links of Harvey's circulatory system by his microscopic examination of the capillaries. Biology and medicine were caught in waves of enthusiasm for experiment and observation, which included a rash of studies in comparative anatomy; the French architect-physician Claude Perrault, who designed the east facade of the Louvre, died from an infected wound received while dissecting a camel. Such discoveries—if not Perrault's— had a cumulatively weakening effect on the power of Aristotle and Galen, as did the mere appearance of new forms of life and new remedies from the newly found Americas. The use of cinchona bark as a specific treatment for malaria, for example, cast Galenic remedies in the shade; so too did the growing emphasis on chemically prepared remedies and salts favored by the Paracelsians.

The attacks on Galen—whether from Paracelsians, Harvey's physiology, new specific remedies, or comparative anatomy—formed part of a more general and sweeping assault on the whole basis of Aristotelian philosophy. Important philosophers in the early seventeenth century, especially Descartes and Francis Bacon (1564–1626), came to the radical conclusion that all past knowledge was uncertain and that the human mind must begin anew on different epistemological principles, whether those of deductive reason and mathematics (as Descartes urged) or of the inductive collection of data (as Bacon argued). In either case authority— perhaps Aristotle's, perhaps Galen's, perhaps Christianity's—must be set aside.

By the end of the seventeenth century the scientific revolution had created a picture of the universe startlingly different from that which had dominated previous centuries. The universe was now an infinite one, hence (by definition) centerless, without a privileged position of the kind once occupied by the earth. The earth was simply one of several planets of a sun, itself simply one of a great number of stars. All the universe acted in conformity with laws that described (with mathematical precision) motions in a soulless geometric space. Man's reason had discovered these laws. What was God's role? For Newton, who more than anyone else had shaped this system, God's presence was both everywhere and necessary to the continuing functioning of the universe. But others—including many who called themselves followers of Newton—came to regard God simply as a great watchmaker, architect, or engineer, a being who designed a perfect machine and then simply let it run. Voltaire, the great French writer, popularized

Newton in the eighteenth century and also poured contempt on the idea that God's providence could be bothered with the small details of earthly life and death. By the end of the eighteenth century the French astronomer Laplace had reduced Newton's system to an entirely self-regulating mechanism; asked by Napoleon to explain the role of God in his system, Laplace replied, "Sire, I have no need of that hypothesis."

Man's relationship to God, therefore, underwent drastic change; the scientific revolution placed great distance between humanity and God's constant providence, at least for the minority of the population numbered among the literati. Man's relationship to the rest of nature changed as well. Descartes, by rigorously insisting on a division between "body" and "soul," removed life and powers from matter. Matter was inert; it moved only if something else pushed it; it had no self-willed principle of activity. "Soul," "spirit," perhaps "mind" lay outside matter, observing it, manipulating it, controlling it, but not part of it. Of course not everyone agreed; Paracelsians certainly did not, for animating powers abounded in their universe. But Cartesianism greatly assisted the notion that the human mind in some way stood outside nature, able to observe it objectively and bend it to the human will.

That distance between humans and the rest of nature related in turn to the new spirit in which nature was investigated. The belief grew that experiments could be performed that would extend knowledge, not simply confirm already-known truths; further, in the extension of knowledge lay the key to improving humanity's lot on earth. Confidence in man's power over nature grew, and that confidence included power over disease. Descartes again:

> It is true that medicine at present contains little of such great value; but without intending to belittle it, I am sure that everyone, even among those who follow the profession, will admit that everything we know is almost nothing compared with what remains to be discovered, and that we might rid ourselves of an infinity of maladies of body as well as of mind, and perhaps also of the enfeeblement of old age, if we had sufficient understanding of the causes from which these ills arise and of all the remedies which nature has provided.[27]

Such optimism about human powers might make appeals to supernatural forces, whether those of magic or religion, both unfounded and unnecessary.

Consequences for Healing Practices

Did the new science have much immediate effect on practices designed to combat disease and promote health? The answer to that question has several layers, which relate to the professional position of healers, to the impact of different new ideas, to the more general effect of the new world view, and to the relationship between the new ideas and the social changes of the sixteenth and later centuries.

By the sixteenth century medicine stood as a dignified art, practiced by graduates of medieval universities. In that century physicians moved in the direction of tighter control over their privileges, forming corporations and "colleges" that asserted such privileges and in some instances won legal recognition of those privileges from governments. The social attitude of many physicians therefore became more conservative, as their positions were buttressed by privilege that they strongly defended. The education of physicians remained that of the medieval university, with heavy emphasis on Galenism, however much "Galenism" had been gradually modified since the thirteenth century. For proponents of the new sciences, therefore, the physicians and their ideas stood as attractive targets. An attack on Galen's ideas—whether from the Paracelsian or Vesalian quarter— furthermore might merge with other attacks by the new on the old. Supporters of the Protestant Reformation might see Galenic medicine as one of the products of the corrupt medieval centuries, when the Romish whore grafted scholasticism onto simple Christian truth. The followers of Copernicanism might see Galenist physicians as allied with Aristotelianism; more likely, the opponents of Galenism, especially the Paracelsians, might become partisans of Copernicanism. By the seventeenth century the use of vernacular languages arose as another issue on which physicians might be assailed; Galileo wrote in Italian, and Paracelsians in both England and France supported vernacular language against Galenic, medieval, university Latin.

But physicians in general remained Latin, Galenic, and professionally privileged, despite these assaults. Some new ideas had an effect on practice, but those effects did not manifest themselves consistently or completely. Some physicians, such as the "English Hippocrates" Thomas Sydenham (1624–1689), proclaimed the supreme importance of clinical observation over theorizing, and then theorized anyway. Harvey's new physiology proved very convincing, but it made little difference to therapeutics and no great impression on the continuance of Galenism at the heart of medical education. Harvey, an Aristotelian physician who wrote in Latin and enjoyed the privileges of his profession, did not find favor with the Paracelsians and other iatrochemists, who showed only erratic concern with the relations between physiology and medical practice. Iatrochemical ideas certainly mattered more to therapeutics in the sixteenth and seventeenth centuries. The advocacy of chemical remedies, many of them prepared from inorganic substances, became an important result of the new science. Much iatrochemical inspiration came from Paracelsus and his followers, but some arose independently from practice that was consciously anti-Galenic and more focused on "practical" remedies, whether botanical or chemical.

Paracelsians were often allied with Protestantism, as in the late sixteenth-century court of Henry IV or with the English Puritans in the seventeenth. These religious and political alliances at times gave rise to periods of unusual medical activity. Charles Webster has shown how Baconian visions of a new medicine, purged of the errors of antiquity, founded on observed truths, leading to a prolonged life in an ideal future, combined with Puritan theology in the revolutionary English decades between 1640 and 1660. A remarkable surge in medical publications—and medical hopes—resulted.[28] That was fine as long as the star of Puritanism was in the political ascendant, but at other times the Protestant-Paracelsian alliance might strengthen the world of the irregular healers discussed earlier. That great range of irregular healers, which in fact dominated the world of practice in early modern Europe, also found common ground with aspects of the new science. Protestants and Paracelsians alike called for a new beginning that would involve an inner "experience," and they urged the importance of "experiments," whether spiritual or chemical. The Paracelsians and other iatrochemists praised the importance of practice over theory and book learning; furthermore, their doctrines shared many of the assumptions of the naturalism that lay behind the wise women and the cunning men of folk medicine.

But in the long run, despite the apparent alliances between Paracelsians and the world of folk healing, the scientific revolution dealt folk healers and their allies a heavy blow. Much folk healing depended on a belief that the healer possessed, in some measure, the power to bend nature to his or her will, or at the very least to be an able suppliant with nature. In the seventeenth century the scientific revolution's dominant thinkers established the idea that the natural world was characterized by unvarying laws that could not be compelled by an individual. Spells, chants, and prayers could not stop the course of natural law; sickness was no more subject to that sort of intervention than was gravitation. The scientific revolution never won a complete victory over the folk healers; as we shall see, folk traditions maintained a powerful hold in the Western world into the twentieth century, and in some ways remained dominant into the nineteenth. But the scientific model, and with it a different concept of "disease," was now on the board. Disease was no longer a punishment from God, escapable only by manipulating the divine will, but a natural phenomenon like the tides against which humans built dikes or the storms which humans kept out with a roof.

The scientific revolution also created a world of specialized learning, which (even in its early decades) some of its adherents attempted to distance from vulgar popular misunderstandings. With the successful assertion of a "scientific method" came new respect for knowledge gained through systematic observation, industrious experiment, and mathematical skill. These methods further emphasized the virtues of public demonstration, reconfirmation by experiment, in short verifiability, all antithetical to the practices of the village magi.

In the long run the new science became part of the currency of elite culture, while "popular" culture adopted it only imperfectly, incompletely, and later. Despite the efforts of a variety of popular lecturers and scientific societies, of educational institutions, university core curricula, and autodidactic schemes, "popular" understanding of the new science remained—and remains—incomplete. Old ways persisted: the vast variety of rural customs and beliefs, the popular recreations that contradicted the sobriety and diligence favored by the early industrial pioneers, and—especially—the aspects of religion and "magic" that symbolized "superstition" to the post-Enlightenment elite culture. Popular religious manifestations appeared at different times and places, with their enthusiastic preaching, their Pentecostalism, their prophecy, their faith healing. The occult sciences kept their hold, or rather shifted their hold to an even broader base in the population.

Even in the twenty-first century mass circulation newspapers still carry the comforts of astrology to numbers—and even proportions—that would have astonished Kepler. Spiritualism inspired both storefront practitioners and elite Societies for Psychical Research. That the president of the United States was reputedly guided through his calendar in the 1980s by astrology was both scandalous to elite scientific culture and not very surprising.

So despite the scientific revolution, the position of what I have been loosely calling "magic" has remained strong for at least some people in the Western world. Since the seventeenth century, empirical healers have survived, even if their connections with and rationalizations from the worlds of magic and religion may have weakened. The costs of orthodox medicine remained high, the availability of physicians unpredictable. Official medicine, despite the new science, only slowly offered superior therapy, and then only for some complaints.

Changes in the social circumstances of learning also occurred. Men of learning found new places in which to carry on their work. Learning, heavily clerical in the Middle Ages, could now be found practiced by laymen in courts and in universities alike. The seventeenth century also saw the foundation of a number of scientific societies. Whatever motives lay behind these foundations, the scientific societies of the seventeenth century symbolized new goals for a new intelligentsia. Those goals were increasingly secular. They might be devoted to the power of the state or to the wealth of commerce; they might also hope to provide social legitimation for thinkers or to provide them with means of income. Both of the latter goals would become more important in the eighteenth and nineteenth centuries as men of science found themselves subjected to the whims of a market economy. For those who provided health care to the population, several different changes might eventually flow. Medicine, like science, might come to be seen in the interests of the state, as governments began to associate large and healthy populations with their own potential power. The pressure of a free market, in a literate society with growing disposable income, might bear on the monopolistic privileges enjoyed by corporations of healers. The claims of religion, exerted over both healing and the careers of healers, would weaken.

But while the economy of early modern Europe might have been moving in the direction of a free market in which power would lie with consumers, the scientific revolution also contributed to the strengthening of the closed elite of medicine. The successful assertion of a "scientific method," at first most convincing in the exact physical sciences, would eventually spread to the life sciences and the healing arts as well. The prestige of the new science made it easier for medical professionals to gain political privileges, conferred by states and organized "opinion" alike. The practice of science was for those fortunate few with the time and means to learn carefully and thoroughly, in what would eventually become a prescribed and lengthy university curriculum. It was not for the unlettered village wise woman, nor was it for the adept who awaited the revelation of truth wrapped in dark mysteries. Science, and in the long run medicine, demanded precise knowledge. Prominent figures of the scientific revolution denounced the closed world of the scholastics and the dead hand of Galen, and so seemingly allied themselves with new social and economic forces. But their legacy was mixed. They created a new closed elite whose specialized knowledge immunized it from the free market at a time when economic doctrine and practice proclaimed the virtues of a competitive society. The Western world's approaches to disease have been caught in the resulting tension ever since.

Six

Disease and the Enlightenment

The scientific revolution of the seventeenth century broadened in the eighteenth into the European-wide current of thought and opinion called the Enlightenment. The ideas, assumptions, and methods of the new science spread to other realms of thought and culture. In the course of the Enlightenment, healers adopted a few new approaches to specific diseases and (more generally) showed the pervasive effects of the new scientific thinking. At the same time some of the most important demographic developments in Western history began. The West's population began to rise, this time proceeding unchecked by any epidemic-driven increase in death rates; this population growth continued unchecked until birth rates slackened with the West's industrial maturity.

In fact the connection between the spread of the new science and the eighteenth-century population breakthrough had more to do with environmental change than with any medical intervention against disease. This chapter will therefore first survey the early modern disease environment and the general Enlightenment precepts that advocated (or effected) changes in it. Although widespread agreement existed about such general points, the Enlightenment was also a period of rapid change, lack of consensus, and even confusion in thinking about disease, its essence, and what should be done about it. The professional positions of healers, especially in times of dramatic political change, reflected that uncertainty, as did Enlightenment responses to specific diseases of importance to the time. A study of two diseases (against which eighteenth-century thinkers made determined attacks) follows, and the chapter concludes with another case which suggests that the triumph of Enlightenment was a very mixed one.

The Early Modern Disease Environment

In many ways the disease environment of the Renaissance and early modern Europe was a continuation of that established in the high and later Middle Ages. Although major changes occurred in the years between 1350 and 1800, it is important to start with the continuities, because so much relative attention has been paid to the new features of the early modern scene. Western civilization remained primarily rural until well into the nineteenth century; only in a few places did urban life predominate. Most people remained, therefore, in areas less likely to be affected by diseases of crowds, especially such airborne diseases as tuberculosis, smallpox, measles, influenza, and diphtheria. To some extent Western people remained isolated, as had their forebears in the early Middle Ages; their diets might be subject to local famines and to the deficiencies of heavy reliance on a few foods. Protein and iron deficiency remained common; scurvy, beriberi, and rickets took seasonal tolls, certainly weakening if not directly fatal. Ergotism presented recurrent problems, especially in damp seasons and in marshy soils. Heavy outdoor labor with metal cutting tools brought wounds, tetanus, and erysipelas. In all these respects the Western countryman of the eighteenth century lived in much the same disease environment as his seventh-century ancestor.

But in some respects the pace of change accelerated between 1450 and 1800. Europe may still have been largely rural but its urban population grew, and more cities could be found on more places on the map. Crowding was a fact of life—and death—for a greater proportion of the populations of England, France, the Iberian peninsula, and portions of Germany, as well as of Italy and the Low Countries. Medieval Europe might have contained five cities (Paris, Venice, Naples, Genoa, and Milan) whose populations exceeded 100,000; a dozen other medieval places might have been called "urban." Between 1500 and 1700 perhaps twelve others (Antwerp, Amsterdam, Rome, Palermo, Seville, Lisbon, Madrid, Messina, Marseilles, Vienna, and most dramatically London) passed 100,000, while the number of smaller cities had also multiplied in proportion.[1] And perhaps more important than their actual total populations were the densities of settlement they represented. By the end of the eighteenth century the City of London, an area within the old walls of about one square mile, contained over 100,000 inhabitants. In 1990 Manhattan, the most thickly populated portion of New York City, had a population density of about 67,000 per square mile in a world of tall buildings made possible by electric elevators. No wonder that in the intensely crowded conditions of the early modern city airborne diseases found the critical mass of population they needed to sustain themselves; one estimate, for instance, suggests that measles needs a population of 250,000 to maintain itself.[2] Whether early modern Western civilization really suffered from "new" diseases or not remains a perhaps-unresolvable question, disturbed as it is by perceptions and shifting terminologies and nosologies (systems of classification) of disease; certainly many seventeenth- and eighteenth-century authorities said that new diseases were among them. But if we leave the question of absolute "newness" to one side, we may recognize instead that whether new or not many epidemic diseases could flourish in early modern Europe more readily than they could have in earlier centuries.

Of these the airborne diseases, especially tuberculosis, smallpox, and influenza, became most important. But the crowded urban conditions also probably created more opportunities for those diseases dependent on fecal-oral transmission. The conditions of water supply and sewage removal only changed for the worse, for the increased populations of the cities continued to use rivers as both sewers and sources of water. In the course of the seventeenth and eighteenth centuries European attitudes toward bathing began to change, as cleanliness of the body slowly gained recognition as a positive trait and bathing ceased to be regarded primarily as a sensual experience. Nonetheless, the opportunities for the spread of dysentery, diarrhea, and typhoid fever probably became more frequent with the increasing urban population.

Health conditions in cities may have improved in other respects, however. Some cities, especially those places within the sight of an enlightened prince's palace, began to benefit from stronger central planning and greater use of such construction materials as stone, slate, and brick. London was massively rebuilt with new materials in the wake of a disastrous 1666 fire. Such rebuilding and city planning may have reduced some crowding, although city densities remained very high. More important, and more likely, were reductions in contacts between people and some disease vectors, particularly the fleas that brought plague and the mosquitoes that brought malaria, and possibly also the lice that brought typhus. Plague disappeared from much of the West in the eighteenth century (see Chapter Three), and malaria's position will receive further discussion later in this chapter. But while new construction may have increased the space between humans and vectors, or may have made less welcoming homes for rodents and insects, the increasing frequency of European contacts with the tropics—especially the "Indies"—brought countervailing risks from the rapid dissemination of occasional imports such as yellow fever.

The disease environment of the early modern period also reflected important changes in the character of European warfare. Through the seventeenth century the technology of violence and the inability of rulers to control it combined to create optimum conditions for the spread of disease. Battlefield wounds and their resultant infections, perhaps accompanied by tetanus or erysipelas, increased with the spread of firearms. Towns faced physical destruction from bombardment and hence a collapse of whatever health and sanitation provisions might exist. For a long time this new power remained to a great extent the privilege of those with money, and much European violence and conquest inflicted on others was controlled either by private interests or by states that hired private armies.

But states increasingly brought the new military technology under their monopoly control, beginning in the seventeenth century and certainly by the eighteenth. Sixteenth- and many seventeenth-century armies most often remained shakily controlled by still-impoverished governments that sometimes could not afford to pay them. They also remained basically unwashed and itinerant, a powerful agent for the diffusion of diseases, of which typhus was the classic but hardly the only example. As the absolute monarchies (and some other states) of the seventeenth and eighteenth centuries became more highly organized, a crucial element of their power lay in their better-disciplined armies; they devoted a considerable amount of their resources to military power, sometimes so much that taxes impoverished and weakened an already-frail class of the poor. But the highly disciplined royal armies of the eighteenth century represented less of a threat of anarchic violence and were less likely to diffuse typhus and syphilis through the population.

Early modern social change held perhaps the greatest long-term significance for the disease environment. Some of this change was rural, some urban, and some resulted from the interactions between town and country. Agricultural change, especially in northwestern Europe (the Low Countries and England, spreading to portions of France and Germany), brought new crops and more intensive cultivation of protein-bearing legumes. The wealth from that "agricultural revolution" entered into a complex symbiosis with other economic forces, especially the developing instruments of capitalism (credit, insurance) as they related to Atlantic-based trade. By the eighteenth century (if not sooner) both town and country in northwestern Europe partook of a market economy, one that had the power to overcome the local famines and "subsistence crises" of an earlier time.[3] To some extent at least the roots of the modern industrial society are found there, and that society ultimately adopted a different family structure which, as Stephen Kunitz has argued, shaped a different disease environment.[4] The impact of later marriages, smaller households, longer terms of breast feeding, and declining agricultural labor by women, however, only became significant in the nineteenth century.

And in the meantime agricultural change might not be an unmixed blessing. Potatoes in much of central and eastern Europe (as well as Ireland) proved a rich new source of calories, but encouraged a dangerous monoculture that allowed the continuing exploitation of a farm labor population growing cash crops for export that benefited landlords. Maize corn likewise brought calories to southern and southeastern Europe, but also added another nutritional disease, pellagra. From the seventeenth century into the nineteenth, the growing cities of the Western world drew their population growth from migrants from the surrounding rural lands, whose own populations were swelled by the stimulus of these agricultural, social, and political changes. New generations of city dwellers constantly appeared, whose immune systems lacked experience with the crowd diseases raging in the cities. The growth and persistence of smallpox and tuberculosis as early modern problems may thus have been related to the social forces creating "modernity."

Enlightenment Conceptions of Disease
Environment

The thinkers of the European Enlightenment generally believed in the importance of environment. Part of this conviction grew from their agreement with the epistemology of the English philosopher John Locke, who (arguing against Descartes) maintained that the human mind, a *tabula rasa* at birth, took form under the impressions conveyed to it by the senses. The environment therefore shaped the mind. This doctrine pleased Enlightenment thinkers in part because it implied the possibility of change. Original sin did not imprison humanity, if Locke was correct; the environment produced minds, so presumably a better environment would produce a better mind, or a better character, or better human institutions. The seventeenth-century conviction of the unaided powers of human reason buttressed this optimistic credo. The human mind could stand alone, without the reliance on authority (sacred or profane) that had previously hampered it.

Eighteenth-century thought about disease partook of these general Enlightenment principles. For several different reasons, Enlightenment thinkers generally believed that the "environment" produced disease, although what "environment" might mean varied considerably. For some diseases a "miasma" was favored. This "bad air" doctrine often ran counter to established beliefs in contagionism, and so contradicted the opinions that had slowly built up around (especially) plague. In the seventeenth century many states had evolved elaborate public health machinery to deal with the contagion of plague (see Chapter Three), but in some eighteenth-century circles that machinery, and the thinking behind it, fell from favor. In part miasmist opinion might have been more sympathetically regarded by those Enlightenment thinkers who emphasized the rights of individuals against the coercive powers of the state; in part contagionist arguments also may have withered because plague ceased to be a major menace in the eighteenth century, and that called into question the utility of the machinery designed to divert it.

The miasma theory may also have been produced by the "new" diseases that pressed in on Europeans. These new diseases included scurvy, syphilis, rickets, and above all the "fevers" that by the eighteenth century bid fair to replace plague as the object of greatest concern. "Fevers" might include typhus, malaria (sometimes subsumed under a more general "ague"), yellow fever, and influenza. Seventeenth-century thinkers produced a variety of causes for these diseases, and while some remained familiarly medieval (divine wrath, plutonic exhalations, unfortunate astrological conjunctions), mechanical and particularly iatrochemical explanations came more to the fore.[5]

One of the dominant issues was the very "newness" of the disease. Could descriptions of these complaints be found in the authorities of antiquity? If Galen or Avicenna knew the disease, then their causes (and their remedies) might still suffice. But if the diseases were genuinely new, did new pathogenic agents cause them? The iatrochemist might see a new *archaeus*, while a mechanist might see a change in the atmosphere, perhaps (particularly after the microscope opened a new world of organisms) its pollution by tiny "worms," as Athanasius Kircher hypothesized about malaria. Mechanical explanations of that kind, applied in particular to the new fevers, might therefore focus attention on the environment.

This connection between the environment and human health, or human disease, found curious echoes in changing conceptions of human cleanliness and of odors. In France at least, the use of water in bathing acquired associations with health by the second half of the eighteenth century.[6] In medieval thought baths symbolized sensual pleasure, while in the sixteenth and seventeenth centuries water was thought a positive hazard, which both opened the pores to invasion and was associated (in bathhouses) with disruptions of public order. But in the Enlightenment bathing with water came to have virtues. Cold water might contract the body's organs and thus harden or toughen them. More than that, water might help banish the unhealthy smells and airs that caused disease. By the 1780s the unhealthy stenches of modern, especially urban, life—the odors of cemeteries, rubbish, cesspools, and sewers—were under attack. Air had become the health issue, the nose was a diagnostic tool, and clean water was the solution to the filthy atmosphere that bred disease.[7]

Visions of human cleanliness, and thought about the "new" diseases, flowed together with the general Enlightenment emphasis on the importance (and the controllability) of the environment, creating a widespread climate for what James Riley has seen as a demographically significant attack on the causes of mortality and morbidity.[8] Through advocacy of drainage, ventilation, lavation, and reinterment, European thinkers (and in some cases governments) assailed many of the vectors of disease without really knowing why their measures had an effect. Riley makes a convincing case that opinion was strongly environmentalist; the effectiveness of eighteenth-century environmental measures is harder to assess, if only because so many variables intrude on any discussion of mortality and morbidity statistics. Riley's argument has another use, too, for it shows the complexities of equating "contagionism" with "statism" and "environmentalism" with *"laissez faire."* Undoubtedly much liberal Enlightenment opinion resisted the infringements on liberty that came with a contagionist doctrine; quarantines and health passes were classic instruments of a heavy state hand.[9] But other Enlightenment thinking approved state action; the cameralist and mercantilist state had enlightened supporters. And an attack on the environment might also interfere with human freedoms. In addition, by the end of the eighteenth century both thinkers and governments had developed a lively concern with the "population problem," which most often meant a fear that a state's population was not growing at the pace of its rivals. Public health, even in the eighteenth century, might ultimately be justified by state power, which could take sustenance from either "contagionist" or "miasmatic" interpretations of disease.

Nosology in Transition: "Fevers"

Thought about "fevers" had other ramifications. The seventeenth and eighteenth centuries marked a period of transition in the ontological views of disease. In medieval thought disease was primarily internal or, as Johanna Geyer-Kordesch puts it, "a process unfolding within the definitions of how the body works and functions." In the nineteenth century, disease became "an entity governed by the laws of an unfolding reaction between microorganism and the body."[10] Seventeenth- and eighteenth-century thinkers moved between those poles. Did fevers represent particular, distinct, disease entities, or did they simply differ from one another (and from other, older fevers such as malaria) in degree rather than in kind? At times, a seventeenth-century authority such as Thomas Sydenham seemed to speak clearly about particular disease entities, but he could also, as Lloyd Stevenson argues, characterize some fevers as more or less gradations, modifications of a basic and generic "fever," produced (in a Galenic argument) by an unnatural source of body heat.[11] Nosological schemes became increasingly complicated. Hermann Boerhaave (1668–1738), the dominant medical figure of his generation, employed both mechanical and iatrochemical explanations in differentiating types of "fever." William Cullen (1712–1790), who enjoyed immense influence in the English-speaking world in his position at the University of Edinburgh, attempted a new basis of simple classification, arguing that all disease stemmed from the nervous system, which received (from the environment) either too much stimulation or not enough.

In this increasingly eclectic and contentious discussion the notion of particular disease entities made headway, partly because of the development of a particular "specific" remedy for a specific fever. This was the bark of the cinchona bush, a medication for malaria. Cinchona was one of several herbal remedies favored by the Amerindians; their Spanish conquerors adopted it and brought it back to the Old World. The Spaniards did not adopt all these herbs easily, for a variety of "pagan" incantations and religious ceremonies accompanied their use. (In the sixteenth and seventeenth centuries, for example, the Spaniards debated vigorously whether they should encourage the use of coca as a stimulant that kept the Peruvians at work or eradicate it as a symbol of blasphemous superstition and anti-Christianity.)[12] The Jesuits brought cinchona from Peru to Europe about 1630, and its use as a specific treatment for malaria spread despite another religious stigma, its association with the controversial missionaries who brought it. Not every physician in Puritan England (for example) can have been happy to prescribe "Jesuitical bark," but even in Protestant states cinchona was widely used by the late seventeenth century. Among the panoply of "fevers," some responded to cinchona and some did not. That fact gave weight to specific classifications.

Doubts remain about the effectiveness of cinchona, for some sort of "malaria" remained a very serious problem in seventeenth- and eighteenth-century Europe. Some areas had "malarial" reputations: the Camargue, the Loire Valley, the Gironde in France; lowland Kent and Essex in England; the north German coast; the Pontine marshes and the Po Valley in Italy; and the Don Delta in Ukraine, to name only a few.[13] Malaria repeatedly assailed those areas (as well as others) through the eighteenth century; fevers devastated Brouage (at the mouth of the Loire), and the marshlands of Kent and Essex were characterized by exceedingly high mortality rates, in which burials regularly outstripped baptisms, until the very end of the century.[14] Even if cinchona had been widely used its effects would have been most uneven, owing to the inconsistent quality of the material. Bark, imported over a transoceanic distance, varied in its age and composition; in addition, an effective dose required consumption of quantities that induced vomiting. In 1820 the isolation of the active ingredient of cinchona, quinine, led to more precise dosages and more effective therapy.

The Craze for Scientific Explanation

The Enlightenment placed vast faith in science, both as the source of explanation and as the method for solving problems. The career of Franz Anton Mesmer (1734–1815), while it lends itself to burlesque perhaps too easily, illustrates the conjunction of a number of different scientific currents of the century, especially as those currents might relate to the healing of disease. Mesmer, an Austrian physician, drew together ideas from both the mechanical and the vitalist strands of the scientific revolution, and also employed the most exciting sciences of the eighteenth century, chemistry and electricity.

Some of Mesmer's appeal as a healer related to the traditions of the microcosm and the macrocosm, and some to the pervasiveness of the ideas of Isaac Newton in eighteenth-century culture. From the microcosm-macrocosm came the notion of harmony between the body and the universe, a harmony necessary for health. That harmony might involve the flow of "fluids" from macrocosm to microcosm or vice versa, and the Newtonian philosophy gave a further scientific imprimatur to belief in such fluids. Although Newton appeared to Enlightenment thinkers as the perfecter of the great world machine, we should remember that Newton (in his *Opticks*) also wondered: "Have not the small Particles of Bodies certain Powers, Virtues, or Forces, by which they act at a distance?"[15] And in his great *Principia*, Newton wrote of a "certain most subtle spirit which pervades and lies hid in all gross bodies; by the force and action of which spirit . . . all sensation is excited, and the members of animal bodies move at the command of the will, namely, by the vibrations of this spirit, mutually propagated along the solid filaments of the nerves, from the outward organs of sense to the brain, and from the brain into the muscles."[16]

Much eighteenth-century thought about both electricity and chemistry rested on those Newtonian speculations. Electricity seemed a certain manifestation of such a subtle elastic fluid, pervading all nature and endowed with manifold and exciting powers. Especially after about 1740, when the electrostatic generator made static forms of electricity more accessible, electrical effects became a staple of popular scientific enlightenment and entertainment. Healers—for example, Nicolas-Philippe Ledru, called Comus—seized on the mysterious fluid, urging the curative powers of electric shock therapy. A number of other subtle fluids caught the popular (and the learned) fancy as well. Magnetic effects illustrated one such powerful fluid. And chemistry, the other great popular scientific attraction, contributed others. For a time the theory of phlogiston, advanced by Georg Ernst Stahl, offered a general explanatory principle of chemical events. Phlogiston, a subtle substance, entered into chemical combinations and produced changes, yet it had no discernible weight. Antoine Laurent Lavoisier, the great French chemist who contributed much to the overthrow of the phlogiston theory, retained a subtle weightless "caloric" as an elemental substance.

Newly discovered gases seemed yet another illustration of wonderful, elastic, subtle fluids; balloons became, like lightning rods, symbols of the new science. Gases, like electricity, might also have medical applications. Thomas Beddoes, who lectured in chemistry at Oxford University between 1788 and 1792, became convinced of the medical utility of gases. In 1798 he opened his Pneumatic Medical Institution near Bristol, where he and his assistant Humphry Davy treated diseases (notably tuberculosis) with a variety of gases without much result, although they did report on the interesting physiological effects of nitrous oxide.

So when Franz Anton Mesmer began applying magnetic forces to heal bodily ills in his Viennese practice in the 1770s, he represented widespread Enlightenment beliefs and hopes. "Magnetism" might be mineral, related to lodestones; Mesmer was convinced that it could be "animal" as well. A subtle magnetic fluid exists everywhere in nature, and the health of the body depends on the natural flow of this fluid through it. The physician should manipulate this flow, reinforcing and directing it when necessary. In 1778 Mesmer moved to

Paris, the undoubted center of the Enlightenment world, and there his ideas and his medical practice created a sensation. He positioned his patients around a large tub filled with iron filings and bottles containing "mesmerized" water. Iron rods connected the bottles to the patients, who thus received mesmerized magnetic fluids; they could apply the rods to afflicted body parts, or form a chain with other patients around the tub, thus increasing the magnetic power with "animal" magnetism as well as mineral.

All this was in line with the science of the day: subtle magnetic fluids, directed and controlled for maximum effect on the body. Mesmer added other elements, including powerful psychological suggestion. Robert Darnton describes the scene:

> Everything in Mesmer's indoor clinic was designed to produce a crisis in the patient. Heavy carpets, weird, astrological wall-decorations, and drawn curtains shut him off from the outside world and muffled the occasional words, screams, and bursts of hysterical laughter that broke the habitual heavy silence. Shafts of fluid struck him constantly in the sombre light reflected by strategically placed mirrors. Soft music . . . sent reinforced waves of fluid deep into his soul. Every so often fellow patients collapsed, writhing on the floor, and were carried by Antoine, the mesmerist-valet, into the crisis room; and if his spine still failed to tingle, his hands to tremble, his hypochondria to quiver, Mesmer himself would approach, dressed in a lilac taffeta robe, and drill fluid into the patient from his hands, his imperial eye, and his mesmerized wand.[17]

These methods resulted in some spectacular cures; Mesmer was enriched by his Parisian practice, and by 1789 the Mesmerist Society of Universal Harmony had branch chapters in two dozen French provincial cities.

Darnton has convincingly shown that political issues were involved in this healing craze, as well as scientific and autosuggestive ones. Mesmer's merits divided established French science from the moment he appeared. The Royal Academy of Sciences and the Royal Society of Medicine both opposed his claims, but some of the medical faculty at the University of Paris came to his defense. Disgruntled intellectuals on the fringes of the establishment took up causes such as Mesmer's as their own, seeing in him a man of truth and ability whose merits, like theirs, had not been recognized by the elite ranks. The royal government, alarmed by the conjunction of radical science and radical politics, attacked Mesmer's scientific credibility, and a prestigious commission was formed for that purpose that included Lavoisier, Benjamin Franklin, and Jean-Sylvain Bailly, later to be a prominent (though moderate) revolutionist. The commission's experiments (1784) ridiculed Mesmer's claims, but by then Mesmer had become a symbol of political liberty and (more important) popular culture and belief apart from the dictates of elite science. Mesmerism survived in part because its cures satisfied many patients, but perhaps also because it appealed as an alternative to official medicine.

What had begun, with Mesmer, as science in the service of healing had become a branch of popular antiscientific culture. Although in the course of the nineteenth century mesmerism became more and more closely associated with spiritualism and hypnosis, a large healing element remained in it. And not all the scientific cure enthusiasms of the eighteenth century finished as parts of a counterculture. Some others forced their way into the training and practice of orthodox medicine and surgery.

Evolution or Revolution?

By the end of the eighteenth century many of the traditional ideas and practices of orthodox medicine had come under question or evolved away from their roots. Although some historians, notably Erwin Ackerknecht and David Vess, have emphasized the sudden changes caused—or at least precipitated—by the great French Revolution that began in the 1780s, others have convincingly argued that the medical changes of the revolutionary period in France were more evolutionary in character, and that much of the "new" of that period was not new at all.[18] The humoral medical traditions of the ancients had been widely criticized since the sixteenth century, and while a single dominant paradigm had not replaced them, they no longer commanded general assent. The professional divisions between physicians and surgeons had steadily eroded, and with them the exclusively literary education of one and the exclusively apprentice training of the other. And medicine gradually spawned specializations. These trends were all clearly under way before the French Revolution, however much events in that great upheaval may have accelerated them.

Although it may be possible to argue, in Stevenson's words, that new seventeenth-century thinking about disease "exhibit[ed] conventionality of an antique pattern" eventually the eighteenth century conceived of disease in new terms.[19] Did calling a patient "scorbutic" differ, Stevenson wonders, from calling him "splenetic"? Perhaps not. But for seventeenth- and eighteenth-century thinkers, scurvy became a separate disease, not a variant on a continuum of splenetic disorders. Specific fevers came to be seen as amenable to the specific remedy of cinchona. Particular mechanical or chemical causes came to be seen as responsible for particular diseases. Even insanity, where the hold of religious or folk explanation was especially strong, came to be seen as a separate disease, with chemical or mechanical explanations related to the nerves.

Some medical education emphasized the new views. At Edinburgh, especially during the teaching of Alexander Monro *secundus* after about 1760, medical training shifted from a systemic view of disease to one that placed more emphasis on disease's particular and local character. This localist approach could be found in medical teaching in London, Copenhagen, Berlin, and Vienna as well. If disease was studied as a discrete series of local manifestations, it was therefore not a phenomenon of the humors that systemically coursed through the entire frame.

So when the French Revolution began, a local and particular view of disease was already at large. Philippe Pinel (1745–1826), an especially influential physician of the Revolution, was an antihumoralist, but still believed in classifying disease on a continuum, according to symptoms. The next generation of French thinkers, during the Revolution, broke away from that view entirely. Xavier Bichat (1771–1802) insisted on the completely local character of disease, which he located in the solid tissues of the body as opposed to the fluids carried throughout the system. François Broussais (1772–1838), a student of Pinel and Bichat, argued the case for local disease even more enthusiastically; when the solid tissues of the body, nourished by digestion and respiration, were over- or understimulated, disease resulted. Since stimulus was largely digestive, Broussais traced most disease back to the digestive tract. (Curiously Broussais, the great opponent of systemic humoral medicine, advocated a thoroughly humoral therapy: bleeding, to drain the overstimulated solid tissue. Under Broussais's influence French physicians in the 1820s and 1830s prescribed a phenomenal number of leeches for their patients.)

The growing strength of the local view of disease related not only to the progessive weakening of Galen but to the changing professional positions and educations of physicians and surgeons. Traditionally physicians had received a university education that emphasized ancient learning; surgeons, less genteel, had entered an apprenticeship that emphasized manual techniques. In the eighteenth century (at least in some places) the divisions between the two began to shrink. Surgeons slowly rose in professional esteem. In France they became more formally organized, with their own collegiate guild, while the meaningful division in French healing practice ceased to be between physicians and surgeons and became that between successful and unsuccessful practitioners.[20] In England the surgeons also rose in status, and in wealth as well.

At the same time the educations of the two moved closer together. Schooling as well as apprenticeship was required of French surgeons from 1772 on. At Edinburgh the medical education of physicians came to emphasize clinical training as early as the time of Alexander Monro *primus* beginning in the 1720s; in the period of his son lectures were given to medical students and surgical apprentices simultaneously. In London the anatomical school of John Hunter (1728–1793) was only the most famous of a collection of private facilities that taught would-be physicians and surgeons alike. With this increasing emphasis on clinical training for physicians came a looser connection with the systemic Galenic tradition and a closer connection between the world of the doctor and the hospital, where pathological experience could be found in its greatest diversity. Although London physicians, in the words of William Bynum, came to see hospital connections as "useful" originally because of the social and professional contacts they offered, once in the hospital the physicians might see its connection with clinical learning more clearly.[21]

Recent historical writing has argued that many of these changes, especially as they occurred in the "Atlantic" worlds of western Europe and North America, were driven by the entrepreneurial character of those societies. Roy Porter (speaking of Britain) and Matthew Ramsey (speaking of France) have pictured worlds in which clients—patients—dominated their relations with healers.[22] Thus the power of old monopolies and corporations was savaged, and patients patronized whatever "worked" for them (however "worked" may be defined). Thus surgeons, midwives, apothecaries, and a wide range of irregular and folk practitioners might flourish, regardless of their qualifications. This entrepreneurial climate also affected the education of healers. Especially in London, competitive private enterprise drove anatomical schools; the Hunters' school succeeded because it offered better teaching, the prestige of the teachers' research, and their evident (and conspicuous) monetary rewards. The demands of clients may also have furthered still another eighteenth-century trend: that toward medical specialization, to be discussed shortly.

Intellectual factors, as well as sociological or economic ones, contributed to the linkages of surgeons, physicians, and hospitals. The same Enlightenment doctrine that urged the importance of the environment also stressed learning by the direct experience of the senses. Locke and his French disciple Condillac had made that point. Pierre Cabanis (1757–1808), a physician and *idéologue* who enjoyed much influence in the revolutionary years, carried it into the medical world. For Cabanis experience and observation were the keys to medical learning; the French Revolution, founding new medical schools on that principle, carried out a well-established Enlightenment doctrine in doing so.

The Revolution, determining that past educational systems had created a society filled with error and superstition, swept all the old educational institutions away and created (at least in theory) a wholly new structure. Medical education was not exempt. In 1792–1794, the peak period of revolutionary fervor, medical universities and institutions were abolished together with the old distinctions between regular and irregular medicine. In 1794 the chemist Fourcroy (himself an active revolutionist) submitted a report to the National Convention that urged the complete reformation of medical education:

> In the Ecole de Santé [the new medical school] manipulation will be united with theoretical precepts. The students will do chemical exercises, dissections, operations, and bandaging. Little reading, much seeing, and much doing will be the foundation of the new teaching which your committee suggests.

> Practicing the art, observing at the bedside, all that was missing, will now be the principal part of instruction.[23]

Fourcroy's rhetoric, addressed to a revolutionary assembly, obscured the extent to which his proposals had already begun to be implemented in European medical training before 1789. But the Convention, impressed, decreed that new medical schools were to be opened on these "practical" principles in Paris, Strasbourg, and Montpellier. In subsequent years hospitals were revamped, more hospitals opened, overcrowding reduced, and hospitals began developing specializations that both contributed to clinical teaching and to the idea of separate disease entities. Some of this occurred under the prodding of the Napoleonic minister Jean Chaptal (1756–1832), another chemist. In 1803 the government, now that of Napoleon's Consulate, took its most significant step when it provided for a uniform state licensing system for physicians and surgeons alike; each was now required to complete four years of medical education and then a state examination. All the old regional monopolies and corporations were abolished, and a clear line was thus drawn between "regular" medical practice and all others. The implications of this for the host of irregular practitioners were considerable (see Chapter Ten).

The period of the Revolution also sped the specialization of French medicine, although the Revolution itself can hardly be made the sole agent for such a broad change. In part specializations emerged from greater knowledge; in part more specialized diagnostic technology (such as the stethoscope, invented almost serendipitously by Laënnec in 1816) made them possible; in part the growth of hospital practice, in large cities that generated a volume of cases, made them professionally feasible; and in part they developed because practitioners and patients alike preferred them. The last point was probably important, especially if the eighteenth and early nineteenth centuries were really periods of wild entrepreneurial competition.

Concepts of disease furthered specialization as well. If a disease came to be conceived as a separate entity, it might be amenable to treatment by a separately trained specialist; if disease was a local phenomenon, confined to one organ of the body, the same reasoning applied. In any case, separate hospitals for venereal disease emerged in the 1780s, for pediatrics in Paris in 1795, and for dermatology in Paris in 1801, while psychiatry was another clearly developing specialty.

Psychiatry's evolution has been particularly seized upon by Michel Foucault, for whom it became a paradigm of modern civilization's *gaze*.[24] The state (and institutions related to it) disciplines its populations by placing them under continuous observation and restraint, first and most obviously in prisons and asylums, then in clinics of all sorts, and finally in the insidious collection of information in the modern computer age. Foucault's ideas, as a whole generation of thinkers has now said, have been immensely influential, and their insights have illuminated much thought about disease. Whether the history of Western care of the "insane" can be as neatly categorized as Foucault wanted to do remains dubious, however. Madness called forth a wide variety of responses, theories, and treatments, and behind those treatments lay a messy collection of motives.

In brief, the eighteenth-century conceptions of madness tended to veer away from traditional ideas, either those based on religion (possession by devils, or religious melancholy) or those associated with humoral imbalances. Instead "scientific" thinkers associated madness with chemical or mechanical causes, especially involving the digestive or nervous systems. Enlightenment thinkers also, not surprisingly, believed in the importance of the social environment. These secular explanations, whether scientific or social, gradually led to different conceptions of the mad, and to different possible approaches to their care. Madness was less often equated with evil or with bestiality; the mad were now conceived as victims, perhaps as children, and the conviction slowly took hold that a cure was possible. Reasons for confining the insane became increasingly complex. Earlier rationales—locking up the dangerous for safekeeping—became mixed with confinement for cure, confinement of those thought nuisances or embarrassments, or (as Foucault emphasized) confinement of the poor, women, and the social victims of modern industrial life. Confusing the issue of rationale still further (especially in Britain) was free enterprise; some of the insane were evidently wrongfully incarcerated by entrepreneurs who profited from their "care." As Roy Porter has skillfully shown to be true in Britain, these responses could all be found in the eighteenth and early nineteenth centuries, with considerable local variations and almost no "central" direction at all, so that there at least Foucault's sudden imposition of an all-seeing gaze by central authority did not occur.[25] In any case, however, care of the insane increasingly came to be seen as a medical problem, in which some hopes might be held out for a recovery: perhaps after application of some remedy, such as opium, chemical preparations, or electric shocks; perhaps after expert "management" of the patient by a doctor specializing in madness, such as Francis Willis, who treated George III of Great Britain in 1788 and 1789.

The Enlightenment Attacks Disease

Smallpox and scurvy attracted considerable European attention in the century, and Enlightenment responses to them illustrate the workings of the new science, at once experimental in method and optimistically ameliorative in spirit.

Smallpox

Smallpox has apparently been eradicated as a human disease. Its last reported case occurred in Somalia in 1977, and in 1979 the World Health

Organization officially announced its disappearance. The conquest of smallpox remains one of the most dramatic episodes in humanity's confrontations with disease. The roots of smallpox eradication are found in the eighteenth century, and the history of smallpox in that period occupies an obviously central place in the relations between disease and the people of the Enlightenment.

Smallpox, a common childhood disease to medieval Europeans, became inexplicably serious for them in the second half of the sixteenth century. At that point smallpox, often in combination with measles, began a series of grim visitations, much more frequent than its occasional serious earlier outbreaks: several thousand children dead in Naples in 1544, an epidemic in Rome in 1569, ten thousand dead in Venice in 1570–71, and numerous contemporary reports from other European places as well, some of them not offering clear diagnoses of the different causes of death. Evidence from the seventeenth century was clearer, particularly from the well-studied London "Bills of Mortality." Ann Carmichael and Arthur Silverstein have shown that those data present a "continually increasing annual background level of smallpox's contribution to total mortality from 1629 onward"; by the end of the century smallpox accounted for about 5 percent of London deaths, a proportion that rose to as much as 12 percent in epidemic years such as 1634, 1649, 1652, 1655, 1659, 1664, 1668, and 1674.[26] That pattern, somewhat stabilized, persisted into the eighteenth century: a steady 5 percent of all deaths were caused by smallpox, the percentage rising in the frequent epidemics.

Children accounted for a high proportion of the deaths; smallpox caused perhaps one-third of all childhood deaths in seventeenth- and eighteenth-century Europe. The incidence of smallpox was very high as well, although morbidity figures are even less certain than those for mortality. In the English town of Chester in 1774, about 1,200 cases of smallpox were reported in a population of 14,700; the investigator, John Haygarth, believed that most of the rest of Chester's population had already had smallpox. Of the 1,200 sick in Chester, 202 died, probably a typical eighteenth-century mortality rate, although in some epidemics that figure might have been considerably higher.[27]

As several historians of smallpox have noted, the disease did not respect rank. Smallpox fatalities repeatedly interrupted reigns and successions. Balthazar Carlos, heir to the throne of Spain, succumbed to smallpox in 1646; his death led to the succession of his half-brother Charles II, feeble in both mind and body, the last Spanish Hapsburg. When William II, prince of Orange and stadtholder of the Netherlands, died of smallpox in 1650, the decentralizing aristocracy returned to power in that country and no new stadtholder was chosen until 1672. The death in 1700 of William of Gloucester, sole surviving son of Anne Stuart, stimulated (together with his mother's impending succession to the English throne) the constitutionally significant Act of Succession of 1701.

The death of Luis I of Spain, in 1724, led to the reassumption of the throne by his father Philip V, who had earlier abdicated. Other notable smallpox deaths included those of Mary II of England (1694); Louis, son and heir of Louis XIV of France (1711); Joseph I, Holy Roman Emperor (1711); Peter II, czar of Russia (1730); Ulrica, co-regent of Sweden (1741); and Louis XV of France (1774). This grim royal chronology illustrates the hold that smallpox had established in Europe by the early eighteenth century.[28]

Smallpox killed, but it also disfigured those who survived it. Seventeenth- and eighteenth-century narratives recount, over and over again, the sad stories of scarred beauty and shattered romance. Poets from the early seventeenth to the late eighteenth century moralized in terms that changed little from Ben Jonson (1616):

> Envious and foule Disease, could there not be
> One beautie in an Age, and free from thee?
> . . . Thought'st thou in disgrace
> Of Beautie, so to nullify a face,
> That heaven should make no more; or should amisse,
> Make all hereafter, had'st thou ruin'd this?[29]

to Oliver Goldsmith (1760):

> Lo, the smallpox with horrid glare
> Levelled its terrors at the fair;
> And rifling every youthful grace,
> Left but the remnant of a face.[30]

A virus, *Variola major*, produced this terror. The virus is one of a group called orthopox viruses, which affect a variety of mammals including cows and monkeys with diseases called (obviously enough) cowpox, monkeypox, and the like. The viruses are separate species, biologically distinct, within the genus of orthopox viruses, but immunities to them overlap. Three of these viruses produce differing forms of smallpox in humans. *Variola major* results in a serious disease, whose results we have seen in America and then Europe. *Variola minor*, much less lethal, causes death in only about 1 percent of its victims. The distinction between these two forms of one disease was only recognized in the late nineteenth century. The third form, *Variola intermedius*, producing (as its name suggests) an illness intermediate in severity between the other two, was first distinguished in 1965. The smallpox viruses, while distinct species, are antigenically identical. The existence of the *Variola minor* form calls into doubt much of the early history of the disease, if only because a case of *Variola minor* smallpox might not have been clinically recognized as smallpox.

Because smallpox is an acute disease, exposure to one form of it confers immunity from subsequent attacks by all the others, and that fact—not perceived in those precise terms—lay behind very early attempts at smallpox prevention. Apparently the practice of inoculation, or variolation, for smallpox began in some misty folk antiquity, the product of empirical wisdom. By the sixteenth century descriptions of the procedure began appearing in Chinese medical texts, and in seventeenth-century China the imperial court sponsored experimental trials of it.[31] The pus from smallpox lesions was extracted and placed—perhaps directly in the nostrils or in the skin by scarification—in the body of the person to be inoculated. A mild case of the disease resulted, or so the inoculator who performed the operation hoped; the inoculated person then enjoyed immunity from further attacks. Certainly medieval and early modern Europeans (at least until the early seventeenth century) deliberately exposed their children to smallpox victims, in the belief that, as many medical authorities argued, smallpox was a natural or even beneficial stage in the maturation process. With that theoretical background, it would not be surprising if some Europeans hastened the coming of smallpox by the practice of inoculation; although the documentation of European inoculation before the eighteenth century is scanty, reports of the practice have been found from the British Isles to Greece. African slaves may have brought the technique to the Americas.

But only in the eighteenth century did the folk practice of inoculation gain the attention of learned Europeans. By that time smallpox had long ceased to be a childhood annoyance and had become a first-rate scourge. Accounts of Asian practices of inoculation appeared in scientific publications in the early years of the century, notably the communication from a Greek physician, Timoni, in the *Philosophical Transactions* of London's Royal Society in 1714. Shortly thereafter the practice came under the large and expanding umbrella of experiment and natural curiosity that characterized eighteenth-century elite culture. Inoculation established its first formal beachhead in England, where it benefited from the patronage of important people: Hans Sloane (1660–1753), fashionable physician; Lady Mary Wortley Montagu (1689–1762), an aristocrat who had herself suffered from smallpox and determined to spare her children and friends from its ravages; and some members of the new Hanoverian dynasty, perhaps with a wary eye on the extinction of their Stuart predecessors. Montagu, resident in Constantinople with her diplomat husband, heard of empiric inoculation in that city:

> There is a set of old women who make it their business to perform the operation every autumn, in the month of September, when the great heat is abated. People send to one another to know if any of their family has a mind to have the smallpox: they make up parties for this purpose. . . . The French Ambassador says very pleasantly that they take up the smallpox here by way of diversion, as they take the water in other countries.[32]

Thus reassured, Montagu submitted her son to the procedure and reported its success to her London correspondents.

Sloane and the surgeon Charles Maitland (who performed the first documented inoculation in England in 1721) persuaded Caroline, Princess of Wales, of the merits of the operation. Experiments followed, at the court's behest, in which six condemned criminals agreed to submit to inoculation in return for their freedom. Unlike the Tuskegee syphilis experiments of the twentieth century, this early example of medical trials on the socially marginal may actually have benefited the subjects, for five of the six criminals easily recovered from the mild cases thus induced, while the sixth showed no symptoms at all, leading to the suspicion that he had already had the disease. A further successful test followed on six orphaned children (another powerless population), and then Princess Caroline, her fears of the obvious dangers relieved, acceded to the variolation of her own children.

This royal patronage set off a brief craze for inoculation in England in the 1720s, but several well-publicized deaths following the procedure added strength to the arguments of opponents. By the end of the decade those arguments, which embodied some mixture of fear of danger, professional caution of physicians fearful for their reputations, and religious worries that inoculation interfered with the will of God, combined to drive out the fad. Meanwhile advocates of variolation had also practiced the art in British North America, notably in Boston, where the Puritan divine Cotton Mather added his formidable voice to its support. A British North American, James Kirkpatrick, a physician from South Carolina, restarted the practice in London in the early 1740s, reporting on its success following an epidemic in Charleston; he claimed that he had developed a safer method. From that point, variolation gradually spread across other elite circles and medical establishments in Europe.

By the middle of the century inoculation had become a cause in the Enlightenment's campaign against ignorance and superstition. A prominent French man of science, Charles Marie de la Condamine, became the great propagandist for inoculation in France, and the philosophes came to his support: d'Alembert, Voltaire, and that great Enlightenment broadside, Diderot's *Encyclopedia*. Tronchin, contributing an article on "Inoculation" to the *Encyclopedia*, praised the technique: "It is therefore incumbent on the faculties of theology and medicine, the academies, the heads of the magistracy, and men of letters to banish the scruples fomented by ignorance and to make the people feel that its own interest, Christian charity, the good of the state, and the conservation of mankind are involved in the establishment of *inoculation*."[33]

Peter Razzell has argued that variolation spread widely enough in the eighteenth century to make an important demographic contribution, at least in Great Britain, Ireland, and British North America. Razzell claims that inoculation was a well-established practice of folk medicine in Britain before 1700, and—more important—that it became very widely used in the years after about 1760, so much so that it led to a decline in the overall death rate of the British population.[34] Much of Razzell's thesis rests on his enthusiastic appreciation of the role of Robert Sutton and his son Daniel, aggressive promoters of inoculation in the 1760s and thereafter. The Suttons popularized a new method of inoculation, involving a much shallower incision to engraft the smallpox matter; the result, according to Razzell, decreased rates of contagion from the inoculated, greatly reduced mortality rate from inoculations, and progressively attenuated the severity of the smallpox engrafted without any loss in powers of immunity. By reducing popular (and perhaps well-deserved) fear of mortality from the procedure, the Suttons increased the acceptance of inoculation and performed it on many thousands of people.

At the same time inoculation became considerably less expensive, as belief in the necessity of "preparation" weakened. Previous to the 1760s, physicians, surgeons, and apothecaries had urged that inoculation be preceded by a period of bleeding, purging, and dietetic treatment, which would bring the body's humors (and the purses of the health professionals) into the proper balance to profit from the inoculation. This preparation considerably increased the costs of the process and thus limited its spread, unless a practitioner who had less allegiance to humoral medicine could be found. The Suttons had their doubts about the humoral theory, and they deserve some credit for lowering costs, but they did not advocate the complete elimination of "preparation." According to Razzell, the chief spur to the reduction of preparation time and costs was the pressure of the market.[35]

Inoculation came to be widely practiced in British rural areas, partly through such enthusiasts as Daniel Sutton and Thomas Dimsdale and partly through the activities of local public relief administration (parishes), whose officials might come to see the expenses of variolation, provided gratis to the poor, as lower than those of public burial of victims and public maintenance of widows and orphans. After 1770, charitable dispensaries funded by philanthropists began extending inoculation to more of the British urban poor.[36] But many city people remained unenthusiastic about inoculation, perhaps because smallpox in crowded cities, more truly endemic, inspired in the population a fatalism which assumed that all small children would get the disease in any case.

Dimsdale acquired particular celebrity when he successfully inoculated Catherine II of Russia (and some members of the Russian nobility) in 1768. Catherine subsequently wrote Voltaire that the opponents of inoculation were "truly blockheads, ignorant or just wicked." Voltaire exulted: "Oh Madam, what a lesson Your Majesty is giving us petty Frenchmen, to our ridiculous Sorbonne and to the argumentative charlatans in our medical schools! You have been inoculated with less fuss than a nun taking an enema."[37]

Such incidents lend support to Razzell's argument about the importance of inoculation. But some points remain controversial. Even a very widespread practice of the procedure may not have produced a level of immunity sufficient to affect mortality rates. Inoculation may have remained dangerous, a vehicle for diffusing smallpox as well as suppressing it. And did smallpox itself account for enough deaths so that any reduction in its severity could have made much demographic difference?[38] Thomas McKeown thinks not; although the work of Carmichael and Silverstein suggests that smallpox was a significant seventeenth- and eighteenth-century cause of death, what proportion is "significant"? Finally, the persistence of smallpox as a serious disease into the nineteenth century calls into question the effectiveness of eighteenth-century preventive measures.

It is tempting to see Edward Jenner (1749–1832) as a characteristic figure in the eighteenth-century relation between medicine and experimental science, because (on the surface, at least) Jenner's development of a smallpox "vaccine" seems an illustration of a determined empirical procedure followed by a medical professional who also manifested a generally wide-ranging curiosity about nature. Just what Jenner did, however, has long been controversial. He certainly changed the history of smallpox inoculation. Jenner, the son of an English country clergyman, took up a surgeon's career, traveling to London to study with John Hunter, who (with his brother William) was perhaps the leading developer of surgical techniques and teaching in Europe. After several years in London Jenner returned to a country surgical practice in western England. Natural curiosity and experimentation had become, in the eighteenth century, part of the world of English country gentility; clergymen, physicians, surgeons, attorneys all might examine nature and publish their observations, in the manner of the classic *Natural History of Selbourne* written by the clergyman Gilbert White in 1789.

For Jenner, this milieu's natural curiosity had been further prodded by his friend and mentor Hunter, an indefatigable experimentalist whose appetite for natural knowledge knew no limits: "Have you any caves where Batts go at night? [Hunter asked Jenner] . . . have you got the bones yet of a large Porpass I wish you had. . . . I have received my Hedge Hogs. . . . Have you any queer fish? . . . Send me all the Fossils you find . . . Cannot you get me a large Porpass for either Love or Money?"[39] Over the years Jenner established a successful surgical practice, both in rural Gloucestershire and in the fashionable spa town of Cheltenham; while he did so he pursued natural knowledge in the miscellaneously curious way suggested by Hunter's requests. Most notably, Jenner made an important contribution to understanding the strange nesting behavior of the cuckoo. He also, over a long period of time beginning in the 1770s, took note of rural stories about a coincidence: that victims of "cowpox" did not contract smallpox. He collected such information slowly and not very single-mindedly, building up some cases of people known to have suffered from cowpox who later resisted smallpox, either from contagion or from variolation (which procedure Jenner himself practiced). In 1796 Jenner inoculated eight-year-old James Phipps, not with smallpox, but with cowpox; he then subsequently attempted to variolate Phipps with smallpox, and observed no smallpox symptoms. In 1798 Jenner resumed these tests, inoculating cowpox in a series of children, passing this mild disease from one to another. When they too resisted subsequent smallpox inoculations, Jenner described these results in *An Inquiry into the Causes and Effects of the Variolae Vaccinae*, and the word "vaccination" entered circulation. Mild, nonscarring cowpox apparently conferred an immunity to lethal smallpox.

Some prominent London medical men took up Jenner's cause. By 1800 physicians in continental Europe were demanding more information and the preparation of cowpox "vaccine." Napoleon became Jenner's admirer, Thomas Jefferson personally vaccinated his own children, the kingdom of Denmark made vaccination compulsory as early as 1810, while in 1802 the British Parliament awarded Jenner the gigantic sum of £10,000, followed by a further £20,000 in 1807.

But controversy enveloped Jenner and his vaccination from the very start, and what Jenner had actually done remains unclear. Derrick Baxby has convincingly argued that great difficulty attends any attempt to identify the true composition of Jenner's "vaccine."[40] It may have been, as Razzell and other anti-Jennerians have argued, simply contaminated smallpox variolae.[41] The present *Vaccinae* virus, now solely the product of the laboratory, is not identical to modern cowpox. Baxby offers the tentative suggestion that Jenner's vaccine and the modern *Vaccinae* were both derived, not from cowpox, but from a now-extinct variety of horsepox.[42]

Of course no knowledge of viruses existed in 1798, and the controversies that accompanied Jenner's "discovery" revolved around other issues. Was Jenner's vaccination safer than variolation? Its proponents said yes; opponents said either that Jenner hadn't presented enough evidence or that his "cowpox" was in fact dangerous. Benjamin Moseley claimed that "cowpox" was really syphilis. Did Jenner show that vaccination was truly effective against smallpox? If so, was its effect permanent? Jenner rashly argued that one vaccination conferred life-long immunity to smallpox, and only gradually did his supporters realize that that was not so. Some other controversy was certainly professional: inoculators resented the challenge to their methods, their esteem, and their business, while disagreements about priority in the "discovery" also arose.

For all the controversy, however, Jenner soon won acclaim as a hero of the human race and a symbol of the march of enlightenment against superstition. Following Denmark's lead, a number of European states compelled vaccination for their entire populations, including Russia in 1812 and Sweden in 1816. Vaccine hospitals and Jennerian societies promoted the practice, while charity schemes evolved to provide the poor with vaccine. In the first decade of the nineteenth century, eager Europeans had carried vaccines to distant corners of the earth: India by 1802, China and the Philippines by 1805.

The spread of vaccination was uneven, however. In rural districts, particularly in the British Isles, empirical practitioners clung to the established variolation method. The credulous could be convinced that catching an "animal" disease—cowpox—might in some way reduce one's humanity, "animalizing" one. Confidence in vaccination was shaken by the gradual realization that one vaccination was not enough; although Jenner's opponents had raised that question from the start, he only reluctantly conceded doubt, and the first systematic revaccination began in 1829, in Württemberg.

Despite the triumphs of scientific medicine that inoculation and vaccination represented, smallpox remained a serious disease in the nineteenth-century West. As such it illustrated two particularly nineteenth-century problems of disease and health: the relation between disease and urban poverty, and the mounting questions about the proper regulatory role of the state. Smallpox persisted in part because vaccination led to an unwise suspension of concern, because poverty might lead to overcrowding, itinerant vagrancy, and lack of access to vaccine, and because the liberal state hesitated to compel vaccination (or anything else) on a free people. Autocratic Russia compelled vaccination early, but lacked the effective bureaucratic apparatus to enforce such a rule; liberal Britain made no such move until 1853, and liberal France not until 1902, as smallpox vaccination became an important symbolic issue in the state's powers over public health. The discussion of smallpox will resume in Chapter Twelve.

Scurvy

The history of the West's confrontation with scurvy parallels its experience with smallpox in several ways. Scurvy, like smallpox, became an important disease in the early modern centuries. In the eighteenth century a workable preventive was "found," although no one understood why it worked. Scurvy became the subject of considerable experimentation; and in the wake of the scientific revolution new explanations of its cause appeared that illustrated the general approaches of the new science.

Scurvy, a disease of nutritional deficiency, arises in populations that consume inadequate amounts of vitamin C, or ascorbic acid. Although scurvy's history is very ancient, it first attracted specific Western attention as a by-product of the great age of exploration that started in the late fifteenth century. Certainly the isolated poor, particularly in the villages of northern Europe, had suffered from scurvy in the winter for many centuries, but the coming of spring annually brought some vegetables (however few) and thus relief. Prolonged ocean voyages posed more extreme nutritional problems, and concentrated them in populations that the governing elites were bound to notice. Magellan's voyage across the Pacific in 1520–21 included a passage of more than three months out of sight of land, between the straits that bear Magellan's name and the Marianas; in the course of that journey, as in the course of many others, scurvy ravaged the crew with its brutal symptoms: skin covered with purple spots, limbs weakened, and gums swollen grotesquely over the teeth in a way that made eating nearly impossible.

As Europeans ventured more frequently on transoceanic voyages (and carried enslaved Africans with them), scurvy became a more frequent companion. And as the economic and political importance of those voyages grew, so too did the problem's perceived severity. Remedies for scurvy were not lacking; if anything, too many remedies existed, all with adherents. The benefits of oranges had been noticed as early as Vasco da Gama's voyage to India around the Cape of Good Hope in 1498, but that was only one in a forest of solutions, and only in the eighteenth century did careful empiricism establish the relative merits of the preventives.[43] That sea voyages suffered from scurvy in the meantime is beyond doubt. The British naval expedition of 1740 commanded by George Anson may serve as a good example. Ordered to venture into the Pacific and attack Spanish possessions and shipping, Anson set sail with six warships and over 1,900 men. From the standpoint of military victories and booty the voyage succeeded immensely, including as it did the capture of a westward-bound (that is, silver-laden) Manila galleon. But when Anson's sole remaining ship returned to Britain in 1744, 1,400 of his original force had perished, about 1,000 of them from scurvy, as against only *4* from enemy action.[44]

Such depredations stimulated theories about the cause of the disease. Humoral medicine believed scurvy a disease of the spleen and thus associated it with an excess of black bile. Humoral therapy therefore urged removal of black bile by purging and attention to diet. Seventeenth-century thinkers in both the chemical and the mechanical camps disagreed, and their beliefs led to competing therapeutic schemes. Mechanical philosophy placed emphasis first on the thinness (or thickness) of the blood, and by the eighteenth century had come to see the atmosphere as playing an important role in scurvy (as well as in many other diseases) . The elasticity of the air, it was believed, related to perspiration and thus to the proper (with a nod in the direction of Harvey) "circulation" of body fluids; cold and wet air, of the sort found on shipboard (and especially below decks) interfered with perspiration and brought on scurvy. Therefore, some eighteenth-century thinkers urged, proper ventilation would prevent scurvy.

Chemical philosophers held to another view. Seventeenth-century iatrochemists such as van Helmont saw scurvy as the product of either excess acid or excess alkali (depending on the symptoms), and so they proposed a chemical readjustment of (to use a modern term) the body's pH, perhaps through diet, perhaps through chemical remedies. This chemical interpretation took a new form in the eighteenth century, with the interest in pneumatic chemistry

stimulated by the discovery of the different constituents of the previously elemental "air." Joseph Black isolated one of the first of the gases, carbon dioxide,
in the 1750s. For a time, through the 1770s, Black's "fixed air" was a sovereign
remedy for scurvy, until—by the 1780s—it was realized that the body produced
"fixed air" all the time anyway. But in the meantime "fixed air" had also been
related to a therapy that had been popular through much of the century: the use
of malt as both preventive and cure. Carbon dioxide was succeeded as a wonder
drug by another exciting product of pneumatic chemistry, oxygen. That gas's
name meant "acid former," for late eighteenth-century thinkers believed that it
was a component of all acids. Therefore oxygen was part of chemical remedies
for scurvy caused by excess alkali.

All these theories, and trial-and-error practices as well, resulted in a wide variety of answers. Spurred by the disasters of Anson's voyage, the British naval surgeon James Lind conducted a sophisticated experiment (the results of which
were published in 1747), in which he tried a number of different scurvy remedies under well-controlled conditions. One of the remedies, the use of oranges
and lemons in the diet, gave the most favorable results. But this experiment, so
decisive to our minds, made little impression on Lind, let alone on others.[45] Lind
and his contemporaries believed that scurvy must have layers of cause, with
some factors "predisposing" victims to the disease; one simple dietetic remedy
could not by itself be sufficient. In the 1740s Lind held to the atmospheric theory, and supported the numerous trials of ventilating ships; when by the 1760s
those trials gave poor results, Lind became uncertain and discouraged. His 1747
essay had not convinced its readers of the powers of citrus fruits; it had not even
convinced its author; but it did leave the field open for continuing trial and error
and experimentation.

That empiricism was followed, in a much less controlled way, by the celebrated
Pacific explorer James Cook, whose voyages between 1768 and 1779 are often
mistakenly said to have shown the way to the use of citrus against scurvy. Cook
carried with him a vast battery of different supposed antiscorbutics—his own
favorites being malt and sauerkraut—and supplied his seamen with all of them.
His voyages were remarkably free of scurvy, but what he had shown was not at all
clear to his contemporaries. As O.H.K. Spate says, "so many nostrums were tried,
without controls, that it was like killing a bird with a shotgun; impossible to say
which particular pellet was fatal."[46] In the year after Cook's death in Hawaii in
1779, the British fleet in the English Channel suffered 2,400 cases of scurvy in ten
weeks, proving that Cook had not established the unique power of citrus fruit.

The successful arguments on behalf of citrus turned out to be empirical, not
theoretical. Gilbert Blane, a British physician with both naval experience and
social connections, approached the subject in a Baconian, collect-all-the-facts
way, and in the 1780s and 1790s gradually persuaded British naval and political

leaders of the virtues of citrus fruits as a prevention and cure of scurvy. In 1795 the British Admiralty bowed to the weight of Blane's persuasions and ordered a daily ration of citrus juice for its crews. But understanding of the cause of scurvy, or of the reasons for the efficacy of citrus, lay in the future.

How Complete Was Enlightenment?

Even in the eighteenth century, the era of science and enlightenment, when human reason exulted in the powers conferred on it by the giants of the scientific revolution, continuities rather than change dominated much of the West's relations with disease. Physicians' therapies, even for those who could receive the finest medical care, remained fundamentally Galenic, as the well-documented and -discussed case of the "madness" of George III of Great Britain illustrates.[47] And epidemic outbreaks made the case for continuity even more clearly. One such epidemic, at the end of the century, brought a prosperous and self-consciously enlightened Western city to its knees.

In 1793 yellow fever fell on Philadelphia, then the capital of the United States, one of the largest (outside London) English-speaking cities in the world, and certainly one of the most "enlightened," the city of Benjamin Franklin. This epidemic began in August, and by September and early October the city had been badly crippled. Although numbers are not precise, it seems likely that 5,000 Philadelphians died in those months, of a total population of about 55,000, while as many as 20,000 others fled the city. Benjamin Rush, a leading Philadelphia physician of the time, estimated that as many as 6,000 residents were ill from the fever at a single time.

Yellow fever is an acute viral disease, which reaches humans through the bites of the mosquito species *Aedes aegypti*. Yellow fever is highly virulent; drastic symptoms of suffering—a sudden onset of high fever, skin hemorrhages, pains, vomiting, and then internal hemorrhages—are often succeeded by death. The mortality rate of yellow fever varies widely, but in some epidemics may approach 50 percent. In the eighteenth century Western civilization began encountering this basically tropical disease more frequently, as European contacts with the tropics multiplied. (A more thorough discussion of European-tropical disease connections is found in Chapter Nine.) For European medical opinion, slowly working its way through arguments about the nature of "fevers," this terrifying disease took its place in that broad category. Philadelphia debates over yellow fever's cause and nature illustrated many of the general themes of such eighteenth-century discussions. Was yellow fever a single unique disease? Or was it located on a continuum of fevers and so a variant (however extreme) of a general type? Was it of essentially foreign origin, carried to Philadelphia by contagion from the tropics? The recent arrival of refugees from French Haiti lent credence to that belief. Or, as many eighteenth-century thinkers believed, did yellow fever arise from a miasmic atmosphere?

These questions roiled the Philadelphia medical community, one dominated by physicians who had received the best education that the English-speaking world afforded. Many of them had studied in Edinburgh or London, and were imbued with the traditions of William Cullen, the Monros, and the Hunters. The city itself had a university, where a medical college had been founded in 1765, the first such institution in British America. The city also had a medical society and the American Philosophical Society, founded under Franklin's inspiration in 1743. Philadelphia's civic pride, which the doctors shared, did not mean unanimity of opinion when the epidemic struck. Some physicians, led by Rush, insisted that the sources of filth in the city produced a lethal miasma; a particular target for this opinion was a rotting heap of spoiled coffee, dumped on a wharf by a ship from the Caribbean. Not all physicians agreed with Rush. William Currie led a party which insisted that the fever had been borne by contagion from foreign parts.

Within the general frameworks of "miasma" and "contagion," other more specific theories of cause flourished: for instance, electric fluids in the air were "invariably fatal" and the large number of lightning rods in Franklin's city, "by imperceptibly drawing off the electric fluid from the clouds," put Philadelphia in peril.[48] Beside these up-to-date scientific speculations, many older beliefs coexisted. The yellow fever was a divine visitation punishing the wicked, perhaps a specific judgment on the sins and errors of the new nation, perhaps a judgment on that urban life abominated by supporters of a commonwealth of free farmers. Echoing very old theories about plague, some believed that fear itself might cause the fever. Especially if contagion was blamed, scapegoats might suffer, with the French refugees from Haiti the obvious targets.

Different theories of cause, as always, called forth different responses to the emergency. Many urged prayer. For many—perhaps 20,000—either miasma or contagion prompted flight from the noxious air of the city or from the bearers of the disease. The Philadelphia experience did add a twist to the old arguments about the presumed effects of a quarantine on a city's commerce. For several centuries European city governments had struggled to control contagious disease in the face of the objections of merchants who saw quarantines as unacceptable interference with trade. In Philadelphia in 1793, however, the merchant community saw the doctrine of miasma as the greater threat, for it might say to the world that fever was "native" to Philadelphia, tainting all the city's products and inhabitants. The state government was thus moved to act—cautiously—on the contagion theory, and it imposed a quarantine on incoming goods and people. Of course other American towns and cities reciprocated, declaring quarantines on movements from the beleaguered capital. Mail from Philadelphia was dipped in vinegar before being opened.[49] But because the contagion theory did not have universal support, a variety of schemes were suggested to clear the miasma. No really systematic cleanup was undertaken, however; the offensive pile of coffee apparently stayed on the wharf for some time, perhaps because those who most feared its effects were therefore most leery to approach it and clean it up. Some citizens fired guns in the streets in the belief that doing so would purify the air.

Many of the city's services collapsed, as those who performed them sickened, died, or fled. The federal government simply closed down; President George Washington retired to his Virginia estate. Much of state government likewise came to a halt. The city administration was kept alive, though barely, by the determined mayor Matthew Clarkson, an ad hoc committee of citizens, and the efforts of Philadelphia's African-American population, who (like the poor in general) could least afford flight. Their actions included the commandeering of property for an isolation hospital and an orphanage, staffing those institutions, raising money for supplies, organizing the burial of the dead, conveying the sick, caring for the destitute, and burning or burying the property of the deceased. The ad hoc committee acted in a clear and long tradition of urban response to epidemics; Renaissance Italian cities had created such committees, before their evolutions into standing boards of health.

Doctors attacked the disease with a wide range of remedies, none of them clearly effective, although recoveries enabled them to claim success. Many of the therapies, regardless of their theoretical connections with modern science, varied little from old humoral traditions. Benjamin Rush, in the midst of the epidemic, became messianically committed to a savage regimen of bleeding and purging, including massive doses of calomel (a favorite mercury-based purge) and venesection that removed up to a quart of blood several times in as many days. His zeal, his prior standing, and his political reputation carried many along with this astonishing therapy, but some doctors disagreed and urged a gentler approach, notably Jean Devèze, a Frenchman who assumed medical charge of the city's isolation hospital. Between the careful Devèze and the heroic Rush could be found a wide range of herbal remedies, purges, decoctions, and suggestions for healthy diets and habits, purveyed by physicians, apothecaries, and a group of empirics whose connection with "official" medicine was even more blurred in North America than it was in Europe (although less so in Philadelphia than in the backwoods).

Political issues affected theories of cause and remedies alike. Rush enjoyed a prominent political as well as medical position. He had been an ardent republican and had signed the Declaration of Independence. When Alexander Hamilton, the Federalist secretary of the treasury, was struck by yellow fever in September 1793 his rapid cure, in the care of one of Rush's medical opponents, acquired political overtones; was "Federalist" medicine superior to that offered by Rush, the friend of Thomas Jefferson and James Madison? Rush himself believed that Hamilton might have accepted his therapies if only their politics had coincided.

The epidemic may have had political effects as well. It broke out in the middle of the most determined attempts by revolutionary France to enlist the alliance of the United States. Some years later John Adams claimed that the epidemic had prevented a revolution led by Citizen Genêt, the French envoy, the goal of which would have been to force Washington to join France's war with Britain or be overthrown. And while modern historians concur with Dumas Malone's view that Adams "exaggerate[d] both the political dangers of the times and the effects of the plague on them," the epidemic certainly resulted in a period of political paralysis as the government dispersed and neither political rallies nor news could come from Philadelphia.[50] Washington and those who supported his neutralist stance more easily maintained an inactive position.

The epidemic also exacerbated internal divisions. Controversy about the merits of Rush's "heroic" therapy intermingled with broader arguments about the nature of American culture. Rush believed that civic virtue and a successful volunteer effort at governance (in conjunction with his therapeutic measures) had saved the day, but others, seeing failure where Rush saw triumph, drew different conclusions. Eve Kornfeld believes that the epidemic weakened Philadelphia's cultural primacy in the new nation; its united and confident cultural community broke apart, and Rush formed a new and rival academy of medicine among his supporters.[51]

The Philadelphia yellow fever epidemic serves as a useful summary of the eighteenth century's disease history. The episode displayed the characteristics of the Enlightenment: its environmentalism, its search for causes in such physical phenomena as the atmosphere and electricity, its eclectic and divided nosological arguments, and its self-consciously "scientific" approach. Much, however, remained from earlier times: appeals to providence, visions of doom, searches for scapegoats, and the overt associations of therapies and political positions. While rationales for therapies had changed, remedies in the humoral tradition persisted in practice. The orthodox practitioners of medicine offered no clear therapeutic advantage over the empirics. If medicine made any contribution to the reduction of eighteenth-century death rates, it did not do so in its response to violent epidemics.

The roles of disease, and the attempts of Western thinkers and actors to control it, remain unclear for the period of the eighteenth century. It is possible that eighteenth-century hospitals, at least in some places in Europe, were not the positive menaces to health that French revolutionaries, determined to make a dramatic case for reform, made them out to be. It is difficult to agree with E. M. Sigsworth that reformed hospitals may have positively contributed to health, however.[52] Although a significant reform in nursing practices was under way in some parts of Germany (see Chapter Ten), it had not spread widely. Physicians and other healers clearly had no stronger grip on the causes of disease at the end of the century than they had at its beginning. Epidemics still baffled everyone. Any possible demographic impact on the death rate from human "medical" action must rest on two bases: the preventive measures that evolved against smallpox, scurvy, and malaria; and the indirect (and still largely uncomprehended) effects on environment, particularly those that interfered with disease vectors such as insects. The jury remains out on the general demographic impact of both those ameliorations.

Seven

Cholera and Sanitation

Cholera occupies a somewhat anomalous position in the history of diseases that have affected Western civilization. It shares many of the characteristics of plague: its suddenness of onset, its horrible symptoms, its high rate of mortality, and its apparent inexorability. For many nineteenth-century people cholera seemed as much a visitation from a vengeful God as plague had seemed to Europeans in 1348. And as they had in 1348 Europeans took flight when they could; as in 1348, they searched for the sinful who had brought on the disease and made scapegoats of them. Social turmoil followed in cholera's wake. But cholera also appeared at a time when science was making more extensive claims of explanation, and when many societies were groping toward the control of disease through social and political action. Cholera's victims might be as helpless as plague's had been, but nineteenth-century thinkers were hardly resigned to that fact.

Cholera's position in historical writing has also been anomalous. For some it qualifies as the great disease drama of the nineteenth century, one that moreover focused attention on the environmental evils of early industrial urbanization. But much recent scholarship has discounted the importance of cholera in either the evolution of etiological theory or the development of sanitary practice, and we have recognized that its demographic impact was slight. It is as though cholera represented the last gasp of an earlier period of disease history. Nineteenth-century thinkers recognized its horrors, but were more concerned with an agenda determined by endemic complaints such as tuberculosis and "fevers," an agenda in which this violent Asian visitor did not find a clear place.

Cholera in 1831

The shock value of the disease came in part from its newness on the Western scene. Cholera had been at home on the Indian subcontinent for centuries. In warm river waters the causative microorganism *(Cholera vibrio)* flourished, reaching humans most often through water, but also carried on infected food or from hand to mouth. Microorganisms passed through digestive tracts and reentered water supplies through excreta. The growth of commerce and communication between India and Europe increased the likelihood of its importation from its Bengal home, and the imposition of British authority on the subcontinent increased the human (and disease) interchanges among regions of India itself. A major cholera epidemic began in India in 1817; from India the disease spread to Afghanistan and Persia and thence into Russia, appearing at Orenburg in 1829. From Orenburg it traveled into the West with remarkable rapidity, considering that the age of steam travel had scarcely begun. Cholera reached the major cities of Russia in 1830, spread to the Baltic in 1831, and by that autumn jumped into England. Northern Europe felt the disease in 1832, as did North America; cholera reached southern Europe, as well as Central and South America, in 1833. As railroads and steamships appeared in subsequent years, later episodes of cholera moved with even greater speed, with especially severe epidemics in 1848–49, 1853–54, the middle 1860s, and the early 1870s. One of the most serious outbreaks occurred as late as 1911, in Naples.

Europeans took fright at cholera's virulence, and with reason. Mortality rates from cholera approached those of plague, for roughly half of its victims died. It is worth noticing, however, that cholera's morbidity rate fell far below that found in the great plague epidemics, and even below that customarily maintained by nineteenth-century tuberculosis. Cholera affected about 35,000 people in Paris in 1832 (in a population of 785,000), for example, and about 17,000 people in Hamburg in 1892 (in a population of 620,000).[1] Cholera is not particularly easy to catch. Although the microorganisms must have been plentiful during the nineteenth-century epidemics, many people probably ingested them without harm, for human stomach acids often kill the organisms before they reach the intestines where the trouble starts.

That trouble could devastate the victim. Cholera came as a sudden, overwhelming attack, most notably of dehydration marked by vomiting and profuse, uncontrollable excretion. The drastic loss of body fluids collapsed the tissues; coagulated blood ceased to flow, the skin turned alarmingly blue, and the heart (or the kidneys) failed, often within a few hours. People perfectly healthy in the morning died by nightfall, having undergone some hours of great agony. And the bourgeois of the nineteenth century found such a death particularly repugnant, for his sensibilities about the grosser body processes were becoming more acute. Cholera could strike down a prim middle-class man away from the privacy of his home, leaving him collapsed in his own excrement on the street or in a railroad car. A more shameful condition was hard to imagine.

The inexplicability of cholera's attack increased its impact on the imagination of the time. Cholera appeared in Europe and America when confidence in the powers of science had been receiving enthusiastic expression for over a century. Although (as Chapters Five and Six have suggested) the new science did not always consistently affect the practice of Western medicine, nineteenth-century European medicine took pride in its status as a "science." It could point to one clear triumph: the reduction of the peril of smallpox through cowpox vaccinations; it had self consciously allied itself with the experimental method; it trumpeted its reliance on observation and eschewed the old Galenic categories as explanations of disease. New and exciting etiologies and nosologies filled the air. Cholera, an alien embodiment of an oriental "other," rebuked that pride. Modern medicine had many different explanations of cholera, but those explanations conflicted. More important, modern medicine offered neither a convincing cure nor good advice on how to avoid it. The physician's therapeutic arsenal relied on a melange of bleedings and purgings that candid members of the learned profession admitted had little effect.

In the 1830s opinions about the causes of cholera reflected more general etiological arguments that had a long history and that were (as the previous chapter has shown) very far from settlement. By the early nineteenth century the conflict between "contagion" and "miasma" was beginning to favor the latter. Progressive opinion, according to Erwin Ackerknecht, saw atmospheric pollution as a dominant cause of disease, partly for political reasons. The contagion doctrines that had gained ground in the late Middle Ages in the wake of bubonic plague epidemics had led (as we saw in Chapter Three) to the creation of health boards, *cordons sanitaires*, and systems of quarantine, what their eighteenth-century advocate Johann Peter Frank called "medical police." To the generations of the American and French Revolutions such state machinery represented unreasonable limitations on the freedom of the individual. Quarantines, as we have seen, certainly disrupted trade and inspired widespread resentment. To some Enlightenment thinkers medical police and the theory of contagion that lay behind them symbolized all that was wrong with the Old Regime: its corruption, its tyranny, its superstition. Further, the liberal-bourgeois background of many physicians predisposed them to this politically motivated anticontagionism.[2]

But politics did not provide the sole argument. A more general environmentalism dominated much of the thought of the Enlightenment. And an apparent lack of evidence also troubled the contagionist theory. "Contagion" meant a direct passage of the disease from one person to another. When the *mechanism*—the physical mode of transmission—could not be shown, contagionism remained an unproved hypothesis. The discovery of microscopic "animalcules," van Leeuwenhoek's "wee beasties," in the seventeenth century promised at first to show such a mode of transmission; but as the eighteenth century went on the beasties resisted indictment for any specific disease. If the beasties couldn't be shown to carry a disease, then how (apart from vital or chemical action at a distance) did it pass from a sufferer to a new victim?

Contagion clearly explained one disease: smallpox. Fluids from a smallpox patient, injected in a healthy person, resulted in a new case. The venereal character of syphilis suggested another mode of contagion. But attempts at inoculation against other diseases in the hope of proving their contagious nature discouraged the contagionists, for in a large number of experiments only a few cases "took." Still weightier arguments derived from experience with some serious epidemic diseases. Europeans experienced yellow fever primarily in the West Indies, but their encounters with the disease elsewhere suggested its seasonal character; why should a contagious disease cease transmission when the weather changed? In the 1793 yellow fever epidemic in Philadelphia the partisans of miasma were strong, and the Barcelona epidemic in 1821 was even more decisive. On the latter occasion the French physician Nicolas Chervin, who had practiced in America and was acquainted with Benjamin Rush, maintained that a "miasma" produced yellow fever. Travelers from Cuba did not bring the disease, as the contagionists argued. It arose from bad air produced by open sewers and other filth. By 1827 the French government agreed and lifted its quarantine laws that applied to yellow fever. Plague, largely absent from western Europe (though not from eastern Europe) since the early eighteenth century, also seemed seasonal in character; plague also affected poorer districts more severely (as would cholera), which suggested the significance of local environmental conditions.

As cholera spread it posed problems for both contagionists and proponents of miasma. If cholera was contagious, why did it suddenly appear in a section of town out of touch with cholera victims? Why did it not affect medical personnel who attempted to care for the sufferers? If a miasma was responsible, why did the disease strike some people in a town and not others? Why did the disease seem to move along routes of human traffic?

When cholera first made its way into Russia the czar's government, acting on vaguely contagionist advice, imposed quarantines and ordered the isolation of victims. The czar, after all, possessed a strong state regulatory apparatus (at least in theory), and political liberalism was no threat to contagionist measures in Nicholas I's Russia. But the Russian state measures failed to halt the advance of cholera, and serious consequences resulted. Elsewhere in Europe the Russian experience discredited contagionist measures such as quarantines and enforced isolation, although they may have failed because the Russian application of them was neither consistent nor complete; the czar's police system was stronger on paper than in practice. And not only did the Russian measures fail to halt the spread of cholera; they led to major social turmoil, when the heavy police presence necessary to enforce isolation led to serious riots in St. Petersburg.[3] Would governments act on the theory of contagion when doing so might be not only ineffective but positively dangerous politically? In a Europe brimming with revolution in 1830–1832, why look for trouble?

Although thinkers in Western countries reacted in a number of ways and with a number of beliefs, a rough consensus emerged in the early 1830s that in a way overrode the "contagion" versus "miasma" debate. Why did cholera strike its victims in such a whimsical way? Nineteenth-century minds rejected blind chance. Cholera's descent on a victim, whether it moved through person-to-person contagion or through some environmental cause, was apparently contingent on some other factor that predisposed certain people to the disease. And while such thinking about "predisposing causes" went back to the medieval plague, it assumed new force in a time when the contagion-versus-miasma debate seemed inadequate. Peter Baldwin has suggested that the debate was overtaken, in different ways in different places, by a general acceptance of a contingent contagionism.[4]

On what was cholera "contingent"? For some the answer remained the Almighty. Fearing a scourge of the entire society, the British government called a national day of fasting and humiliation, although it did so only after a fanatic member of Parliament embarrassed his colleagues with his prophecies of national desolation. President Andrew Jackson vetoed a similar proposal in the United States, holding that such a resolution violated the constitutional separation of church and state. But attempts to see in cholera a general divine punishment were weakened by the particular incidence of cholera. In 1348—when half the population was affected—a general curse seemed more plausible than it did in 1832. Did God single out individuals, or at most social groups? And if so, on what basis? In America, for example, were African Americans or recent immigrants the targets of His wrath?[5]

More common were associations of cholera with individual immorality or irreligion. The *Wesleyan Methodist Magazine* reported: "On the Christmas day, two men (one of whom was a notorious dog fighter) were fighting in a public house, in a state of intoxication, near the Wesleyan chapel, and that too during the time of worship there. One of them died of the cholera in a few hours after, and the other in two days!"[6] And the question of immorality of course opened a Pandora's box of possibilities, for immorality too often lay in the eyes of the beholder. Did immorality mean drunkenness? Licentiousness? Failure to observe the Sabbath? Blasphemy? Or might "immorality" include such characteristics as laziness, imprudence, or stupidity?

With the last-named traits we move (perhaps insensibly) from the realm of moral conceptions of disease toward theories of social causation. English village churches that observed the day of fasting and national humiliation collected money to relieve the suffering of the poor. Henry Hunt, the British radical, pointed out that one-third of the population fasted almost every day of the week.[7] When cholera invaded France in 1832, studies of its incidence showed meaningful statistical correlations between poverty and the disease. René Villermé (1782–1863), a pioneer medical statistician, used the evidence from cholera to bolster his arguments that poverty, not environmental "miasma," was the true cause of disease. But what caused poverty? For the laissez-faire thinkers of the Manchester School, individual failure produced poverty, and the solution to poverty therefore lay in individual achievement: work hard, abandon dissolute habits of drinking and womanizing, save and do not spend. Villermé himself, who pointed out the human problems of the industrial system and thus criticized much Manchester thinking, could offer little more in the way of solution. Public health and the avoidance of disease, he said, were clearly social problems at heart, not environmental ones, but his remedy was the education of the poor into better habits.[8] To some observers in America, the habits of the poor violated God's natural laws, and so virtue—and health—might be gained by education in those natural laws.

Before the completion of Villermé's important studies—almost before cholera even appeared—Europeans and Americans had associated cholera with social class and economic background. Whether one held a doctrine of "contagion" or "miasma" made little difference: slums propagated cholera, whether because they polluted the atmosphere or brought their dwellers into proximity with others. In Britain, France, and the United States the governing and middle classes feared cholera as a threat to social stability, for it might provoke the anger of the lower orders, it might spread to others, and measures against it might disrupt the economy. Such fears added weight and perhaps bile to the faltering and uncertain measures of public health undertaken in 1831 and 1832: cleansing of streets and districts, isolation of victims, quarantines. The St. Petersburg experience was repeated, as in many places such measures sparked countering fears in the poorer classes. Cleansing and isolation interfered with traditional patterns of life, and the poor feared attacks on those traditional ways. Those fears related to many issues. The poor feared doctors as representatives of another class and as purveyors of remedies often nauseous or painful, and so they resented legally mandated confinement in isolation hospitals in the hands of doctors.

In Britain the fear of doctors in 1831 gained a particular edge from the recent and horrible revelations of the case of Burke and Hare, Edinburgh criminals who murdered the homeless poor and sold their bodies to anatomical lecturers who paid and asked no questions. Small wonder that an Edinburgh crowd "pelted the medical men with mud and stones, shouting 'medical murderer,' 'cholera humbug' and 'Burkers' " at surgeons who tried to treat a cholera victim, or that a crowd in Manchester cried, "To the hospital, pull it to the ground" on their way to attack it.[9] In Britain and France alike the poor could hear Malthusian voices who seemed to urge the purging of excess population. The drastic symptoms of cholera brought "poison" to the popular mind; were the governing classes engaged in a dreadful plot to reduce the numbers of the poor? Variations on that theme appeared elsewhere. In Russia, for example, the St. Petersburg rioters might blame the foreign physicians who dominated the medical community there, or perhaps the Poles, then rebelling against Russian rule; in Russian Poland, cholera could be seen as a poison spread by the Russians.[10] National and/or class resentments boiled over in St. Petersburg, Moscow, Warsaw, Paris, Edinburgh, Glasgow, and Manchester. Hospitals, doctors, government functionaries, the police all found themselves under attack. And—for the governing classes—such disorders proved the ignorance and superstition of the lower orders.

Meanwhile physicians grappled with other possible "contingent" causes. In places as far apart as New York and Hamburg, doctors emphasized the importance of maintaining morale, in the belief that a despondent state of mind predisposed one to cholera. Many doctors shared—or gave voice to—the more general beliefs that the disease stemmed from sin, poverty, dirt, or some combination of them; but nowhere did a precise consensus emerge, and a wild garden of therapies flowered. Calomel, for example, frequently prescribed as a powerful purgative, was both a common choice and (we would now think) a catastrophic treatment for dehydration, one that led Norman Howard-Jones (in 1972) to call nineteenth-century cholera therapy a "form of benevolent homicide."[11]

But despite the lack of consensus, the experience of cholera did contribute to some shifts in medical thinking, most notably in conceptions of discrete disease entities and their relationships to human physiology. As we saw in Chapter Six, some medical thinking by the early nineteenth century maintained that diseases were local in character, not systemic as ancient Galenism had held. Despite these new ideas, a pathology that emphasized disorders of the humors, or fluids moving through the whole system, had deep roots in Western thought. Associated with such a pathology was a conception of diseases along a continuum, in which (for example) one suffered from a greater or lesser imbalance of black bile. According to this view one might have a little cholera, or a lot of it. But if disease was a specific malady, associated with a particular "poison" or external agent and affecting a particular organ of the body, then either you had cholera or you did not. In the nineteenth century, eclectic and uncertain nosological ideas gradually moved toward the specific, discrete conception of diseases. French thought, in the revolutionary period, had especially leaned in that direction. Broussais—not surprisingly—saw cholera as an inflammation of the gastric tract, brought on by ingestion of a specific poison found in the environment. To Broussais (and to other French physicians, many of whom did not otherwise agree with him) the significance of cholera lay in its specificity, and not in whether it was or was not contagious. But in some other places cholera did not play an important role in medical thought; thus British medical opinion gave more attention to the continuing problem of "fevers" than to the episodic cholera.[12]

The Gospel of Sanitation

For some, cholera's Asian origins meant a concern with "Asian" environments, particularly with the poverty, crowding, and dirt of India. But the environmental problems might not be imports. The great cholera epidemics and the explosive growth of industrial cities in the Western world certainly coincided. In the early nineteenth century British cities offered the most dramatic examples of that growth, but by the 1880s others had joined them (see Table 7.1).

More important than raw numbers, however, were the circumstances of much urban growth. Housing construction proceeded with great speed and with accompanying great carelessness: flimsy buildings, ill-ventilated and ill-heated,

_____ Table 7.1 _____
City Populations: 1800, 1850, 1880

	1800/1801	1850/1851	1880/1881
Great Britain			
Birmingham	71,000	223,000	401,000
Edinburgh	83,000	194,000	295,000
Glasgow	77,000	345,000	587,000
Leeds	53,000	172,000	309,000
Liverpool	82,000	376,000	553,000
London	1,088,000	2,491,000	3,881,000
Manchester	75,000	303,000	341,000
Continental Europe			
Berlin	172,000	419,000	1,122,000
Budapest	54,000	178,000	371,000
Lyons	110,000	177,000	376,000
Moscow	250,000	365,000	612,000
Munich	40,000	110,000	230,000
Paris	547,000	1,053,000	2,269,000
St. Petersburg	220,000	485,000	877,000
Turin	78,000	135,000	254,000
Vienna	247,000	444,000	726,000
United States			
New York	63,000	696,000	1,912,000
Philadelphia	81,000	388,000	847,000

Sources: C. M. Cipolla, ed., *The Fontana Economic History of Europe*, vol. 4, *The Emergence of Industrial Societies* (London: Collins, 1973), 750; B. R. Mitchell, *Abstract of British Historical Statistics* (Cambridge: Cambridge University Press, 1962), 24–27.

provided very overcrowded living space. In some cities, such as Liverpool, over-crowding often involved quarters below street level, where water constantly seeped in.

Arrangements (or lack thereof) for the disposal of excrement bedeviled these cities, and the large number of large animals in the cities exacerbated that problem. Most human wastes found their way either into leaky cesspools or directly into street drains. Water-flushed toilets, an invention of the eighteenth century, were still rare, a decided mark of status, and in any case simply conveyed the wastes out of the house into the same cesspools or street drains. Cesspools leaked into the surrounding soil; when they were cleaned (perhaps only yearly) their contents wound up in rivers or were sold to "night-soil" contractors to be stored in a dump that oozed into the water table. Sewers, where they existed, were constructed on the ancient model: large tunnels into which streets drained, large enough to accommodate the men who cleaned them and hence large enough to allow the formation of great stagnant pools. City water supplies came from a variety of sources, including private contractors; most often the contractors used either local ground water (in which sewage might mix) or local rivers. Most urban rivers were simply appalling, and as the century went on they got worse. Trash, sewage, animal (and human) bodies befouled them, as did a growing mixture of industrial pollutants.

What Hans Zinsser said of early modern warfare—that it provided ideal conditions for a gigantic natural experiment in epidemiology—might with equal justice be said of nineteenth-century cities and their environments.[13] Waterborne diseases such as typhoid fever and dysentery (and of course cholera) ran riot. Overcrowding, poor ventilation, and general dirt favored typhus and tuberculosis; air pollution caused nausea, and hence poor digestion and inadequate nutrition, as well as discouraging clean clothes and the provision of ventilation. A growing panoply of industrially related diseases added other health problems: asthmas suffered by miners, cutlers, and potters; necrosis ("fossy jaw") associated with match manufacture; bleach workers exposed to chlorine; rubber workers exposed to naphtha; and the widespread industrial use of poisonous lead and arsenic.[14]

In addition to the conviction that the "environment" might be responsible for disease, nineteenth-century thinkers inherited from the Enlightenment a predisposition to use quantifiable evidence. The great sanitarians of the 1830s and 1840s—René Villermé, Lemuel Shattuck, and Edwin Chadwick—shared a belief in statistics. All believed in the power of civilization to eradicate disease. Each received a stimulus, or at least evidence, from the early cholera epidemics. As we have seen, Villermé used the 1832 Paris experience to show correlations between mortality and poverty; he was convinced that (as William Coleman puts it) death was a social disease. Since for Villermé the root cause was poverty, not the environment, he perhaps should not be called a sanitarian at all. His remedies did include some environmental action against urban congestion, for he urged a return to small-scale manufacturing and the settlement of workers on small plots of arable land. More important, his arguments became crucial to the French thinkers called (by Coleman) *le parti d'hygiène,* a diverse group of intellectuals and empirical investigators who flourished in the years after 1825. Criticizing Rousseau's view that civilization had led to degeneration, they assiduously collected facts about hygienic conditions in the conviction that civilization created the power to solve hygienic and public health problems.[15]

Lemuel Shattuck (1793–1859), a Boston publisher and genealogical scholar, became interested in community statistics. In 1841 he published an analysis of the vital statistics of Boston that demonstrated the declining health of the town. For this Shattuck found a moral cause; disease, he believed, was "a penalty for deviation from moral behavior," and could be avoided by a regimen of "Godliness and cleanliness."[16] But the return of the cholera in the late 1840s helped to convince him that, although disease remained fundamentally a moral problem, the state must intervene to protect public health. A Massachusetts legislative commission that he chaired (1849–50) blamed the environment for deteriorating health, saw social factors as responsible for environmental change, and urged state responsibility for eliminating social and environmental evils by regulating or eliminating wastes and undertaking central water and sewer systems. Although Massachusetts did not act on this report for two decades, Shattuck had planted the sanitationist flag in the United States.

Of all the sanitarians Edwin Chadwick stands foremost, perhaps because his voice came from Britain, the pioneer industrial society. Chadwick (1800–1890), a disciple of the philosopher Jeremy Bentham, initially approached the problems of disease from the standpoint of political philosophy in the service of state bureaucracy. In 1834 the British Parliament mandated a sweeping change in the government's provision of poor relief, and Chadwick took an important position in the bureaucracy responsible for the new relief system. In Chadwick were balanced the conflicting strands of Bentham's philosophy. At times that philosophy endorsed the idea that a society's greatest happiness could be attained by assuming that each individual could best judge his own interests (and thus that government was best which governed least). But at other points individuals' judgments had to be educated or in some way directed by the society as a whole (and thus an enormous regulatory camel might nose into the laissez-faire state's tent).

The poor-relief reformers of 1834, working on the first of these assumptions, hoped to make the receipt of public relief unpalatable to the recipient, thus getting the state out of the welfare business and aiding a free labor market; individuals should be left to seek their own best interest with their employers, without the intervention of an artificial state welfare system. Chadwick agreed, and as a

_____ *Table 7.2* _____
Average Ages of Death in City and Country, England, 1842

Social class	Manchester (city)	Rutland (countryside)
Professional persons; gentry	38	52
Tradesmen; farmers	20	41
Mechanics; laborers	17	38

Source: G. M. Young and W. D. Handcock, eds., *English Historical Documents. 1833–1874*
(New York: Oxford University Press, 1956), 779. This work contains a convenient collection of
Chadwick's 1842 *Report*: 772–793.

bureaucrat sought to reduce state welfare costs. When a local government authority illegally spent funds to improve sanitation, Chadwick wondered if such action might in the long run reduce costs by preventing epidemic disasters. In the name of lowering state expenses, Chadwick launched an inquiry, at the right hand of which were two extreme "miasmist" physicians, James Kay-Shuttleworth and Thomas Southwood Smith. This inquiry resulted in the *Report on the Sanitary Condition of the Labouring Population* (1842), the single greatest classic of the sanitation movement and one that outsold well-known novels.[17]

Whereas Villermé had argued a causal connection between disease and poverty, Chadwick's *Report* found the major correlation to be between disease and dirt. The best-known illustrations of the *Report* contrasted the health of rural areas with the sickness of the great industrial towns (see Table 7.2). In a famous sentence Chadwick proclaimed "that the annual loss of life from filth and bad ventilation is greater than the loss from death or wounds in any wars in which the country has been engaged in modern times."[18] Chadwick was impressed by the differences between bucolic Rutland and teeming Manchester; Villermé would have looked at the same table and noticed the differences between gentry and laborers. Villermé's perspective raised awkward questions about the justice and wisdom of capitalist society, and Villermé shied from some possible answers. Chadwick's view threatened no such embarrassment. No fundamental restructuring of the class system would be needed; society simply had to clean itself up. G. M. Young said of Chadwick: "Born in 1800, in a Lancashire farmhouse where the children were washed all over, every day, the mainspring of Chadwick's career seems to have been a desire to wash the people of England all over, every day, by administrative order."[19]

For Chadwick the key to a clean society lay in the provision of integrated water-and-sewer systems for towns. The prevention of disease therefore became the responsibility of engineers, not of physicians (whose abilities Chadwick distrusted), and certainly not of socialist revolutionaries (whose hand Villermé unwillingly reinforced). Chadwick insisted on a "fully articulated" water-and-sewer service, embodying a steady supply of piped fresh water to each dwelling, house drainage, street drainage, and main sewers connected to each dwelling. The hydraulic force of the water supply constantly pushed wastes and sewage along. Flush toilets were crucial, and so too were sewer pipes of a narrow diameter, laid in steep gradients, through which the flushing water could forcefully propel wastes. The sewage should be carried out of the town, and there (Chadwick believed, following the ideas of the German chemist Justus Liebig) turned into fertilizer.

How to build such a fully articulated service? The money, expertise, and power that would be needed to override vested interests could come only from government. Such a system would require a massive construction project in every city, at great cost. It would strain the rights of private property, for what good would be a sewer system if property owners were not compelled to join it? It would confront overlapping and even competing local authorities, especially in Britain; in Birmingham three different sets of commissioners existed for drainage and four for surveying, all intensely jealous of one another. The Benthamite Chadwick therefore—in the name of public health—advocated a single local authority, acting under guidelines set by the central government's expertise. Chadwick, though an arch-anticontagionist, was hardly an antistate liberal in the conventional Manchester sense.

Chadwick's *Report* was an impassioned piece of propaganda, which appealed both to a desire for political stability and to fears of such horrors as cholera. Water and sewer engineering works could be seen as tools of social control, and while they eventually involved huge capital outlays, they also represented what Christopher Hamlin has called "arguably the greatest 'technical fix' in history," one that avoided the larger questions of poverty.[20] In 1848, the British Parliament approved a Public Health Act that re-created the Central Board of Health that had fallen into desuetude after the waning of the 1832 scare; more than that, the 1848 act empowered local boards of health to enforce drainage, build sewers, compel the servicing of cesspools, pave and clean streets, deal with nuisances, inspect lodging houses and burial grounds, control the water supply, and raise local taxes to pay for it all. Chadwick's vision had passed into legislation. Some cities showed earlier interest in such Chadwickian activity than others, but in the second half of the century cities both in Britain and elsewhere gradually took up the sanitation cause. The sewer and water systems of Paris and London ranked with the greatest engineering projects of a century that elevated engineers into a cultural pantheon. In London, sewer construction began after yet another cholera outbreak in 1853–54 provided a spur; main sewer lines there were completed in the 1860s, but the entire system took decades. The municipalization of water supplies similarly stretched over the years.

Chadwick's emphasis on water-and-sewer systems stemmed from a conviction in the miasmatic origin of disease, a doctrine couched in general terms for much of the eighteenth and early nineteenth centuries, concerned with the environment in toto, with particular attention to the "atmosphere" as the cause of trouble. The filth of streets and in rivers was feared because such conditions affected the surrounding air. Attacks on filth undertaken by health boards aimed at the improvement of atmospheric quality; water or ordure might be targets not in their own right but as contributors to a totality of environmental pollution. Thus the British authorities argued in 1849 that polluted streams gave rise to atmospheric corruption. In the course of the 1850s, however, some thinkers became convinced that water in and by itself might be the carrier of disease. In 1854 John Snow, a London physician, carried out what may be seen in retrospect as a classic epidemiological investigation. He studied two adjoining districts of London, very similar in their social and economic compositions, one of which suffered a far higher incidence of cholera than the other. The districts were served by different water supplies. Cholera, Snow argued, was therefore a waterborne disease.

Although Snow made some converts to his view in subsequent years, many observers still fit his findings into the framework of a more general environmentalism. The different water supplies affected the immediate atmospheres of the two adjoining areas differently. The miasma theory, that is, could argue that even closely adjacent neighborhoods might not share the same airs and vapors. But Snow's arguments became part of a slowly developing focus on water itself. In the 1850s the condition of the Thames, London's river, became an important political issue for reasons that had more to do with national image than with a view of water as the specific bearer of disease. British politicians, arguing that the filth of the Thames reflected poorly on pride of an imperial people, determined on an at least semicollectivist body of regulation to clean up the river.[21]

Chadwick's advocacy of a complete water and sewer system should be seen in that perspective: a general environmentalism, in which some greater emphasis was being accorded to water, for a mixture of aesthetic and practical reasons. In subsequent years Chadwick's campaigns made headway partly because of that confluence of general environmental beliefs with concern about water. Another cholera visitation in 1866 stimulated more argument. Snow and his allies, notably William Farr and Edward Frankland, pressed their view that polluted water produced cholera. But questions remained unanswered, particularly about the actual mechanism of pollution carried by the river. Where was the cholera "poison" to be found? If the water carried a poison, why did it not affect everyone who drank it?

One of the first European cities to build an "articulated service" was Hamburg, and that city's experience introduces us to the evolution of thought about cholera in the years when general miasma gradually gave way to emphasis on water. After a disastrous fire swept through Hamburg in 1842 a British engineer named William Lindley, a Chadwick disciple, carried the gospel of sanitation and anti-contagionism to the city fathers. Prodded by Lindley, the German port constructed a water-and-sewer system according to Chadwick's principles.[22] Hamburg became a shining beacon to the sanitationists. Yet in subsequent decades European perceptions of disease in general and cholera in particular underwent changes as evidence appeared for contagion mechanisms. Hamburg suffered a catastrophic cholera epidemic in 1892, and that disaster illustrated both the uncertain state of etiological theory and the continuing importance of political factors in responses to diseases.

By the 1850s sanitationism dominated approaches to public health. Three different champions had come forward to build on Chadwick: John Simon, Florence Nightingale, and Max von Pettenkofer. To Chadwick, disease arose from a corruption of the air, in turn generated by the exhalations of filthy waters, sewers, ground, and organic matter; thus disease should be attacked by the systematic cleansing of the (especially urban) environment. Relatively little emphasis fell on personal hygiene, and Chadwick's anticontagionist views discouraged such state measures as quarantine and isolation of individuals. John Simon (1816–1904), an able surgeon and pathologist, was most responsible for carrying out Chadwick's program in Britain, initially as the first "Medical Officer of Health" for London (in 1848) and then as chief medical advisor (with several different bureaucratic titles) to the central government between 1855 and 1876. Although his etiological views gradually shifted away from Chadwick's dogmatic anticontagionism, Simon took the lead in chevying the complex world of British local government along, propagandizing the cause of sanitation, offering central government loans to local governments for sanitation projects, and sending expert central government inspectors into the provinces. For Simon, as for Chadwick, what was at stake was not state action, but what sort of state action; neither was a laissez-faire liberal, although anticontagionism was central to their beliefs.[23]

Florence Nightingale (1820–1910) achieved a legendary position in world public opinion in the 1850s as a result of her activities in the Crimean War (1854–1856), when she reorganized the military nursing services. From that time forward she was revered, especially in the English-speaking world, as the Lady with the Lamp. If secular nineteenth-century society had saints, she headed the list. Nightingale's role in the professionalization of nursing will be discussed in Chapter Ten. Here I note her role as an important sanitary reformer. Shortly after her return from the Crimea, Nightingale fell ill, and believing herself at death's door, she lived as an invalid for fifty-three years. Possessed by a sense of urgency, she commissioned, cajoled, and commanded studies of public health conditions, studies undertaken by her followers and coordinated by her.

If anything her belief in the miasmatic origin of disease exceeded Chadwick's, as she applied her energy and intelligence to sanitizing first British army quarters and then the Indian subcontinent.

Max von Pettenkofer (1818–1901), a Munich medical scientist, hygienist, and nutritionist, introduced a complex and sophisticated explanation of cholera's cause in the 1850s and 1860s. Cholera, he concluded, shared both contagious and miasmatic aspects. A contagious ("x") factor might come from human excreta, but particular soils and ground waters (factor "y") had to act on that contagious matter before cholera resulted, and for Pettenkofer the soils and ground water were the crucial elements. Pettenkofer became the most influential sanitarian of his generation, especially in Germany. Rather like Villermé and unlike the English sanitarians, he placed more emphasis on personal hygiene and less on the intervention of the state's regulatory apparatus. He urged individual effort and education, in the best nineteenth-century liberal tradition.

Whether sanitarians demanded bureaucratic expertise (as did Chadwick) or looked to individual efforts to expunge filth (Pettenkofer) or poverty (Villermé), one message dominated: a clean society would be a healthy society. "Cleanliness is next to Godliness," a sentiment ascribed to both Francis Bacon and John Wesley, became a nineteenth-century cliché, especially for the middle classes of Western society. Personal and community cleanliness became a symbol of civilization, and their absence represented barbarism. Of course, as Richard Evans has pointed out, the middle and upper classes possessed certain advantages: it was far easier to stay clean in larger houses with servants and perhaps fewer children than in small, crowded, servantless quarters.[24] The gospel of cleanliness might therefore be seen as part of a self-justifying class ethic, but its strength in mid-nineteenth-century opinion about disease was nonetheless real.

Sanitationism in the 1860s was clearly allied with science. It had elevated a new class of technical experts to a position of authority: statisticians, meteorologists, engineers, and chemists such as Liebig (enticed to a professorial chair in Munich by Pettenkofer). Even if the understanding of disease was not yet clearly in the hands of physicians, it had apparently been taken from the hands of theologians once and for all. As Charles Rosenberg has noticed, American thinkers in 1832 saw cholera as either a punishment from God or a consequence of the neglect of God's natural laws. By the epidemic of 1866 God had nearly disappeared from American thinking about cause, and the New York Board of Health—created in response to that cholera visitation—had sweeping Chadwickian powers to clean the city.[25] Perhaps because the Civil War had accustomed Americans to heavy state intervention, public authority assumed more power. Did that happen in part because the miasma doctrine wound up placing more responsibility for disease on society as a whole? If disease was a product of individual moral failure, then society bore no responsibility. Villermé's conclusion—that poverty was the problem— placed a great potential burden of responsibility on society, but he shrank from its implications and urged individual efforts to escape poverty. A doctrine of dirt and miasma could place blame on dirty individuals or groups, thus preserving the liberal ideal of individual initiative and responsibility; but it opened the door to social action as well, for an entire community might be affected by the irresponsibility of those who fouled the ground and water that all must use.

Cholera and "Germs"

By the 1860s another scientific view of the cause of cholera (and of disease in general) had reappeared: the "germ" theory. We should not assume that this theory was self-evidently true in those years, and it did not assume a position of dominance for some decades. Could a tiny microorganism produce such drastic effects as the symptoms of cholera? It seemed improbable, and that difficulty of relating huge effect to trivial cause was only one of a number of arguments raised against the theory (see Chapter Ten). But if microorganisms *did* cause disease, then an explanation of contagion might be at hand. The germs simply traveled from one person to another. Could the transmission be shown? In 1876 Robert Koch traced the life history of the organism responsible for anthrax, a disease of cattle and sheep; Koch cultivated the organism in his laboratory and with it transmitted anthrax to previously healthy animals. By 1882 Koch had isolated and traced his first human disease microorganism, that of tuberculosis, and in 1884 he announced that the causative agent of cholera had been found. Yet still the argument left miasmists unconvinced.

The case of Hamburg illustrates the difficulties facing the germ theory.[26] Hamburg's city government retained considerable local autonomy within the federated German Empire, a legacy of its long history as a free city. All through the nineteenth century Hamburg's government was among the most liberal in Germany, as a merchant oligarchy held political sway. Contagion theories found little support in Hamburg; health boards, with their quarantines and isolations that interfered with trade, had only advisory powers there. Hamburg did not require smallpox vaccinations until after a serious smallpox epidemic in 1871, long after compulsory vaccinations had been adopted in many other states, including liberal Great Britain. Hamburg spokesmen consistently downplayed the menace of cholera. The ideas of Pettenkofer, with their emphasis on individual responsibility and personal hygiene, found particular favor there.

When Koch and his followers announced the discovery of the cholera microorganism in 1884 the germ theory gained many followers, especially in Germany, where national pride in Koch's achievements might have been a factor. Koch was a strong proponent of state action: quarantine, state-directed disinfection, careful policing of the water supply, isolation hospitals. Richard Evans argues that Koch's ideas fit into a growing tendency for state intervention in the society and the economy, especially in Germany in the 1880s, the decade of rising tariffs, campaigns against socialism, and the beginnings of the German Empire's welfare-state legislation. An active state public health machinery might also give the imperial government a justification for overriding the local powers of governments such as Hamburg's.

By the same token Koch's ideas constituted a political threat to state governments, and Hamburg feared the centralizing power of Berlin, dominated as it was by statist Prussians. In the 1880s and early 1890s doubts still existed about the role of Koch's germs in causing cholera, and Hamburg's elite seized on those doubts. Koch—and before him his teacher Jacob Henle—had laid down what became the ruling postulates of bacteriology. The "Koch postulates" said: (1) that the organism should occur in every case of the disease, (2) that the organism should occur fortuitously in no other disease, and (3) that after being isolated from the ill person and grown in laboratory cultures, the organism could induce disease in another subject. For obvious reasons Koch and his followers had not applied the third postulate to their cholera organism. Another weakness existed as well. One of the great triumphs of the germ theory was its application to prevention by means of "vaccination," or the development of attenuated doses of causative bacteria that would, when administered, confer on their recipients immunity from the full-blown disease. Such vaccines had been produced by Louis Pasteur for a number of animal diseases, but Koch's attempts at an effective vaccine for his first human disease germ, tuberculosis, repeatedly failed. Was the germ theory flawed? Hamburg's political and medical establishment had some reason to distrust Koch's cholera solutions.

Hamburg, as we have seen, possessed a proud water-and-sewer system. Unfortunately its water did not pass through a sand-filtration process, so that if sewage, carrying a deadly bacterial load, washed upstream to the source of the water supply, the town could be infected. That happened in 1892. Those circumstances weakened the apparently straightforward case for John Snow's view of cholera as a waterborne infection, and gave Pettenkofer's picture of disease appearing after water fermented the soil some credibility. The mere provision of an "articulated service" provided no guarantees, especially if the sewers emptied into the same river from which the water supply was drawn.

But what was to be done? Koch was certain: kill the microorganisms in the water and stop their transmission from those already suffering from the disease. Hamburg officials were not persuaded, since stopping transmission meant quarantine, isolation, and disinfection. When cholera broke out in Hamburg in August 1892, almost certainly brought to the city by emigrants in transit from the Russian Empire to North America, a fatal period of hesitation ensued; the city fathers, fearing an adverse effect on commerce, hesitated to pronounce an epidemic, and the bacteriological tests that Koch advocated to confirm the presence of the disease proved difficult to perform. Koch, with the pressure of the imperial government in Berlin behind him, eventually arrived on the scene and compelled the adoption of his remedies as the epidemic worsened. The 1892 epidemic provided a convincing demonstration of the germ theory, for areas of Germany that followed strict quarantine and isolation procedures escaped Hamburg's fate. Those areas included the adjacent city of Altona, in Prussian territory.

On the heels of the Hamburg epidemic the German Reichstag debated a comprehensive Epidemics Bill that would confer on the imperial government the powers that Koch had assumed, de facto, in Hamburg. The debates on the bill occasioned continuing argument between Koch's supporters and the miasmists, led by the now-venerable Pettenkofer. When his arguments were rejected by a committee discussing the bill, Pettenkofer performed the most radical medical experiment of the nineteenth century: he obtained a culture of cholera bacilli from Koch's laboratory and swallowed it. Severe diarrhea resulted, but Pettenkofer survived; one of his assistants then repeated the experiment before a large group of witnesses, with the same result. The germ itself, said Pettenkofer, could not cause the fatal cholera; other factors—soil, water—must interact with it. But these bizarre experiments did not contain a swelling contagionist, germ theory tide; by the end of the century medical opinion was overwhelmingly contagionist, miasmists were on the professional margins, and the germ theory had had many triumphs.

Paradoxically the German Epidemics Bill did not pass until 1900; the Reichstag lost interest when the shock of the Hamburg cholera epidemic wore off, and the bill only passed in response to fear of bubonic plague, which had revived in Asia in the 1890s. The plague organism had been identified by Yersin and Kitasato in 1894, and although its path of infection was not positively traced for some years, in 1898 Simond suggested the involvement of rats and fleas in a chain of contagion. Cleansing and disinfection might therefore interrupt this terrible scourge. With that spur the bill passed and the German government assumed new powers. Medical officers could compel quarantines that sealed borders, order disinfection of private property, and forcibly isolate individuals in hospitals. The simple provision of a water-and-sewer system—the contribution of the engineers—no longer seemed adequate. The bacteriologist, the new expert, must analyze the water the engineer provided and the sewage he washed away, as the state undertook to monitor waters and wastes.

The German Epidemics Law of 1900 may serve as the terminus of the convoluted tale of cholera and the sanitation movement. A cholera scare contributed to the bill's formulation, but not to its final passage. Its provisions, and the arguments that surrounded it, encapsulated the overlapping etiological theories of the nineteenth century, for while contagionism lay behind the powers it conferred on the state, those powers recognized that contagion passed through the environment and not just through immediate person-to-person contact. When the Epidemics Law passed, furthermore, the waterborne infections that attracted epidemiological attention were rapidly ceasing to carry their former menace. The campaigns for pure water and safe sewage disposal had their effect; in many cities by the 1870s, 1880s, and 1890s, typhoid fever, dysentery, and cholera were becoming rare. The belated enlistment of bacteriology perfected the engineers' campaign, but the germ theory played a complementary role, not a primary one.

Cholera provided dramatic episodes of disease in the nineteenth century. The shock of cholera, and indeed of other diseases, at times added urgency to the demands of the sanitationists, but many other factors aided them as well: city fathers' reluctance to spend money on improvements might be overridden by civic pride, the gospel of cleanliness acquired an evangelical zeal that had little to do with disease or etiological theories, and the power and prestige of scientific professionals and experts increased over the century, regardless of the theory they advocated. The prestige of engineers and chemists aided anticontagionism in mid-century; by the end of the century the lab-coated bacteriologist symbolized science.

The triumphs of sanitation (and germ theory) may conceal from us the failures of the nineteenth century. The causes of infant mortality had hardly been addressed at all, and it remained very high in 1900. Although some nineteenth-century thinkers had associated disease with poverty, a culture of poverty still existed in almost all countries in the West. Urban overcrowding, inadequate nutrition and hygiene, and a general lack of community preventive care all meant that influenza and a variety of "fevers" still ran rampant. Tuberculosis waned in some areas (for reasons to be discussed in the next chapter), but the major medical attacks on its causes lay in the future. Compulsory school attendance, becoming more common, created new opportunities for such diseases as polio and diphtheria. Attempts to compel notification of illness to authorities had only begun: in Great Britain in 1889, in Germany in 1900, for example. Governments remained loath to admit the presence of some diseases in their territories. In 1911 the Italian government launched a remarkable (and remarkably successful) campaign to deny that the cholera epidemic ravaging Naples existed at all.[27] Air pollution and the pollution of waterways were virtually untouched. Although some were beginning to recognize industrially related diseases, the regulation of hazardous materials in manufacturing processes remained very spotty.

But while an imposing list of failures certainly existed, the nineteenth century also marked the age when Western thinkers became convinced that any scourge, even one as terrible as cholera, could be met and defeated. That important conviction would inspire assaults on a broad spectrum of diseases in the twentieth century. As long as those assaults proceeded under the banner of "science," they might win general assent. Questions of poverty and social attitudes loomed over the remedies for other diseases, however. Tuberculosis, the true plague of the nineteenth century, slackened not when—or because—a causative microorganism was found, but as a result of changes in social conditions and beliefs.

Eight

Tuberculosis and Poverty

In the nineteenth century more people in the Western world died of tuberculosis than of any other epidemic disease. The "White Plague" generated enormous fears, for good reason. Yet for all its importance, and all the attention lavished on it, tuberculosis presented a tangled picture to nineteenth-century thinkers, who could not agree on its causes. Of great antiquity, tuberculosis appeared in different symptomatic guises, inspiring a great variety of etiological theories and an even greater variety of therapies, while different social and political beliefs became associated with those theories and treatments.

Twentieth-century microbiologists gained a firmer grip on the causes of tuberculosis, which (we now believe) has a number of manifestations and may be caused by two different organisms: *Mycobacterium tuberculosis* or *Mycobacterium bovis*. The first of these (although it may infect other animals as well as humans) passes from person to person, most often via the respiratory system. The second infects most domestic animals and reaches humans when they consume the products of such diseased creatures. The bacteria lodge in many possible places in the human frame. *Mycobacterium bovis* often finds its way into glands and joints, and one group of symptoms that results is called scrofula, the medieval "King's Evil" (see Chapter Two). Although *Mycobacterium tuberculosis* may also infect different parts of the body, when it settles into the lungs it may produce pulmonary tuberculosis, known earlier as "consumption" or "phthisis." Many people infected with *M. tuberculosis* do not develop "consumption" at all, however, and many others only show consumptive symptoms after a long period of infection. A large number of others do develop such symptoms, and it was that pulmonary form of the disease—"consumption" or "phthisis"—which attracted particular nineteenth-century attention. But for all that apparent simplicity and certainty, the history of tuberculosis remains unusually complex even in the context of past epidemics. The rhythm of its past severity has not yet been convincingly explained, so that even with a surer grasp of its "cause," we cannot be certain why it savaged the early nineteenth century and abated in the late nineteenth and early twentieth.

Early History

Tuberculosis in humans has an ancient history, revealed by paleopathology. The Hippocratic writings of the ancient Greeks discuss consumption at length. Some evidence—scanty to be sure—suggests that its ancient and medieval incidence varied more or less directly with population density. Thus classical Roman civilization, relatively urban, may have suffered high rates of tuberculosis, while the medieval West, rural and thinly settled especially in its early centuries, offered fewer opportunities for contagious respiratory infections. The resurgence of tuberculosis in the West, accompanying the urban growth of the twelfth and thirteenth centuries, may have affected the incidence of that other great mycobacterial killer, leprosy (see Chapter Two). Certainly by the early modern period of European history tuberculosis had resumed a place among the major epidemics, and in that period (coinciding with the scientific revolution) a diverse collection of explanations of phthisis arose.

Those explanations rested, first of all, on an understanding of the sensible symptoms of the disease: shortness of breath, coughing, blood-flecked phlegm, progressive weakness and debility, and loss of skin color, all of which only became characteristic of the disease in its later stages. The persistence of such complaints in the same family encouraged notions about the hereditary character of consumption, notions that had found expression as early as Hippocrates and that the chronic nature of the disease perhaps strengthened. The prolonged presence of a victim of a chronic disease may burn images into the memories of onlookers, and these may be recalled when others in the same family recapitulate the symptoms. But not all early modern theorists accepted the hereditarian explanation. Others, attracted to the general notion of contagion that gained credence in the sixteenth and seventeenth centuries (see Chapter Three), applied that to consumption as well as to plague. The consumptive, like the leprous the victim of a chronic complaint, posed a long-standing threat by her simple existence; that sense of danger, perhaps intuitively felt by neighbors, was given theoretical justification by the doctrine of contagion. Both these hypotheses—heredity and contagion—remained popular into and through the nineteenth century and affected responses to the tubercular.

With the improvement of anatomical knowledge between 1500 and 1700 came an awareness of consumption's pathological signs, especially the lesions or "tubercles" formed in the lungs. That knowledge led to other etiological ideas, especially those that saw such lesions as the product of some form of irritation, perhaps caused by physical agents such as improper food or ingested matter, perhaps the product of muscular (or even nervous) exhaustion. Such beliefs led in turn to therapeutic suggestions: change diet, change environment, rest, avoid stress. Whether tubercular lesions represented one disease or a panoply of them formed part of the larger pattern of nosological uncertainty discussed in Chapter Six.

Tuberculosis and Romanticism

These general etiological views—heredity, contagion, and irritation of tissue whether physical or psychological—informed Western responses to tuberculosis in the age of "romanticism," when the disease seemed to threaten the well-born and the gifted. Between the late eighteenth century and the mid-nineteenth, a variety of cultural circumstances led literate observers to associate pulmonary tuberculosis with the upper and middle reaches of society, and the disease acquired an air of fashion. In reality, of course, most of its victims belonged to the lower orders, but its associations with misery and poverty only became more widely acknowledged later in the nineteenth century.

Romanticism remains an elusive historical construct, but I will assume here that it may represent a net of cultural practices and beliefs that had particular importance between the late eighteenth and mid-nineteenth centuries. Those practices and beliefs included an emphasis on emotions, mystery, and spontaneity as opposed to the Enlightenment's practice of reason, an interest in the remote (whether in time or space), and a glorification of the beauties of nature; politically, "romantics" could be either radically revolutionary (glorying in bold breaks with tradition and in the virtues of the common man) or very conservative (viewing aspects of especially the medieval past with favor). Such tendencies, perhaps "endemic" (in Lilian Furst's words) at all times in some thinkers and artists, became "epidemic" for many between roughly 1775 and 1850.[1] Some of those tendencies (certainly not all) related to the themes of health, disease, and death. Romantics, H. G. Schenk argues, suffered a "malady of soul," a *Weltschmerz*, as a consequence of religious frustration; for them the "bonds of allegiance and belief" to and in religion had been weakened by rationalism, leaving a nihilistic preoccupation with the "dark side of life," a fascination with sleep, death, "utter extinction." Schenk holds that this weariness of life was deepened— though not primarily caused—by the physical suffering and early death that came to many of the leaders of romanticism.[2]

Tubercular experience may also have reinforced a more specific "romantic" view of disease and its causes. As Hermione de Almeida puts it, "rivalling theories of disease and its treatment could and did flourish [see Chapter Six], and the Romantic fascination with the 'energizing' ambiguity of illness found ample domain."[3] Romantic thinkers, de Almeida argues, believed disease to be always present, part of a continuum of energy that included life itself. An inexorable chronic condition such as consumption confirmed such a belief, especially for a poet as well informed as John Keats, who had studied medicine, observed consumption in his family, and then suffered (and died) from it himself.

Certainly a remarkable collection of cultural figures, many of them "romantics," succumbed in relative youth between 1775 and 1850 (see Table 8.1). Little wonder that death was a favorite romantic theme, especially the death of the young, or that romantic writers and artists focused on tombs, sorrowful weeping willows, and the heart-wrenching ruins of decayed monasteries. Autumn, as René and Jean Dubos noted in their classic study of tuberculosis, came to rival spring as the poet's favorite season: the autumn of melancholy and falling leaves, not autumn the season of jolly harvest.[4]

Some of the lives of those in that formidable list (Table 8.1) became paradigms of romantic tubercular suffering: Novalis, Keats, Chopin, and the Brontë sisters. Consumption's victims slowly and chronically declined, gradually wasting away, becoming fragile and pale. Seeking relief they traveled to warmer climes or undertook sea voyages. Such travels often took them to the Mediterranean, where notions of the contagiousness of disease in general and tuberculosis in particular remained more influential than they did in northern Europe. The tubercular travelers thus met hostility that added to the pathos of their stories: Keats, feared by his Italian landlady; Nicolò Paganini (1782–1840), the violin virtuoso, thrown out of a house in Naples; Chopin shunned on Majorca; François René de Chateaubriand, the French author, unable to sell his carriage in Rome because he had allowed a consumptive to ride in it. Consumptive northern European artists who stayed home may have thus contravened medical advice, but their compatriots, apparently less terrified of contagious disease, may have spared them such ostracism. The composer Carl Maria von Weber, in the last stages of consumption, was lionized by concertgoers in London and literally embraced by his musical admirers, one of whom lent a shoulder to help Weber to his carriage.[5]

Such experiences contributed to a romantic view of the effects of tuberculosis. A wasted pallor acquired a fashionable beauty; whitening powders replaced rouge; the Pre-Raphaelite artists of England, in the mid-nineteenth century, exaggerated the thinness and paleness of their female subjects.[6] Keats saw love and consumption as closely related products of similar causes; his "La belle dame sans merci," de Almeida maintains, serves as an "emblem of the destructive aspect of love, of frustrated creative endeavor, and of death by consumption," at one and the same time.[7] Romantic, pathetic literary sufferers abounded: *David Copperfield's* Dora, *Dombey and Son's* Little Paul, *La Dame aux Camélias's* Marguerite Gauthier, *Scènes de la Vie de Bohème's* Mimi. The last two entered the operatic repertoire in Verdi's *La Traviata* and Puccini's *La Bohème*. Perhaps

_____ Table 8.1 _____

Deaths at an Early Age, 1776–1849

*Ludwig Christoph Hölty, German poet	1748–1776
*Johannes Ewald, Danish poet	1744–1781
Wolfgang Mozart, Austrian composer	1756–1791
*Joseph Michael Kraus, German-Swedish composer	1756–1792
*Karl Philipp Moritz, German author	1757–1793
*Novalis (Friedrich von Hardenberg), German poet	1772–1801
*Philipp Otto Runge, German painter	1777–1810
*Cecilia Tychsen, bride of Ernst Schulze	1794–1812
*Ernst Schulze, German poet	1789–1817
*Karl Solger, German philosopher	1780–1819
*Friedrich Gotlob Wetzel, German author	1779–1819
*John Keats, English poet	1796–1821
*Percy Bysshe Shelley, English poet	1792–1822
Erik Johan Stagnelius, Swedish poet	1793–1823
J.L.A.T. Géricault, French painter	1791–1824
George Gordon, Lord Byron, English poet	1788–1824
*Franz Horny, German painter	1797–1824
*Carl Maria von Weber, German composer	1786–1826
Franz Schubert, Austrian composer	1797–1828
*Wilhelm Waiblinger, German poet	1804–1830
*Victor Meyer, German sculptor	1807–1831
*"Napoleon II" ("King of Rome"), son of Napoleon I	1811–1832
Vincenzo Bellini, Italian composer	1801–1835
Karel Mácha, Czech poet	1810–1836
Mariano Jose de Larra, Spanish author	1809–1837
Aleksander Pushkin, Russian poet	1799–1837
Giacomo Leopardi, Italian poet	1798–1837
Mikhail Lermontov, Russian author	1814–1841
*Nicholaus Becker, German poet	1809–1845
*Alphonsine Plessis, French actress	1824–1847
Felix Mendelssohn, German composer	1809–1847
*Emily Brontë, English author	1818–1848
Edgar Allan Poe, American author	1809–1849
*Anne Brontë, English author	1820–1849
* Frédéric Chopin, Polish composer	1809–1849
*Sándor Pëtofi, Hungarian poet	1823–1849

_____

Source: The major source for this table is Erich Ebstein, *Tuberkulose als Sckicksal* (Stuttgart: Ferdinand Enke Verlag, 1932).
*Suffered from tuberculosis

the memory of Paganini, playing as one possessed while in the throes of consumption, lent credence to the sopranos who filled an opera house with their voices despite their characters' tubercular lungs.

Tuberculosis conferred therefore a kind of beauty; men, according to René and Jean Dubos, strove for a fashionable emaciated look, a fashion to which even the corpulent Alexandre Dumas *père* aspired.[8] In addition, some in the early nineteenth-century also associated consumption with genius. Sensitive souls seemed prone to consumption. Did consumption impart a nervous force to the mind? Did it lead to a frantic urge to accomplish something great before the shadow fell? The empirical evidence for such causal connections was not very convincing, however, and here as in other respects tuberculosis defied nineteenth-century attempts to generalize about its causes or effects. As the Duboses point out, four of the six children of Thomas and Frances Trollope died of tuberculosis between the ages of twelve and twenty-three, showing no sign of literary gifts. The two other children—Thomas (1810–1892) and Anthony (1815–1882)—were prolific authors, as was their mother. The Trollope authors never manifested consumptive symptoms.[9]

The Decline of the Nineteenth-Century Epidemic

Romantic views of tuberculosis may obscure the real demographic importance of the disease, the greatest epidemic killer in the nineteenth-century West, and one that affected far more of the poor than the romantically creative. In the first half of the nineteenth century mortality rates from tuberculosis probably ranged between 300 and 500 per 100,000 population in most Western countries. When England and Wales had about eighteen million people (in 1851), over 50,000 people died there of tuberculosis annually, compared with the 40,000 cholera victims in the worst single cholera year, 1849. Cholera epidemics appeared as spikes on a graph, but those spikes rarely (if ever) rose above the high annual level of tuberculosis deaths.

In the second half of the nineteenth century the mortality of tuberculosis began declining in most of western Europe and North America. This decline occurred in different places at different times and rates. The industrial pioneers, England and Belgium, whose mortality rates had risen above 300 (per 100,000), were the first countries whose rates then fell below that appalling figure: Belgium in the mid-1860s, England about 1870. (Some places—bucolic Ireland and Switzerland, thinly settled Australia and New Zealand—may never have been that high.) Between about 1890 and World War I rates fell below 200, again chiefly in the most advanced industrial states: Italy in 1891, Belgium in 1892, England in 1894, the Netherlands and the United States in 1901, Denmark in 1902, Germany in 1906, Scotland in 1909, Switzerland in 1914. In 1921 the mortality rate from tuberculosis dropped below 100 in the United States and Denmark; the Netherlands followed in 1925, Belgium, England, and Germany in 1926, Scotland in 1928, Italy in 1933, Switzerland in 1935.[10]

Exceptions to the pattern existed, however. In Ireland the tuberculosis mortality rate did not peak until the late 1890s, declined only slowly until about 1908, and then—while it fell more rapidly—remained above 100 until after World

War II. Norway's experience mirrored Ireland's, although its mortality fell below 100 by 1937. In east-central Europe—Austria, Hungary, Czechoslovakia—tuberculosis mortality remained very high (and perhaps even peaked) in the first decade of the twentieth century, fell below 300 by 1914, surged upward again in World War I, and then dropped rapidly after the war. But like Ireland they all remained over 100 until after World War II. In France, something of an anomaly in western Europe, rates remained well over 200 during World War I and fell below that number only in 1920.

The decline in the tubercular death rate, accomplished before the dramatic reductions that followed antibiotic treatments after World War II, poses some of the thorniest problems in the disease's history. Those problems are ultimately those of explanation: did deliberate human measures contribute in some way to loosening the hold of tuberculosis? If so, how decisive were those interventions? Or were all such human responses overshadowed by more general changes in the social and economic condition of the poor? Or did tuberculosis decline for reasons entirely exogenous to any human actions, whether deliberate or inadvertent?

Because etiological views about tuberculosis remained in conflict for much of the nineteenth century, disagreement persisted about what possible measures could have a beneficial effect. As the century went on (and the disease's mortality started to fall) many thinkers came to view consumption more clearly as a social problem, or as the product of social problems, and to tie it less clearly to romantic sensibilities. Associations of tuberculosis and romantic suffering did not disappear; the consumptive images of Thérèse de Lisieux (in real life) and Sarah Bernhardt (on the stage) remained a part of late nineteenth- and early twentieth-century French conceptions of tuberculosis.[11] The romantic view of the creative, artistic tubercular sufferer persisted outside France as well; Puccini's *La Bohème* was, after all, first performed in 1896. But that opera may also illustrate the point that more often slums, not literary salons, yielded the prototypical consumptive. Mimi may have a beautiful voice, and the characters may live in a creative Latin Quarter, but they are also poor and cannot afford medical treatment. Tuberculosis might accordingly confer shame, not cachet. The new perspective almost certainly reflected a more accurate demographic understanding than the old, for tuberculosis had always been a disease that ravaged the poor. But with it came a further burden of stigma, which associated poverty and tuberculosis in a symbiotic relationship of individual failure.

Nineteenth-century etiological arguments about tuberculosis, centering on either contagion or heredity, remained uncertain in part because neither explanation seemed entirely satisfactory. Too many members of "consumptive" families remained free of disease; descent from a tubercular parent did not inevitably lead to consumption, and sharing a house with one apparently did not either.

Those circumstances led—naturally enough—to an emphasis on "predisposing" causes that might explain why the basic cause (be it heredity or contagion) could overcome the resistance of some and not others.

It might be well at this point to consider modern explanations of tuberculosis. The causative "germ," whether *M. tuberculosis* or *M. bovis*, lodges in the human body. Immunological reactions shortly begin, and a walled-off "tubercle" results that contains the bacillus and prevents its further spread through the body. The person so infected may now be said to "have" tuberculosis, if by that word is meant a positive reaction to a tuberculin test; but in many cases no clinical symptoms ever develop, so that if the tuberculin test were not administered no assumption of tuberculosis would ever be made. In some individuals, however— and here the etiological puzzles arise—the body's immune systems fail to contain the spread of the bacillus, and different clinical manifestations of tuberculosis result, sometimes rapidly, more often much more gradually.

Some people apparently enjoy more resistance to tuberculosis than others. Their resistance is not to the initial infection, for bacilli make their way into the body (through either respiration or ingestion) without much interference. Resistance rather arises when the body's immunological defenses respond to the invasion. Many possible variables have been suggested to explain different powers of resistance. In the nineteenth century "predisposing" causes included diet, stress, dirt, general bad habits, and—for those who denied the primacy of one or the other—heredity and contagious contact. In some form modern discussions still debate some of those causes as possible explanations of varying tuberculosis mortality and morbidity.

Pulmonary tuberculosis undoubtedly found favorable conditions for spread in the nineteenth century, in both Europe and North America, if only because of the rapid increase of population and its dramatic urbanization. Cities grew explosively; more than that, they experienced remarkable congestion, especially in the earlier decades of urban growth, before the cities began their expansion into the suburban hinterland. Dwellings crowded together; within dwellings lived more people per room. Urban and industrial life also meant more crowded workplaces, whether in the factory or in the office. The spread of compulsory schooling, and its extension to older age groups of children, promoted congestion in another setting as well. The sooty and sometimes noxious air that characterized the early industrial city, especially in those economies fired by coal, may have increased confined life and discouraged ventilation; who would willingly open a window to the grime and the smells? All these circumstances increased the likelihood of respiratory infection.

And it remains possible that many nineteenth-century city dwellers also lacked defenses once respiratory infections took hold. Diets, especially of the urban poor, were high in fats and carbohydrates (yet perhaps low in calories), low in vitamins and proteins. Sugar (in various forms) supplied a disproportionate and growing share of working-class calories.[12] Alcohol consumption was high; British per capita consumption of spirits was 1.11 gallons per year in 1831, five times the comparable 1931 figure, while 21.6 gallons of beer were consumed per capita, also much higher than the 1931 amount.[13] Those figures, impressive as they are, probably understate actual consumption, for they take no account of extralegal production. French consumption of alcohol, largely wine, may have been even more formidable than British. Men got a larger portion of food and drink (for better or for worse) than did women, who were especially likely to be denied adequate protein and vitamins. As long as urbanization and industrialization meant a decline in nutrition—if in fact they did—populations may have been less able to resist the spread of *M. tuberculosis* within individual human frames.

Stress may have added to dietary weakness. Some modern historians—following some commentators of the period—have drawn vivid pictures of the disorientation resulting from moves from village to city, and from agricultural (or craft) labor to factory work at the pace of a tireless water mill or steam engine.[14] Until the migrants to the cities evolved their own culture, with its network of friends, relatives, and customary social supports, stress may have been very severe. "Stress" is of course hard to evaluate, especially in the past. The surge in tuberculosis mortalities that accompanied both World War I and World War II might have been due to "stress," but it more likely was produced by the crowding together of people—troops, internees, prisoners, factory workers—and resultant heightened chances of contagion that those conflicts afforded.

To assert that the early decades of industrial urbanization were marked by poor diets, high levels of stress, and a general decline in standards of living, especially for working people, steps into a historiographic minefield of considerable power and antiquity. One authority warns that "Any search for a single answer to the question of what happened to the standard of living [in Great Britain] between 1700 and 1850 is unrealistic," and scholars have increasingly focused their attention on particular components of "standards of living."[15] On the one hand, some evidence suggests that British wages in the late eighteenth and early nineteenth centuries may have risen faster than pessimistic estimates assumed, which if true might reduce the period of industrially related vulnerability to tuberculosis.[16] But the fact that the average heights of British birth cohorts declined between 1820 and 1850 suggests that environmental pressure and perhaps nutrition were unfavorable for health. As Roderick Floud and Bernard Harris put it, "any wage increases that did occur were bought at a high price in terms of health and mortality."[17] And many of the "optimistic" wage studies lean on national aggregates, which (as Maxine Berg and Pat Hudson note about similarly based population estimates) may "conflate opposing tendencies in different regions, sectors of industry and social groups."[18] Studies of human heights

reinforce that point: urban people were consistently shorter than their rural counterparts, and people of lower socioeconomic status were shorter than those further up the scale. A later example may illustrate the dramatic contrasts in
tuberculosis rates that could be found in different sections of the same city. In
1926 the tuberculosis mortality rate in the affluent eighth arrondissement of Paris
was 75, while in the poor thirteenth arrondissement it was 306.[19] Clearly poverty
and class mattered, and clearly their significance might be masked by national
aggregates.

The phenomena first seen in Britain played themselves out later in other countries. British cities grew most rapidly in the first half of the nineteenth century.
French cities—Lyons, Marseilles, Paris—showed their highest rates of growth
between 1850 and 1880; and in the following decades (1880–1910) the cities of
Germany, Austria-Hungary, Russia, Italy, and Scandinavia grew most rapidly
(see Table 8.2). The chronology of industrialization was similar. In France the
period from 1850 to 1875 may have been analogous to 1800–1840 in Britain;
Germany may have followed France by a decade, Italy's surge occurred at the
end of the century, and Russia's had hardly begun by the outset of World War I.
Urban overcrowding and the pains of intensive industrial take-off, therefore,
spread their way across Europe, outward from Great Britain and generally from
the northwest to the east and south.

Nineteenth-century thinkers also considered "race" another possible predisposing cause, in effect an extension of belief in the power of heredity as an
explanatory principle. Were some social groups, whether of blood or of class,
more prone to consumption? Were the Irish more likely victims simply because
they were Irish? In fact some groups may have been more at risk, and the circumstances of early industrialization and urbanization—apart from the environment—may have made them so. The body's ability to resist tuberculosis, to
contain the invading bacilli in a tubercle, may in part depend on inheritance;
repeated exposure leads to increased powers of resistance and inheritable immunity. Especially in the early decades of industrialization, large migration from
rural areas fueled city population growth. The newcomers moved from areas of
low density and congestion, where tuberculosis bacilli were rarer, to a much
more disease-laden environment. For at least a few generations the immigrants
formed a virgin population for the tuberculosis organisms. Hence the suspicion
that the rural Irish were especially susceptible might have had a basis for a time;
and indeed, the incidence of tuberculosis morbidity and mortality continued to
rise in Ireland down into the early twentieth century, long after it started to
decline in areas that became urban earlier.

Racial explanations of tuberculosis received a particularly strong hearing in
the United States, where the considerable differential between tuberculosis rates
for whites and blacks lent credence to such theories. In 1910, when the national

_____ Table 8.2 _____
Percentage Rates of Urban Growth, 1800–1910

City	1800–1850	1850–1880	1880–1910
Great Britain			
Birmingham	230	72	31
Edinburgh	134	52	36
Glasgow	348	70	34
Liverpool	359	47	35
London	140	78	52
Manchester	304	13	109
France			
Lyons	61	112	26
Marseilles	76	85	53
Paris	93	116	27
Germany and Austria			
Berlin	144	168	85
Breslau	90	140	88
Cologne	94	50	256
Dresden	62	128	148
Hamburg	2	120	221
Leipzig	110	137	295
Munich	175	109	159
Vienna	80	64	180
Russia and Poland			
Moscow	46	68	142
St. Petersburg	121	81	117
Warsaw	0	152	240
Italy			
Genoa	20	50	51
Milan	42	33	86
Naples	28	10	46
Rome	14	71	80
Turin	73	88	69
Scandinavia			
Copenhagen	26	85	97
Stockholm	22	82	102

Source: Complied from figures in Carlo M. Cipolla, ed., *The Fontana Economic History of Europe*, vol. 4, *The Emergence of Industrial Societies* (London: Collins, 1973), 750.

tuberculosis mortality rate was 160, American blacks suffered 446 tuberculosis deaths per 100,000; and while the 1940 figure for African Americans had fallen to 128, the overall rate had then reached 46.[20] At the beginning of the twentieth century, when most African Americans still lived in the largely rural South,

American medical opinion about their health was dominated by the views of southern physicians, who led the development of theories of "inherited susceptibility," part of a more general view that Africans were destined to be losers in the struggles of natural selection. Only slowly, in the early decades of the twentieth century, did environmental explanations of the high tuberculosis rates among African Americans make headway against such "genotypical" beliefs.

Congestion, poverty (and the resultant overcrowding and poor nutrition), and migration of vulnerable rural populations to cities all combined to spur nineteenth-century increases in tuberculosis incidence. But social and economic change eventually had ameliorating influences as well. The Victorians came to place great emphasis on the virtues of fresh air and ventilation, in part because of general beliefs in the miasmatic origins of some diseases, in part because of dislike of industrialization itself and a desire (especially strong in Great Britain) to restore the purer and simpler life of a preindustrial past. The conviction that ventilation in general benefited health led to assaults on such early urban housing evils as "back-to-back" construction and cellar dwellings. Gradually cities adopted building codes, undertook slum eradication, and began providing municipally funded housing for the poor. Nowhere was the task of slum clearance complete, or quickly or easily done; the barriers erected by vested interests, demographic pressure, and persistent poverty and unemployment were difficult to overcome.

But it is possible that by the early twentieth century even the urban poor lived in less congested and better ventilated quarters than they had earlier. In the more advanced industrial societies at least, city populations were becoming more suburban, and less dense, by the end of the nineteenth century. The proportion of greater London's population that could be called "suburban" rose from 13 percent in 1861 to 25 percent in 1891; in Paris, while the population of the city proper increased 50 percent between 1861 and 1896, the remainder of the city's *département* grew 203 percent.[21] And as industrial economies matured, many— though certainly not all—of the working class graduated into more highly skilled trades to service the increasingly sophisticated industrial plant. For these upwardly mobile workers better wages might translate into better housing; some statistics suggest that between 1875 and 1910 the proportion of the population of German cities living in one-room dwellings gradually fell, while the proportion enjoying two rooms gradually rose.[22]

Improvements in diet also gradually occurred, a point repeatedly emphasized by Thomas McKeown in his numerous writings. McKeown, concerned with explaining the rapid growth of the European population in the nineteenth and early twentieth centuries, believes improvements in nutrition played the key role in the reduction of mortality from epidemic disease in general and from tuberculosis in particular. The decreasing severity of epidemics in turn accounts for population growth, which McKeown attributes to declining death rates, not increasing birth rates.[23] Some factors certainly lend support to McKeown's argument. Total calories available per capita may have increased in Europe over the nineteenth century, thanks in part to the spread of potato cultivation and in part to the opening of rich grain lands elsewhere, especially in North America. Transoceanic imports of cheap grains, especially in the years after 1870, forced many European farmers to abandon cereals and turn to fruits, and that circumstance (accompanied by the development of preservation businesses such as canneries) meant greater variety in diets. Some evidence also suggests that by the end of the century some Europeans (especially in Great Britain) consumed more meat and fish than they had earlier, perhaps because of improvements in transportation and preservation. And as Richard Steckel and Roderick Floud notice, early stages of industrialization did not necessarily result in periods of declining stature. In countries that industrialized later in the nineteenth century, the environmental stresses reflected in British (and American) statures might be counterbalanced by such nutritional gains, and by real improvements in sanitation and public health.[24]

Better nutrition benefited only some, of course; Walter Minchinton, who also argues a case for general improvements in diet through the nineteenth century, quickly adds that "throughout these years the very poor were badly fed," while alcohol consumption remained high and sugar use continued to increase.[25] And although urbanization and transportation improvements may have promoted greater dietary variety, the removal of populations from immediate access to the fresh food supplies of farms had some adverse consequences: the greater the time consumed by transportation of foods, the greater the loss in nutrient values. Real questions remain about the degree to which diets improved for the mass of nineteenth-century Europeans, and those questions may have particular force in the relations between nutrition and tuberculosis mortality. Direct connections do not link tuberculosis and dietary deficiencies, as they do for instance with scurvy; diet may be only one of a number of variables that explain an individual's resistance to the effects of the tubercle bacillus.

All arguments about the role of improved social and economic conditions obviously depend heavily on the actual timing of improvements in standards of living, especially for the urban populations. Dating dietary and housing changes for sufficient numbers of city dwellers may be difficult. F. B. Smith, who dismisses the active roles of medicine in the reduction of tuberculosis, emphasizes another point: that in Britain the disease declined meaningfully when the birth rate of the mass of the population began falling.[26] Only then could the working classes better their standards of living (specifically their housing and nutrition) and thus more strongly resist the inroads of tuberculosis. Birth rates in different European states peaked at different periods in the nineteenth century, but in most cases (with the exception of Russia and perhaps some of the Hapsburg lands) those rates were declining by the century's end. In Germany the birth rate peaked at 39 births per thousand population per year in the 1870s, and by the period 1911–1913 it had fallen to 28. England and Wales also peaked in the 1870s, at 35.5, and by 1911–1913 the rate there had fallen to 24.2. Italy went from 37.5 in the 1880s to 32 in 1911–1913; Sweden's peak, 34.5, had been as early as the 1820s, and by 1911–1913 had declined to 23.5. The birth rate in France declined steadily throughout the century; over 30 at the beginning of the century, it had fallen to 19.5 just before World War I.[27] Ultimately, then, the incidence of tuberculosis may have varied directly with the birth rate. But the consistently low French birth rate and high tuberculosis mortality show the insufficiency of birth-rate explanations.

These "standards of living" arguments concentrate on exogenous factors, certainly nonmedical ones, to explain the declining mortality and morbidity from tuberculosis that began in the nineteenth century. The exogenous point of view may also include the argument that tuberculosis rates may follow a cycle of their own, undisturbed by any human action, medical or social. A relatively virgin population suddenly exposed—whether by migration of people or microorganisms—will suffer high rates through several generations. But inherited immunity builds up in the survivors, while (in the best natural selection manner) the particularly susceptible die, perhaps without offspring. In the increasingly more resistant population the morbidity and mortality rates fall, and that may have occurred in urban Western civilization between roughly 1860 and 1940.

Active Social and Medical Responses

Did conscious human action (medical or otherwise) contribute to falling tuberculosis mortality rates? Perhaps. In the years between 1850 and World War II the menace of tuberculosis certainly spurred vigorous and changing responses, some of them (even such a skeptic as Smith agrees) ultimately important in altering the balance between people and the White Plague.

The sanitation movement of the nineteenth century, discussed in the previous chapter, did not take particular aim at tuberculosis. But many of its emphases coincided with the uncertain and complex etiological ideas that attempted to explain consumption. Sanitarians held that a variety of environmental factors, probably working in combination, produced disease. Tuberculosis was attributed to a variety of causes: bad air, bad habits, heredity. The sanitation movement made attempts to control such possible tubercular agents as industrial and civic pollution. Soot and smells discouraged open windows, ventilation, and fresh air. Studies in the 1890s showed the correlation between high tuberculosis rates and some especially dusty environments such as those around grinding machines. Perhaps dirty air, especially air laden with particles, provided the irritant that provoked the tubercular lesions of the lungs. In addition, the sanitationists' emphasis on the general reformation of the manners of the lower orders might have some particular applications to consumption, and some believed that if the poor suffered from tuberculosis they had only themselves to blame. Who, after all, produced the dusty and dirty environments?

Other nineteenth-century responses grew from the belief that consumption was hereditary. As René and Jean Dubos point out, such beliefs were strengthened by the recurrence of tuberculosis in prominent families, such as that of the Brontë sisters, Ralph Waldo Emerson, and Henry David Thoreau.[28] The hereditary view gained more credence, however, because of its potential for association with class; the poor might be seen as trapped in an inescapable loop, condemned to consumptive weakness and hence poverty by the inexorable force of heredity. Such arguments also helped excuse medicine (and society in general) from responsibility for a disease that frustrated both explanation and cure. Hereditarian arguments acquired more scientific varnish in the 1860s and the 1870s, as Darwin's theory of evolution by natural selection (published in 1859) fed interest in the importance of inheritance.

These hereditarian beliefs about tuberculosis also coincided with the pressing questions of "national health" and "national deterioration" that arose in the late nineteenth and early twentieth centuries, especially in France and Britain. In the French case such fears grew out of the disastrous Franco-Prussian War (1870–71); subsequent French medical and public health efforts seemed obsessed with the presumed causes of national failure, which included tuberculosis, venereal disease, and alcoholism, and strong hereditarian arguments surrounded all three.[29] In Britain the "eugenics" movement associated with Francis Galton (1822–1911) led to ideas about selective breeding that might discourage the tubercular from conceiving children. Doctors in the 1880s advised many consumptives against marriage, while that decade also saw a rising number of abortions among tubercular women.[30] (Although eugenic arguments were thus employed, women may also have associated pregnancy with "stress," which supposedly increased one's susceptibility to tuberculosis.) The embarrassing Second Boer War of 1899–1902 gave national worry about "deterioration," expressed by such thinkers as Karl Pearson, a particular focus.

By the end of the nineteenth century, however, sanatoria had become the most widely heralded response to the problems of tuberculosis. The enthusiasm for sanatoria had a number of historic roots; several different establishments might claim to have been the first tuberculosis sanatorium. For example, in the 1790s the prominent English Quaker physician and philanthropist John Coakley Lettsom opened a facility for the victims of scrofula at Margate on the Kent coast, moved to do so by his observation that fishermen rarely contracted scrofula. In the conflicting etiological beliefs of the eighteenth century, different consumptive sufferers followed different advice about what sort of "air" would give relief; many of the romantic generations made pilgrimages to the south, especially to the Mediterranean, perhaps for its warmth, perhaps for its sea air. The pure air of the mountains became more popular by the middle of the nineteenth century; the Swiss town of Davos acquired a particular cachet for the scrofular and consumptive, especially if they could afford the trappings of an expensive resort. Herman Brehmer, credited by the Duboses with work that "marked the turning point in the treatment of tuberculosis throughout the world," opened his tuberculosis sanatorium at Görbersdorf (Silesia) in 1854.[31] Brehmer was convinced that pulmonary tuberculosis led to progressively weaker circulation, and that exercise in the fresh air of the mountains could work a cure by reversing the process. After a time he changed his mind about the virtues of exercise for his consumptive patients and instead advocated rest, but still in the pure mountain air.

The advocates of sanatoria remained ambivalent for decades about the relative merits of exercise and rest, although the advocates of rest generally won more favor. That approach certainly dominated the early sanatoria in the United States, where Edward Livingston Trudeau popularized the concept. Trudeau, a young physician, despaired of a cure when he contracted tuberculosis and moved to the Adirondack Mountains of New York, apparently to live out his years in a place he loved. The remission of his symptoms convinced him that mountain air and rest had worked a cure, and he opened the sanatorium that would become a widely copied model at Saranac Lake in 1884.

Sanatoria appealed for a variety of reasons. If stress exacerbated tuberculosis, sanatoria provided a respite from the pressures of modern life. If "bad air" caused consumption, the mountains offered "good air." In the sanatorium the diet of sufferers could be improved. Generally the sanatoria fed their patients protein-rich menus, laden with milk, eggs, and meat; at Lawrence Flick's sanatorium at White Haven, in Pennsylvania, the superintendent reported (in 1901) that "one man had 17 glass [sic] milk and 8 raw eggs yesterday and another 14 and 8," and that "all who take 15 glasses are allowed a cup of tea for supper."[32] Interest in the virtues of the sanatoria related to the profound anti-urban and anti-industrial sentiment that existed in the nineteenth century; the influence of cities, the homes of dirt, drink, disease, and depraved habits, could be overcome in the pure Alpine or Adirondack air, where protein could be supplied in heroic quantities and a vigilant staff could correct bad habits of work and life.

The doctrine of contagion lent other strengths to the sanatorium movement. Some of the pioneer advocates of sanatoria were deeply convinced of its truth, even before bacteriological arguments emerged that called the multicausal explanations of the sanitationists into question. A mechanism for tubercular contagion became clearer in the 1860s when Jean-Antoine Villemin transferred tubercles, and with them disease, from one animal to another and even from one species to another. Robert Koch (1843–1910)—who will receive more complete discussion in Chapter Ten—presented a thorough "history" of the tubercle bacillus in 1882, which seemed (at least to some) to provide a convincing path of contagion for tuberculosis. Following his "postulates," Koch removed such tubercle bacilli from a sick animal's tissues, grew a separate culture of the bacilli, and then introduced them into a healthy animal and made it sick. But contagion, despite this impressive demonstration, remained a controversial idea in the field of tuberculosis as well as that of cholera (see Chapter Seven), for it denied the many causes that sanitationism addressed.

The political implications of contagion theory seemed unpalatable, especially to the liberal temperament and ideology of the nineteenth century. Tuberculosis presented particularly serious political issues both because of its wide extent and because of its chronic character. If contagion were accepted, tuberculosis victims—many thousands of them—might have to be isolated for years, at enormous cost. Would the enlightened modern age revert to the medieval leprosaria? Who would pay for them? Leprosy provided frightening parallels as another chronic disease, believed contagious, whose victims were not just isolated but stigmatized. Could consumptives be trusted with useful work? If so, how to make the workplace safe for others? Would families lose their places in community and society, perhaps unfairly? In addition to these very old objections to contagion, other opposition arose from the contemporary social and political position of physicians, increasingly sensitive and jealous of their professional prerogatives. Would contagion policy, mandating notification and isolation, take authority out of their hands and place it with public health officers, creatures of a state bureaucracy? Would physicians be required to report cases of tuberculosis to public authorities? If so, the patient's trust in the confidentiality of her physician would shatter. The interference of public officials further implied that someone other than the physician knew what was best for an individual patient, a notion becoming increasingly offensive to physicians as their professional power and self-confidence grew. Little wonder, then, that many physicians insisted, long after Koch's supposedly conclusive demonstration in 1882, that Koch's bacilli might be only a secondary cause of a disease whose true origin lay in heredity, bad air, dirt, or irritation of the lung tissue.

These different anticontagionist arguments especially appealed to physicians and officials in France, where sanatoria did not flourish. French opinion remained strongly attached to a multicausal approach to public health, especially as it related to the supposed causes of national decline (tuberculosis, venereal disease, and alcoholism). Regarding tuberculosis as a simple product of a microorganism denied the importance of many public health measures; it also meant acceding to a "German" theory, and both Koch's bacillus and sanatoria were tarred by the same xenophobic brush.[33]

But the contagion theory made headway, and in doing so provided another raison d'être for the sanatorium: to segregate the sick from the healthy. And those who did not accept the centrality of the contagion doctrine might find still other reasons for solving the tuberculosis problem with the sanatorium. Those who took a moral view of the disease could seize the opportunity to reform the habits of the patients, which might be a desirable middle-class goal regardless of etiological theory. The virtues of exercise remained dubious, but for some sanatoria directors "graduated labor" would supposedly stimulate "inoculation of patients by their own bacterial products," as well as prevent working-class patients from becoming lazy and losing the habit of work in the restful atmosphere of the sanatorium.[34] Linda Bryder paints a dismal picture of life in British sanatoria in the early twentieth century. The sanatorium was a "total institution" not unlike a prison, in which patients lived lonely and isolated lives, rejected by the local population. Superintendents imposed strict discipline, especially regarding contact between the sexes and the consumption of alcohol, and they dismissed patients' complaints (about unpalatable food or uncomfortable quarters) as further symptoms of disease. When one patient exercised his right to leave, his sanatorium superintendent remarked, "Tell your widow to send us a postcard."[35]

In Britain the disciplinary aspect of the sanatorium had, in any case, been anticipated by another institution: the workhouse. In 1834 the British Parliament had ordered a reform of the system of public relief of the poor. From that date forward—at least in theory—those poor in need of public relief could receive it only by residence in a "workhouse," where conditions might discourage applications from all but those in genuine need of assistance. Among those in genuine need might be numbered the sick poor, and as the nineteenth century wore on workhouses under public control came to approximate public hospitals, in which a high proportion of the patients suffered from tuberculosis, a wasting, chronic disease that made work (and hence self-sufficiency) difficult.[36]

Certainly both sanatoria and workhouses, as well as the tuberculosis dispensaries that spread rapidly in Britain after about 1909, proved powerful instruments for intruding into the private lives of individuals, as did home visits and "march pasts" conducted by public health authorities and nurses. Barbara Bates, a recent student of early American sanatoria, describes the rugged regimen and spartan existence they imposed on their patients. She also notes that sanatorium directors had to keep business considerations in mind: one physician was "desirous that the summer boarders about to arrive shall not find . . . patients who have been here so many months without being cured, as it would be a discouragement to them. It is simply a matter of business and convenience."[37] Really ill patients should therefore be discharged. Did patients carry changed routines—of sobriety, fresh air, bathing—into their everyday post-sanatorium lives? Bryder thinks not; more likely they developed anger, both at the officious behavior of their keepers and at the stigma assigned them by contagionist (or hereditarian) fears. The other close student of British sanatoria, F. B. Smith, concurs.

But while habits may not have been changed by institutional discipline, facilities such as workhouses and sanatoria did isolate consumptives from the rest of the population. Leonard Wilson, strongly dissenting from McKeown's views that direct human agency had little to do with the reduction of tuberculosis mortality before World War II, argues that the isolation of poor consumptives in British workhouses was crucial. Adopting the early twentieth-century views of Arthur Newsholme, Wilson presents a case that questions McKeown's evidence and thus the conclusions of social historians such as Bryder and Smith who in effect accept McKeown's arguments about the inefficacy of conscious human response. Enough poor consumptives were isolated to make a difference, Wilson maintains, and their isolation coincides chronologically with declines in British tuberculosis mortality.[38]

Unresolved questions remain, however. Were enough British poor immured in workhouses to make enough of a difference in mortality rates? The evidence of the effectiveness of the 1834 workhouse system is very spotty indeed; the custom of "outdoor" relief, awarded to applicants outside the workhouse, did not end after 1834. Anne Digby's study of the administration of the poor law in Norfolk suggests the continuing problems. She argues that in 1870 "two-thirds of the sick poor in England and Wales were [still] treated in their homes," and that "as late as 1896 only eight Norfolk unions [out of twenty-two] had separate infirmaries or infectious wards."[39]

In addition, Wilson argues that the British workhouse position was unique, which explains why Britain led the way in declining mortality. German rates started to fall in the 1880s, following the rapid acceptance of Koch's theories by German opinion and the subsequent acceptance of the necessity of isolation. But how is the Belgian situation to be explained, since if anything the initial mortality decline there preceded that of the British?

Wilson's argument also assumes that the reduction in mortality was the result of a reduction in infections, made possible by isolating the healthy from the sick. But some evidence also suggests that even after tuberculosis mortality fell, infection rates remained high. In 1909 von Pirquet applied Koch's tuberculin test to 1,100 Viennese children, none of whom showed any clinical signs of tuberculosis; 70 percent of them tested positive anyway, so that a high proportion had at least been infected by their tenth birthday.[40] Even later, at a time and in a place where mortality had fallen more dramatically, tuberculin tests were given to overwhelmingly middle-class American college students in the middle 1930s. Results varied widely from one college to another, but of over 12,000 male students tested, about 39 percent were positive; about 33 percent of 6,600 women were positive as well.[41] Had a reduction in mortality followed a reduction in infection, as Wilson assumes? Or had it followed an increase in resistance to the bacillus?

In Britain the enthusiasm for sanatoria began to wane after about 1920, partly because their benefit was difficult to demonstrate; as Smith argues, measuring their rates of successful cure remained guesswork, largely because of the chronically elusive character of pulmonary tuberculosis. A sufferer might be released from an institution "free" of consumptive symptoms, but how long would she remain so? Could the sanatoria keep track of their former patients at all? Bates, reflecting on American evidence, raises still other doubts about the effectiveness of sanatoria. At the least, since all the sanatoria advocates and proprietors had interested motives, the data they supplied must be suspect.[42] Despite those questions, sanatoria did not so much vanish as lose their position as society's principal response to tuberculosis, except perhaps in the United States and Germany, where sanatoria had taken a particularly strong hold. In the 1920s other remedies and responses appeared, which seemed to make the sanatoria obsolete: chemical remedies, surgical procedures, a growing attack on milk-based tuberculosis and *M. bovis*, and continuing efforts to find a vaccine that would prevent the disease or even cure it.

In the nineteenth century tuberculosis attracted a wide variety of nostrums, and that often bizarre collection of remedies persisted and even extended in the early twentieth century. Some were offered by quacks, others by legitimate medical practice; of the latter, a variety of gold salts became particularly popular in the 1920s and 1930s, while vaccines remained controversial. Smith makes an interesting point: that quack remedies and treatments found special favor with women, especially with domestic servants, whose fear of dismissal (and whose working hours and poverty as well) prevented them from seeking orthodox medical advice.[43] And quack remedies may have avoided some hazardous side effects, which could not be said of "gold therapy."

Surgeons, filled with new confidence in the late nineteenth century as a result of the successful application of anesthesia and antiseptic methods (see Chapter Ten), also advanced claims to cure tuberculosis. In the 1880s the Italian surgeon Carlo Forlanini pioneered the technique of lung collapse, in which a gas (or air) was injected into the chest cavity between the lung and the chest wall, thus collapsing the lung. Believing that this procedure would allow the infected lung to rest, other surgeons gradually adopted it; by the 1920s and 1930s lung-collapse therapy was another popular and self-consciously "modern" treatment, in addition to (or instead of) gold salts. Other more dramatic surgery appeared as well, notably the removal of infected lobes of the lung, or even of the entire lung itself.

In addition to providing ammunition for the sanatorium movement, Koch's "germ" explanation of tuberculosis gave rise to vigorous campaigns against public spitting, conducted by both voluntary societies and governments. It also inspired a hope that a vaccine might be found. By laboratory manipulations of cultures of the microorganism, some dosage or concentration might be found that would immunize the subject from future infection (as did "vaccination" proper, with smallpox), or would actually counter the effects of an infection already under way (as—apparently—did Pasteur's treatment for rabies, to be discussed in Chapter Ten). By 1890 Koch's laboratory had produced such a substance for tuberculosis, called tuberculin and hailed as a great triumph of modern scientific medicine when it appeared. Koch believed that tuberculin could act as a cure for tuberculosis, at least in certain of the disease's stages. Finding which stage proved a problem, for at some points the use of tuberculin proved rapidly fatal. Although tuberculin ultimately failed as a cure, it proved diagnostically useful. Skin reactions to tuberculin demonstrated whether a person had previously been infected by the tubercle bacillus.

A preventive vaccine developed from the bacillus was clearly another goal of this heroic age of bacteriology. The most celebrated of these appeared in its initial guise in 1906, the product of two Pasteur disciples, Albert Calmette and Camille Guérin. Their vaccine, an attenuated strain of *M. bovis*, acquired the name of Bacille-Calmette-Guérin, and was generally called BCG. It had a very controversial history. For some years Calmette and Guérin experimented with the inoculation of different animals, especially cattle. In 1922 they began administering BCG to humans, and its use spread widely in France, Poland, Spain, Scandinavia, and Quebec (Canada)—mostly places where French cultural influences were strong. It met resistance in other countries, notably in Great Britain, where (as Smith and Bryder agree) physicians specializing in tuberculosis did not want their routines disturbed and so raised clouds of objections to it. Adopting the vaccine would pose administrative difficulties; the patients wouldn't like it anyway; the quality control and standardization of the vaccine were untrustworthy. Then in 1930 a disaster occurred that strengthened the opponents' case. Seventy-one of 323 babies in the German city of Lübeck died (and many others became gravely ill) after being inoculated with "BCG" (actually a heavy dose of tubercle bacilli), and a predictable outcry against the vaccine arose.[44] Despite its impressive statistical success in the countries that used BCG, its opponents continued to distrust it until the 1950s, by which time other and more dramatic weapons—antibiotics—had come into use.

Another important preventive approach developed in the early twentieth century as concern with bovine tuberculosis grew. Villemin, in the tradition of very old associations between human and animal diseases, had inoculated tuberculosis from one species to another in the 1860s. A few others followed such connections, and then in the 1890s the American Theobald Smith clearly isolated *M. bovis* and showed its differences from *M. tuberculosis*. But what degrees of immunity from, or resistance to, different bacterial species did different animals enjoy? Were humans little affected—or not affected at all—by bovine tuberculosis? Could human tuberculosis be regularly transmitted to cattle? In 1901 Koch lent his great prestige to the belief that the animal tuberculosis could not infect humans, and vice versa, but that declaration ran counter to the assumptions of existing public health advocates, who had commenced a zealous attack on infected milk and meat as part of their broad-fronted war on multicausal tuberculosis.[45] In 1911 a British Royal Commission agreed that Koch had been mistaken and that milk from tuberculous cattle posed a danger to humans who consumed it.

That belief now joined hands with practices already under way. Pasteur, back in the 1860s, had shown that microorganisms caused fermentation and the accompanying souring of milk (and of wine), and that such living agents of fermentation could be killed by heat. Would the same heat also kill *M. bovis*? The process of heating, "pasteurization," initially undertaken to prevent the souring of milk (and the conversion of wine to vinegar), slowly spread as a method of cutting the transmission of bovine tuberculosis to humans.

Resistance to pasteurization of milk could be substantial, sometimes stemming from simple conservatism of habits and such important cultural issues as the "taste" of the milk, and sometimes from more directly vested interests of dairymen and even some physicians. Likewise, attempts to eliminate tubercular cattle threatened important interests, for landowners and farmers still wielded much political and economic power in most countries. Tuberculin tests revealed that (for example) between 20 and 30 percent of the cattle population of the eastern United States were infected; did eradication of bovine tuberculosis mean the slaughter of millions of beasts?[46] Agricultural interests rose up in fear (as they did again in the British bovine spongiform encephalopathy crisis in the 1990s), and taxpayers faced huge compensation claims if a government decreed such a massacre in the name of public health. Different American states individually began various measures in the 1890s, involving banning the importation of infected breeding cattle, free tuberculin testing, and some compensation to farmers who agreed to the destruction of tubercular animals; but the expense of such programs, especially in light of Koch's dismissal of the menace of bovine tuberculosis, brought many of them to a halt.

But the 1911 British report symbolized a change of views. In the United States a remarkable display of the power of the gospels of public health and scientific medicine followed, in which the acolytes of those gospels were aided by cultural assumptions about milk; "clean milk carried a freight of meanings," as Barbara Rosenkrantz puts it.[47] So inspired, a vast and largely successful federal campaign to destroy tubercular cattle began in 1917. In five years the incidence of tuberculosis in American children was one-half that in their British counterparts, although the causal connections between that fact and the cattle campaign remain murky. In Scandinavia similar success was attained not by slaughtering infected animals, but by the more labor-intensive system of isolating them from contact with others. In Britain political resistance to either the American or Scandinavian systems proved much stronger, and rates of nonpulmonary tuberculosis (such as scrofula) remained much higher there throughout the 1920s and 1930s. F. B. Smith, calling this a "massive waste of national resources," adds that the tuberculosis rate in British children would have been even higher if British milk consumption had rivaled American.[48] Perhaps for the same reason— low per capita milk consumption—bovine tuberculosis remained a less serious issue in southern Europe.

Reducing bovine tuberculosis and its spread to humans, both through pasteurizing milk and through culling of infected herds, may have accounted for some decline in tuberculosis rates, but only after about 1920, only in some places, and not in respect of pulmonary tuberculosis. Vaccines, notably BCG, likewise had no effect before the 1920s, and thereafter only locally. The sanatoria—and such other systems of isolation as the British workhouse infirmary—certainly spread earlier, but their impact on tuberculosis morbidity and mortality remains unclear, both because much of their regimen seems of dubious value and because they touched only a minority of tuberculosis victims. Sanatoria (and workhouses) did more or less effectively isolate tubercular patients, and so they reduced the chances of continued contagion. When surer techniques of diagnosis developed in the early twentieth century—first the tuberculin test and then the chest X-ray—the utility of sanatoria as isolation wards increased; but those diagnoses, and effective isolation, followed the decline in tuberculosis incidence that was already long under way.

Much of the explanation of that decline, which began in the nineteenth century, therefore necessarily relies on environmental and social changes. The regulation of workplaces, beginning first in Great Britain in the 1870s, led to the required use of masks and the provision of ventilation, particularly in such industrial dust environments as stone-cutting, brass-working, and abrasives-making. More important, housing improved after the horror-filled first generation of industrial cities; homes became more spacious and sanitary, even if only marginally so. Gillian Cronje has suggested that such improvements in housing may account for the more rapid decline in tuberculosis incidence among women that characterized Britain after about 1860.[49] It may be more difficult to make a case for improved diets among the nineteenth-century working classes, but reduced birth rates certainly made several important contributions: healthier women, healthier babies, greater possibility of improving a family's standard of housing and diet alike, perhaps less stress. It is therefore likely that the decline in incidence of tuberculosis in the second half of the nineteenth century was chiefly caused by increasing individual powers of resistance, for which several environmental and social factors must receive credit.

Those individual powers of resistance may have been further strengthened by heredity, as exposure stimulated antibody activity in successive generations. And as the number of clinical cases began to decline, so too did the number of contagious agents in the population; by the twentieth century the proportion of the population infected (whether "clinically" or not) also began to fall, meaning a further decline in clinically observed cases. When to the deliberate medical ameliorations of the 1920s and 1930s were added the remarkable effects of antibiotics (especially that of streptomycin) in the years after World War II, tuberculosis retreated even further.

That apparent conquest of tuberculosis will receive more discussion in Chapter Eleven. But I should here note that the rhythms of rising and falling tuberculosis incidence continue. Persistent poverty and urban overcrowding combine with rapid international and intercontinental migration to bring little-exposed populations into new and dense urban contact. For example, the incidence of tuberculosis rose again in the United States between 1985 and 1993, and while that increase has subsequently been reversed, tuberculosis (including new strains resistant to antibiotics) now makes its way in populations across the world whose inherited powers of resistance may have atrophied or whose entire immune systems may have been compromised.

Nine

Disease, Medicine, and Western Imperialism

By the end of the nineteenth century Europeans had achieved an unprecedented mastery of the rest of the globe. This mastery included a remarkable expansion of the area settled by Europeans, the extension of European trade and transportation routes to all corners of the earth, and the imposition of European control (of different sorts) on almost all land areas not actually settled by Europeans and their descendants. All of those aspects of European domination had important consequences for the history of disease, its diffusion, and its effects on different world communities, including their ability to resist the continuing spread of Western power and influence. Although in some respects that European dominance had begun in the sixteenth century, its most dramatic manifestations occurred in the nineteenth, and so this chapter largely concerns the "long nineteenth" century between the French Revolution (1789) and World War I (1914).

In the course of that century the world's population literally became more European. The percentages may seem insignificant, but they reveal an interesting shift in the world's balance of population power. In 1800 Europe contained about 21 percent of the world's people; by 1900 the proportion had risen to about 25 percent. In raw numbers Europeans had more than doubled in those hundred years, growing from about 187 million to about 400 million. Much of that increase occurred in the second half of the century, for in 1850 the Europeans still numbered only 266 million.[1] This remarkable surge of population was even more dramatic than those numbers suggest, for while Europe's population grew it also sent forth millions of others; during the nineteenth century perhaps thirty-five million Europeans left their native continent to settle permanently elsewhere, the great majority of them leaving after about 1840. This swarming of Europeans

created large areas of the world in which Europeans and their descendants constituted a substantial or even overwhelming majority of the populations, as was
true of the United States, Canada, Argentina, Australia, New Zealand, and
Uruguay. Substantial European communities settled elsewhere as well, sometimes (as in South Africa) maintaining themselves segregated from other inhabitants, at other times (as in Brazil and elsewhere in South and Central America)
intermingling with peoples both American and African. For European domination of the world did not simply mean the migration of Europeans; it also meant
the massive transplantation of other peoples, in some cases forcibly, in others
voluntarily, from one continent to another in response to European-directed
demands for productive labor. The most obvious example was, of course, the
monstrous traffic in slaves from Africa (largely its west coast) to the Americas,
which began in the sixteenth century and continued into the nineteenth. But as a
combination of conscience and self-interest drove Europeans (and their
American descendants) to abandon that nefarious trade in the nineteenth century, other significant movements of people occurred, often motivated by
European demands for labor. Thus the modern states of Fiji, Guyana, Mauritius,
South Africa, Surinam, and Trinidad have large populations of South Asian
descent. And within both Africa and Asia large internal migrations also
responded to European labor demands.

These movements were accomplished with much greater speed and ease by
the end of the nineteenth century than at any previous time, and for that facility
of movement the steam engine was largely responsible. Steam railways revolutionized land travel with both their speed and their reliability. Much of their early
construction was in Europe and North America, which in 1840 had over 98 percent of the world's mileage; nearly 80 percent was in Britain and the United
States.[2] And while much railway building occurred in other continents later in
the century, the effects of the railway remained greatest in Europe and areas
(Australia, Canada, Argentina, the United States) dominated by European immigrants. In those places the railway spread settlement, sped the exploitation of
natural resources, and moved food supplies in a way that leveled the ancient
regional imbalances (and resulting local famines) that had characterized earlier
Western (and every other) history. Effects on nutrition and hence on health were
complex. Movement of food to different areas became easier, and so both quantity and variety of foodstuffs can only have improved (at least in theory). But
while large populations in cities may now have been supported by adequate calories, they might also receive inadequately preserved goods that had either lost
some of their food value or become infected by harmful molds in the course of
storage and transport. Outside areas of European settlement, railways may have
had less impact on the disease pattern, although in India extensive railway
construction did contribute to unifying that subcontinent's biological systems.

In Africa and much of the rest of Asia and South America, railways affected disease more by contributing to larger social and economic dislocations.

The steamship may have had more immediate importance for moving diseases, their vectors, and their victims to virgin territory. Until the 1860s the sailing ship held its own, but after that decade the weight of a combination of new technologies made the steamship economically superior. The iron hull, such as that of the pioneering *Great Britain* (1843), allowed ships to surpass the structural limits on size that wood construction imposed, and it also permitted the design of ships whose lengths (in proportion to their beams) were far greater. Greater speed resulted, especially with the application of the screw propeller (the *Great Britain* again) and the compound steam engine. For example, steamships so equipped traveled from England to Mauritius in 1865 without refueling.[3] Multiple propellers, triple (or even quadruple) expansion steam engines, and steel hulls, all in use by century's end, added to the steamship's advantages. A sailing ship's voyage across the Atlantic might vary considerably; in the middle of the nineteenth century an average sailing packet might make the crossing eastbound in three weeks, with the westbound voyage slower. The first steamship crossings in 1838 were accomplished (westbound) in eighteen and fifteen days, and by 1879 the crossing had fallen to seven days.[4] In the sixteenth century the movement of smallpox across the Atlantic by sailing ship may have depended on a tragic combination of difficult to predict circumstances, but the late nineteenth-century steamship made the transfer of plague from the coast of China to much of the rest of the world a dramatic certainty.

Europeans increasingly exercised both political and economic control over the world in which they had revolutionized transportation. The extent of Western political control in other continents, imposing in 1850, had become breathtaking by 1900, when nearly the entire land area of the globe was claimed and controlled by Europeans or their American descendants; only Ethiopia, Liberia, Turkey, Persia, China, Japan, and Siam maintained independence, and in some of those cases the claim was more titular than actual. European flags flew over most of Africa, South, Southeast, and Central Asia, and all of Oceania. European economic domination was perhaps even more impressive, extending as it did into the reaches of even the nominally independent states; Bernard Porter observes with some justice that politically independent Argentina was "as much a British 'colony' as Canada," and was "Britain's perfect satellite economy: a willing servant who did not need to be enslaved."[5] The Western world was the source of the overwhelming bulk of foreign investment in the nineteenth century; at the outbreak of World War I Britain, France, and Germany alone accounted for 76.7 percent of the world's foreign investments (a number that would fall to 50 percent by 1938). In 1850 92.5 percent of the world's registered shipping (admittedly incomplete figures) carried either European or American flags, and in 1913 that percentage was still 90.5. This shipping symbolized a domination of world trade in general: 78 percent of such trade in 1840 was in European hands, 80 percent in 1880, and still 69 percent in 1913.[6]

European travel and settlement, the reshaping of non-Western societies by European political and economic influence, and the revolutionary impact of Western transport on international and transoceanic intercourse all had numerous and important consequences for the world's disease history. By the end of the nineteenth century most Westerners regarded their impact on world disease complacently or even proudly. Where Western trade and conquest went, so also went Western science and medicine. Especially after the power of the germ theory asserted itself in the last two decades of the nineteenth century, Westerners were convinced that they could master the diseases of the world, at least for their own benefit (enabling them to settle or reside where they chose), and perhaps for the natives' preservation as well. Western medicine, and its power over disease, became a justification for the expansion of Western imperial power and an illustration of the superiority of Western culture. Subsequent medical history agreed, focusing on the triumphs of Western biomedicine and sanitation over "tropical diseases" such as malaria, yellow fever, and cholera.

More recent scholarship has argued that the relations between Western expansion and the world's disease history were far more complex than that suggested by a simple model of enlightenment extending into darkness. Some writers have seen the power of Western medicine as a "tool of empire" (in Daniel Headrick's phrase), which made possible penetration and settlement in areas previously closed to Europeans by disease barriers and enabled European employers to keep native work forces healthy. Thus Philip Curtin has shown that European troops, for whom assignment to the tropics was earlier a sentence of death, benefited from a "revolution in tropical medicine and hygiene."[7] A more subtle version of the "tools of empire" argument focuses on the ways in which medicine became part of the West's assertion of cultural supremacy, an assertion sometimes accepted by non-Western peoples as well. David Arnold summarizes such points: disease enabled Western colonial powers to contrast their science with the "fatalism, superstition and barbarity of indigenous responses"; western "tropical medicine" became a specialty that studied primitive environments, and disease proved the social and moral inferiority of non-Westerners.[8] Western medical power could convince the indigenes of their own inferiority; thus Western medical ideas displaced the traditional practices of healing in Tunisia.[9]

Another view of Western biomedicine simply rejects any notion of "triumph" altogether, arguing instead that Western expansion and domination in the nineteenth century meant new opportunities for the spread of disease; far from a triumph, Western imperialism was a disaster in disease history. Certainly the expansion of Europeans brought them into more frequent contact with diseases that they had previously rarely met, and faster transportation made the transmission of those diseases back to Europe and North America more certain. Diseases could travel both ways in the nineteenth century as well as in the sixteenth, so that Europeans brought their diseases to other parts of the world too. And perhaps more important, when Westerners made the world their common ground they facilitated the movement of disease in many ways. Western conquest, colonization, and development might impose changes on physical infrastructure that not only facilitated the movement of disease but created new (and perhaps more favorable) environments for disease vectors. Conquest itself often meant military occupation, which brought both venereal disease and the conquerers' concern with the health of their troops. Conquest and economic development or exploitation resulted in the movement of people to new locations where they met new microorganisms, were subjected to the disease stresses of an urban area, or found their resistance weakened by difficult working conditions.

In some ways Western colonial powers responded vigorously to diseases in their overseas territories, but their motives for doing so were mixed and the vigor of their responses varied widely. They certainly desired to protect Western troops and administrators from the ravages of disease; they hoped to maintain the health and thus the productivity of the native work force; they wished to deflect international criticism from the more sordid aspects of empire. Many Westerners held deep humanitarian convictions, which they joined with a faith in the efficacy of Western science and medicine to improve lives. But in other ways, scientific medicine provided a vehicle for thorough social and political control of fractious colonies. And the sense persisted that Western lives mattered more than those of the subject peoples; if wars on disease threatened to cost too much, the health of the "natives" might be ignored.

In fact both the "triumph" and the "disaster" schools overstate their cases. At least until World War I biomedicine and sanitation had only inconsistent success against yellow fever, malaria, plague, and cholera. By the late twentieth century some of the subsequent successes began to seem temporary, as Chapter Eleven will show. Certainly Western influence changed disease environments, often for the worse, but sometimes for the better. And just as the effects of Western biomedicine on disease fell short of some enthusiastic claims, so too did the use of medicine as a "tool of empire." Western assertions of medical superiority bolstered many egos and helped shape "constructions" of non-Western societies, but those non-Western societies and indigenous healing systems were sometimes more resilient than they appeared. Lack of resources, or internal conflicts and contradictions in goals, sometimes frustrated Western intentions to reform a colonial disease environment.

Europeans Bend the Disease Environment

The improved means of European travel soon proved their power as facilitators of disease. And just as it did in the fourteenth century, plague afforded a dramatic example of a disease in motion along human trade routes. As its fourteenth-century march had proceeded slowly across land and then jumped by sea from the Crimea to Sicily, so the nineteenth-century pandemic crept across Asia and then—carried by steamship—spread over the world in a few years.

After its waning in Europe in the late seventeenth century, plague had remained or became endemic in several portions of Asia, including (by the late eighteenth century at the latest) the Chinese province of Yunnan, which underwent considerable urbanization in the early nineteenth century.[10] The great Muslim rebellion that began in 1855 resulted in nearly two decades of internal turmoil in Yunnan, in which plague epidemics coincided with military massacres, famine, and considerable emigration. Although troop movements and emigration may have spread plague to other areas of China, trade routes were decisive in the more rapid diffusion of the disease. Opium and tin moved from Yunnan to coastal points only very slowly, but plague spread along those routes in the years between the rebellion and the 1880s; the disease reached Beihai, on the Gulf of Tonkin coast, by 1867. Then in the late 1880s the steamship intervened, replacing the slow junks that had moved goods along the Chinese coast. Towns near Guangzhou (Canton) were infected in 1892, and in 1894 plague broke out in both Guangzhou and neighboring Hong Kong. In Canton about 40,000 people died of plague in four months of 1894, while an unofficial observer estimated 12,000 deaths in Hong Kong by 1895.[11] From those international ports the disease spread rapidly both along the Chinese coast and to other places, especially savaging India, where six million people died of plague between 1896 and 1908. Plague reached Madagascar in 1898, and a reservoir of infected rodents quickly became established there; that island nation has had plague deaths annually since.

By 1899 plague had spread to such distant points as Honolulu, San Francisco, Egypt, and Paraguay, with steamships the efficient conveyers of the microorganism and its vectors. In Honolulu plague especially affected the Chinese quarter, a large part of which was destroyed when the burning of infected houses got out of control.[12] In San Francisco plague arrived on the same ship that had earlier brought it to Honolulu; although that ship arrived in June 1899 (with plague aboard), no further cases appeared in the city until September 1900, suggesting that plague had first moved from the infected ship to the city's rodent population. Plague's appearance among the city's people precipitated "one of the most scandalous events in the history of U.S. public health." When the Board of Health ordered a sanitary cordon around the city's Chinatown, business interests and some newspapers denounced the very idea that plague could be in the city; the governor of California, Henry Gage, called it a "scare" and proposed that "it be made a felony to broadcast the presence of plague."[13] A major political struggle ensued, with the Board of Health and city government, most doctors, and the university medical schools lined up against the governor, most merchants and newspapers, rail and shipping interests, and the Chinese population, all of whom denied the presence of plague. In 1901 a federal commission was appointed to override the state government and force a disinfection of the Chinese parts of the city. (Californian capacity for denial persisted. When plague broke out in the Mexican district of Los Angeles in 1924 the city's newspapers called the disease "malignant pneumonia.")[14]

Among the places that plague reached (in 1899) was Japan, whose nineteenth-century history well illustrates the power of Western pressure and steam transportation. Japan seemed relatively free of a number of diseases down to the middle of the nineteenth century. Although it was not entirely isolated from trade with other Asian countries in the Tokugawa period, as an island state it enjoyed a natural *cordon sanitaire*, and its governors tightly controlled the few ports of entry. No evidence of plague in Japan has been found before 1899; Ann Bowman Jannetta points out that Japan, unlike mainland Asia, was not on the caravan routes that had been the traditional means of diffusing plague. But when "a commodity trade . . . linked infected Chinese ports with Japanese ports, we have clear evidence of plague in Japan."[15] Japanese isolation had also kept typhus out and cholera at bay. Jannetta finds no evidence of typhus before the 1890s, and indeed the Japanese language had no word for it. Cholera did reach Japan in 1822, as part of its first spread from India, but when that outbreak died out Japanese quarantines held the fearsome visitor away in the years of the 1830s and 1840s when it so impressed the Western world. The collapse of Japanese isolation, in the face of American and other Western pressure in the 1850s, opened the way for a serious cholera epidemic in 1861–62.

The islands of Oceania experienced the clearest episodes of "virgin soil" diseases in the nineteenth century. Early European contacts brought a panoply of new viral diseases: influenza to Tahiti in 1772 and Fiji in 1791, smallpox to Guam as early as 1688. Tuberculosis followed Europeans to Fiji by 1791, dysentery to Tahiti in 1792, syphilis to Tahiti in 1769 and to Hawaii in 1779. But more frequent contacts in the nineteenth century combined with significant movements of laboring populations to intensify disease diffusion. In the 1860s Polynesian laborers returned home from work in Peruvian mines, bringing a new wave of smallpox with them. Chinese and Melanesian laborers carried leprosy to Hawaii in the 1830s, to New Zealand in the 1850s, and to New Guinea in 1875. In the same year a serious measles epidemic devastated Fiji, and measles spread to Vanuatu and the Solomon Islands as well. Still another pattern of migrant labor brought disease to Fiji in 1879, when Indian laborers carried a fresh smallpox epidemic as well as cholera. The Caroline Islands were struck by influenza, smallpox, and whooping cough; the Marshalls by influenza, syphilis, and dysentery, some of it brought by Chinese laborers; measles, influenza, and whooping cough all reached the Cook Islands.[16]

In addition to transporting infected humans and their microorganisms, steamships could also be efficient carriers of disease vectors. Thus a serious malaria epidemic struck Mauritius in 1866, after *Anopheles* mosquitoes arrived there by ship; similarly *Anopheles gambiae*, not native to Brazil, made its way there by sea, reaching the city of Natal in 1930.[17]

Nineteenth-century transportation also brought together different subpopulations within a single country, and changed the biological environment as it did so. The previously isolated island populations of the Philippines began converging in cities and traveling from island to island, and separate disease environments broke down there. The network of railways built by British capital in India greatly magnified the problems associated with the subcontinent's already formidable traffic in pilgrims. Cholera, smallpox, tuberculosis, malaria, dysentery, and diarrhea followed them around, and pilgrim traffic may also have contributed to the rapid and catastrophic diffusion of plague in the years after 1896.

Western penetration also meant ecological changes. Plantation agriculture could have immediate effects on a disease environment. For example, in Egypt the demand for raw cotton encouraged the country's westernizing ruler Muhammed Ali to introduce "perennial irrigation" north of Cairo, and later British influence and investment finished that job by cleaning irrigation canals and building the Aswan Dam. The result was a nearly ideal environment for bilharzia, a parasitic disease carried by snails.[18] As British and Afrikaner settlers pressed toward the Limpopo river valley in South Africa, their firearms reduced the game population, reducing in turn the *Anopheles* mosquitoes and tsetse flies that had made the valley a center of malaria and trypanosomiasis (sleeping sickness).[19] Other ecological changes showed the complex interrelation of human and animal diseases; when rinderpest found its way into the Philippine cattle population in the late 1880s, the decline in cattle led mosquitoes to turn to secondary hosts—humans—and an increase in malaria followed.[20] Political change too could have ecological and hence disease consequences. Belgian rule in Congo redrew territorial boundaries and with them traditional agricultural arrangements that had limited the contact of humans and the tsetse fly. When the traditional patterns of cultivation broke down the incidence of African trypanosomiasis rose.[21]

But the most complicated and far-reaching effects of Western imperialism on disease environments stemmed from the social and economic changes that accompanied Western control. In the wake of Western domination came enlarged urban populations, difficult working conditions, increased population mobility, and many of the stresses of modernization. At the same time existing social structures and values were systematically discounted or dismantled, and with them much of the traditional routines of healing.

Urbanization created new foci of disease in many parts of the Western imperial world. In Southern Rhodesia (Zimbabwe), cities, mining compounds, and mission schools all became important centers of influenza, and the movement of labor to "pass offices" (where identities were checked) was a mechanism for influenza's transmission.[22] In Indochina the growth of urban areas under French rule was accompanied by spreading Western viral diseases and tuberculosis.[23] In South Africa, where Westernization was relatively complete, a full complement of Western urban health problems combined with the massive social disruption of "conquest." The great mineral discoveries in that country—diamonds in the late 1860s and gold in the 1880s—led to dramatic concentrations of people, heavy labor at great hazard in mines, and impoverishment of much of the countryside as labor was pulled off the land. The resultant poverty opened the door for epidemics that continued into the twentieth century. The health problems of a mining culture spread far over the globe: the terrible working conditions of the phosphate mines of Nauru led to beriberi, influenza, typhus, and dysentery, and the riches of the mines led to the eventual high per capita income of independent Nauru and the problems of obesity and hypertension that accompany it.[24]

Social and economic change led of course to migrations as well, some of which I have already noted. In Congo labor-intensive exploitation of ivory and rubber took men out of primary food production as well as uprooting people from their homelands, although Maryinez Lyons discounts the importance of the latter factor in the region's disease history.[25] The growing demand for sugar in Zululand encouraged the migration of Indian labor to that South African territory, and this in turn fueled a malaria epidemic in the 1920s. All through East and Central Africa in the late nineteenth century the movement of people working as porters and bearers for the conquering European armies disrupted local health systems and spread new diseases.[26]

Simple "modernization" often had unforeseen disease consequences. The construction of dams for irrigation and electric power in Africa created conditions for the spread of schistosomiasis, while the extension of cash crops into the Tanzanian economy made demands on female labor that in turn increased perinatal mortality.[27] In India irrigation and road building created ideal environments for *Anopheles* mosquitoes and hence for malaria. In the Philippines the conversion of land to cash crops forced the population to rely on imported—and milled—rice from Indochina and Siam, rice lacking the vitamin-bearing husks that guarded its consumers from beriberi.[28]

Intellectual and cultural pressures accompanied these tremendous effects on the environment. Western medicine contradicted, and/or rode roughshod over, other healing systems. The spread of smallpox vaccination illustrates that phe-nomenon. Such vaccination met widespread resistance, often on grounds similar to those found in European societies themselves. Many Indians believed that smallpox was caused by goddesses, and so religious remedies were needed; local practices of variolation offered another alternative to vaccination. Sub-Saharan Africa likewise had traditional variolation methods that opposed colonial vaccina-tion. And in French North Africa (especially in the years before 1860) vaccina-tion was seen by Muslims as a "threat to cultural integrity" and as a scarification with ritual (and alien) significance.[29] In some cases vaccination simply made very slow progress, owing not only to such cultural conflict but also to internal weaknesses in colonial administration.

Western rule also meant attempts at establishing a sanitary regime whose fea-tures might conflict with a myriad of other beliefs, both Western and non-Western. Attacks on rats might be resisted by Hindus in India, despite the conviction growing after 1900 that the animals played an important role in plague transmission. North Africans perceived French sanitationism as saying that all the Arab world was dirty and inferior, and they widely resented and resisted it. The American acquisition of the Philippines in 1898 preceded a public health "campaign" for which military metaphors seem if anything understated. And everywhere the march of Westernization and modernization put inevitable indi-rect pressure on traditional healing modes. Urbanization might—as it did in Africa and Oceania—take males in particular out of the reach of traditional vil-lage healers as the migration of labor to mines and distant plantations proceeded. Miners in Rhodesia found themselves transplanted away from the protection (or revenge) of their territorial gods.

Western ideas themselves did not always wholeheartedly support either sani-tationism or biomedicine in the colonies. No doubt the enormous pilgrim traffic of India posed serious threats for public health, and no doubt the railway sped and magnified that traffic. But should that traffic be controlled? The idea of a bureaucracy to control traffic conflicted with some of the most deeply held beliefs of the British rulers; a thalassocracy benefited from facilitating the movement of people, not hindering it. Health policy may have been a tool of empire, but it was often underfinanced; colonial regimes were often loath to spend money.

Illustrative Examples

Western "imperialism" is a slippery topic for generalizations, and so too are its consequences for disease. Many different variables came into play: topography, climate, the disease environment before Western domination, the length of time between first contacts with the West and domination by it, and (most diverse of all) the nature of the West's social and economic impact. The four examples that follow illustrate different themes and hence suggest something of the complexity that must attend any answer to the question: how did Western imperialism affect the rest of the world's disease history?

Fiji

The Fiji Islands afford a clear example of the workings of a well-documented "virgin soil" epidemic, an onslaught of measles in 1875.[30] The first European to see the Fiji Islands, Abel Tasman, did so in 1643; William Bligh, cut adrift in a launch by the *Bounty's* mutineers in 1789, sailed through the islands and returned in 1792 to chart many of them. By that date epidemics had probably begun attacking the Fijian people. Population estimates vary widely for the period before the assumption of British rule in 1874, but early estimators talked both of declining numbers between 1800 and 1870 and of epidemics. An epidemic of 1791–92 may have been pulmonary of some sort, perhaps tuberculosis; acute dysentery struck in 1802–1803, with perhaps even more serious effects than the measles disaster of 1875; an influenza epidemic occurred in 1839.

Unclear documentation clouds the relation of these disease episodes to contacts with Western peoples. Certainly such contacts intensified as Western traders arrived to exploit first the sandalwood of Vanua Levu and then the trepang found in the surrounding waters. Christian missionaries followed closely; by about 1850 Wesleyan Methodists, the most active and successful, had established their circuits over most of the Fiji Islands. By the middle of the nineteenth century this Western presence had contributed to political and economic upheaval in the islands; intermittent wars between local chiefs punctuated the introduction of plantation agriculture by Western entrepreneurs (cotton in the 1860s, then sugar). The plantation owners began importing indentured labor, first Melanesians from Vanuatu and the Solomons, then Indians. When Great Britain assumed sovereignty over Fiji in 1874, therefore, the islands had already experienced both an intensified human contact with distant places and peoples and considerable changes in their traditional economy and society.

But Fiji had apparently not experienced measles until January 1875, when HMS *Dido* arrived at Levuka, then the capital of the principal Fijian chief, Cakobau. Cakobau himself, and his sons, were returning on the ship from a state visit to Sydney; there Cakobau had contracted a case of measles, and his sons became infected on the return voyage. An ideal situation for the diffusion of an epidemic awaited them. Despite the illness on board, no quarantine greeted the vessel. For ten days after the *Dido* arrived, Cakobau entertained subordinate chiefs, explaining the arrangements that he had made for the cession of Fijian sovereignty to Great Britain; eventually eight hundred Fijian dignitaries met Cakobau, then returned to their homes. As Andrew Cliff and Peter Haggett note, "it is hard to imagine a diffusion hierarchy more calculated to accelerate spread of the virus," and spread the virus did. It was a situation involving an "unusual number of people who have come long distances, who meet in loose concourse, who then return to all parts of Fiji where they are met in their turn by local groups." Measles, together with the political news, "spread hand-in-hand downward through the layers of the social hierarchy."[31] By the middle of February measles had spread over most of the Fiji Islands, with the peak of the epidemic wave moving from Ovalau and Bau (where the *Dido* made its first contacts) in March to the rest of the chain in April. The epidemic ended by early June 1875, except for some continuing cases in far-outlying islands.

In those few months Fijian society came to a nearly complete halt. Estimates of total deaths have ranged from 27,000 to 50,000, out of a population estimated at 135,000; Cliff and Haggett, combining that population estimate with the "official" mortality rate of 27 percent, suggest that 36,000 deaths may be a reasonable figure.[32] The magnitude of the human disaster was felt as far away as London, where Lord Carnarvon, the colonial secretary, told the House of Lords that "a very large proportion indeed of the population have perished," and mused on the fact that "diseases which have, comparatively speaking, little effect upon civilized populations produce most disastrous results in the case of Native races, and just in proportion as the race is remote and isolated so are the ravages of the disease violent."[33] As had happened in similar catastrophes elsewhere, the epidemic's scale magnified its severity, as society ceased to be able to care for the sick. An 1893 British report recalled that in 1875 "whole communities were stricken at one time, and there was no one left to gather food or carry water, to attend to the necessary wants of their fellows, or even, in many cases, to bury the dead"; the same report spoke of the "apathy and despair" of the people. To relieve their fever some Fijians lay in water, or exposed themselves while wet to cooling breezes.[34]

Subsequent measles epidemics in Fiji illustrate both the diminishing effects of a disease in what had ceased to be virgin soil and the clear importance of steam transportation in disease diffusion. The next serious measles visitation was in 1903 and resulted in about 2,000 deaths; in 1910–1914 another attack killed 344, but deaths from subsequent measles epidemics were very few, although large numbers of cases often resulted. The disease had been domesticated as a relatively mild (and largely childhood) complaint. Those most affected might have been (as in 1936–37) Polynesian migrant workers from Tonga and the Gilbert and Ellice Islands, who lacked the immunities that Fijians had developed.

Cliff and Haggett have clearly shown the impact of steam navigation on the later conveyance of measles to Fiji. Measles is a highly contagious viral infection that passes directly from person to person. Its victims are infectious for nine days after the onset of symptoms; symptoms manifest themselves after a latent period of eight to twelve days. These epidemiological facts show that the shortest chain of transmission (from the onset of one case to the onset of the next) is eight days, made possible when a victim makes contact with another when symptoms first appear and the new victim's infection appears after the minimum latent period eight days later. The longest chain of transmission is twenty-one days, accomplished when the initial victim makes contact in the last, ninth, day of his infectivity and the disease lies latent in his contact for twelve further days. The average chain of transmission, Cliff and Haggett suggest, is fourteen days.

India was a continuing source of measles for Fiji, for between the subcontinent and the islands a regular stream of migrant labor flowed in the late nineteenth century. Between 1879 and 1916 eighty-seven voyages carried 61,000 laborers from India to Fiji. Sailing ships dominated the early years of this traffic. To reach Fiji from India they sailed to the south of Australia, catching the favorable winds of the "roaring forties." The resulting voyages took an average of seventy days, at times as many as ninety, or time for five or six measles "generations" to move through the ship's company. This immigrant traffic was carefully monitored, for a surgeon accompanied each ship and noted the voyage's disease history. No sailing ship from India reached Fiji with measles; although a number left India with cases, the disease always exhausted the available susceptibles in the course of the long voyage. But steamers traveled between India and Fiji much more quickly, in part because they could steam directly through the Torres Straits to the north of Australia. An average steamer trip was thirty days, not seventy, two or at most three "generations" of measles. Steamers carried more passengers, which increased the list of potential susceptibles. And the records of ships' surgeons show that steamers, unlike sailing ships, did reach Fiji with active measles cases in the years after 1884 when the use of steamships began for such voyages. As it turned out the effect of steamship-conveyed measles from India was not great, for when the ships arrived they were quarantined (a process that began to be enforced after the 1875 epidemic), and most of the infected Indian immigrants would join a community of compatriots who had already been exposed to measles. But the power of steamships as diffusers of disease can be precisely demonstrated by the example.[35]

The Philippines

Although Fiji's 1875 experience with measles coincided with a rising level of Western power and influence, its disease environment remained relatively uncomplicated by Western impositions of social change, political control, or biomedical intervention. The experiences of the Philippines in 1899–1902 were quite different, for there outbreaks of three of the classic epidemic diseases (plague, cholera, and smallpox) accompanied a war in which the United States— a new Western ruler—was imposing its will on the Philippines. A dramatic illustration of the full panoply of an interventionist state, mobilized in the name of conquest (whether of human or microbial enemies) resulted.[36]

The Philippine Islands had a long history of contacts with the West as well as with the civilizations of mainland East Asia. Spain asserted a theoretical claim early in the sixteenth century, and by 1571 the Spaniards had founded the settlement of Manila on Luzon. From that time until the late eighteenth century Spain basically regarded the Philippines as the "mere raft for barter, silver against silk," its intermediary between the silks of China and the silver of Mexico.[37] In those years, therefore, Philippine society was relatively little affected by the Spanish presence at Manila, although its position as an entrepôt made it part of a wider disease world. But in the late eighteenth century Spain began to diversify its economic uses of the Philippines, and in the next hundred years the islands were enmeshed in a more complex system of international trade as Spanish interests developed Philippine plantation agriculture: sugar, tobacco, hemp, and indigo. Ken DeBevoise has argued that the health of Filipinos suffered, as cash crops replaced subsistence and garden agriculture and the local diet declined to rice, sugar, fish, and little else. Further, an increasing proportion of the Filipinos ceased being smallholders, becoming first tenants and then landless migrant laborers, bandits, domestic servants, or prostitutes; the gulf widened between the successful few and the unfortunate many.

By the late nineteenth century the population of the Philippines may have been particularly susceptible to the ravages of epidemic disease. In the summer of 1896 an insurrection against Spanish rule began, led by Emilio Aguinaldo. The Spanish government managed to dampen that fire, if not extinguish it, by late 1897, only to be led into a war with the United States in the spring of 1898. That "splendid little war" was brief, and the Americans wound up in possession of the Philippines as well as other pieces of Spanish imperial territory. During the war's course Aguinaldo proclaimed Philippine independence; when Spain ceded the islands to the United States in December 1898 he and his followers refused to accept the transfer of their yoke from one Western master to another. A rebellion against American rule in early 1899 continued until at least early 1901 (when Aguinaldo was first captured and then swore allegiance to the American regime) or perhaps early 1902 (when the fighting actually ceased). In the midst of this insurrection plague appeared in the Philippines, part of the epidemic that began spreading from China in 1894, and as plague waned a cholera epidemic began in March 1902. And all the while both Spanish and American rulers also wrestled with smallpox, which enjoyed a surge in the turmoil of war.

The 1902 Philippine cholera epidemic was especially severe, although it was hardly the first to reach the islands. It arrived from Hong Kong or Canton, perhaps accompanying a trade in vegetables from those Chinese ports. The resultant Philippine death toll has been estimated by Rodney Sullivan at over 200,000, although Reynaldo Ileto opts for a more conservative 109,000. Those two students agree on much else, however, especially on the vigor of the American "military" response to this epidemic, seen by Ileto as a "chapter in the Philippine-American War" and by Sullivan as part of a more general attempt to "Americanize" the Philippines.[38] Cholera stimulated American fear of Philippine "filth," and the American government determined to impose American standards of sanitation and cleanly civic behavior on the islands. In the short run quarantines and isolations were imposed, in which military authority could and did override traditional commercial objections to quarantines, traditional resentment at the burning of the houses and other property of the sick, and traditional social taboos against cremation. The gospel of sanitation was preached, sometimes with considerable condescension:

> Do not despair
> ... The only remedy that's sure
> Is, after all, the water cure;
> Don't shoot 'em,
> Loot 'em,
> Cuff and boot 'em,
> But lead 'em firmly to the tub
> And make 'em scrub.
> Despite their howls
> And growls;
> Teach 'em the use of soap and towels.
> For cleanliness once understood,
> Creates a higher brotherhood,
> It makes men willing to be good;
> ... Remember, while there's soap
> There's hope.[39]

The results were ambiguous. The Americans had, they believed, waged a successful campaign against the onset of plague in 1899, and they could also glory in their striking success against malaria and yellow fever in Cuba (to be discussed later in this chapter). But the military assault on cholera in the Philippines disrupted harvests and thus weakened Philippine diets, while the concentration of people in camps created favorable conditions for the spread of malaria and dysentery. Both Sullivan and Ileto argue that the American struggle with cholera paralleled earlier Spanish efforts in both its intentions and in its results. Both the Spanish (in the cholera epidemic of 1882) and the Americans (in 1902) intended "to consolidate their colonial state, to suppress forms of disorder and irrationality, and institute modes of mass surveillance."[40] And the possibility remains that neither the Spanish nor the American measures affected the course of cholera very much. Both epidemics, 1882 and 1902, ran similar courses, despite the apparently much more successful (or at least active) American assaults in the latter year. Did cholera burn itself out without regard for human intervention?

The American attack on smallpox was a clearer success. Smallpox had long bedeviled the Philippines, and the Spanish government had mounted serious vaccination campaigns against it. The Spanish encountered the general problems that disrupted many Western attempts to extend vaccination to colonial possessions, or indeed to their home populations. Governments often lacked effective means of compulsion, and even where such legal means existed colonial governments (especially) often lacked the money to mount an effective vaccination campaign. They too frequently employed underpaid or unpaid vaccinators, who were typically poorly trained and poorly motivated. Vaccines used in colonial medicine were too often attenuated, inert, or contaminated by bacteria, so that they either conferred inadequate immunity from smallpox or actively spread other diseases. Vaccination as a response to smallpox often countered traditional beliefs about the disease's cause; many Filipinos, for example, saw spirits as responsible for smallpox and believed that appeal to them was more in order. Others positively feared vaccination. Was vaccination simply dangerous to health? Did it usurp the activities of local healers?

For all these reasons the Spanish efforts to vaccinate the Philippine population remained incomplete, and smallpox persisted in the islands. American efforts were more successful, perhaps in part because the new rulers were initially stimulated by the urgency of a war and employed the power of military government. As DeBevoise reconstructs the situation, an unusual proportion of American troops may have arrived in the Philippines with strains of smallpox (especially *Variola minor*), and the disruptions of war increased opportunities for contagion.[41] The continuing hostilities, from 1898 to 1902, gave rise to flight by many fearful civilians, regional overcrowding, and the inevitable widespread fraternization between American troops and Filipinos, all of which contributed to an ideal epidemic situation. The American authorities, fearing first for the health of their troops (another common colonial issue), began a massive vaccination of the civil population, and it met surprisingly little resistance. Perhaps after decades of Spanish efforts vaccination was more familiar; perhaps, as DeBevoise speculates, its administration contrasted with the harsher anticholera measures and so was less resented. Ileto notices that the resistance stimulated by the anticholera measures led American authorities to make some accommodation to Philippine customs and folk healers. And the Americans simply had more resources than the Spaniards had had. So although a serious smallpox epidemic flared in the Philippines in 1918–19, by 1929–30 endemic smallpox had disappeared from that country, the first place in Asia to achieve that goal.

India

The "Crown Jewel" of the British Empire, India occupied an unusual (if not unique) position on the European world horizon.[42] By the early nineteenth century Britain had gradually gained control of a subcontinent that contained some of the oldest, most populous and complex, and richest civilizations in the world. In this conquest the possibility of eradication of the indigenes and their replacement by European settlers could never remotely arise; European migrants could never be more than foam on the surface of oceanic Indian society. Within the subcontinent a vast panoply of traditions and languages coexisted, maintained by peoples who had rarely been politically united and then usually by the yoke of one "foreigner" or another, of whom the British were the latest and most effective. British rule, therefore, had to make its way through a dense thicket of local beliefs and customs. It also confronted two great religions, Hinduism and Islam, and a number of others with substantial followings as well.

Western cultural influence spread only gradually and incompletely in this "conquered" territory. Although the British imprint was ultimately very deep, the cultures of India were not thrust easily aside. Indigenous elites retained considerable power; in some regions of India they retained at least titular political control. The economic impact of the West took a somewhat unusual form as well. Many other imperial places simply saw their economies overwhelmed by the West, which converted their lands to plantations and exploited their mineral and human resources. India was certainly "exploited" by the British, but the imposition of new products and the breakdown of economic structures proceeded much more gradually, and the whole land of India never became a plantation for the production of export cash crops. In part because India assumed an unusual importance in British imperial thinking and policy, economic change included a significant measure of capital infrastructure, itself another contributor both to gradual economic changes in India and to effects on the disease environment.

That environment clearly differed from that of isolated Pacific islands such as the Fijis, of outlying archipelagos such as the Philippines, or of thinly settled continental expanses such as much of North America. Many diseases had been at "home" for many centuries in India, where their causative organisms flourished in the warm moist climate and where they could feed on (and interchange among) the numerous humans and their even more numerous livestock, especially cattle. India was obviously not "virgin soil" for European diseases; more often it played the role of exporter, not importer, and Europeans certainly perceived it as a dangerous disease environment. Those perceptions themselves affected imperial disease history. And the complexity of Indian society meant that the relations of the British rulers with indigenes filtered through a number of levels: the British government of India itself enjoyed a varying measure of freedom of action from the dictates of Westminster, while within India that government faced different local elites which might themselves be at cross-purposes, or might be at absolute loggerheads with more humble elements of society. All this meant that in India huge gulfs might yawn between imperial policy (about some disease issues, for instance) and what actually happened in the country. India superbly illustrates what Mark Harrison calls the "limited scope and effectiveness" of imperial disease policies.[43] That the control of health and disease became a "tool of empire" has become something of a historical cliché; India tests the limits of that cliché very severely.

Cholera. The imperial government's confrontations with cholera, a disease long "native" to India, illustrate both the complexities of imperial health policy and the interrelation of disease with the evolving Indian society. In the eighteenth century the British had generally shown some respect for Indian traditions and ways of life, including Indian approaches to disease and health. Enlightenment notions of disease that emphasized the importance of environment were applied by Europeans to India, with the result that Indian conditions were held responsible for Indian diseases such as cholera; Indian remedies might also therefore be better informed. This environmentalist view persisted long into the nineteenth century, although British respect for Indian traditions did not. British evangelical Christians and British utilitarians agreed (especially from the 1830s on) that India's customs should be rationalized and civilized, that is to say Westernized. Much of the enthusiasm for making India into a Greater Britain diminished after the Sepoy Rebellion of 1857; its events, many of them weighted with symbolism that affected Britons and Indians very differently but equally deeply, convinced many British that India was beyond redemption and that British rule could aim only at lofty trusteeship of the unregenerate barbarians. The 1857 rebellion had other effects as well: it made British authorities very leery of provoking a reprise, and it made them determined to safeguard the health of their troops, their front line against another Kanpur massacre.

Attempts to better the health of the British troops in India reflected both the enthusiasm for sanitation of the 1860s and the Anglo-Indian conviction that Indian diseases were the products of Indian environments. Cholera was a disease of "locality." Army cantonments and "civil lines" were carefully sited, conditions of barracks were modified, drainage and water supply received attention, reforms of nutrition and drinking habits were pursued. Some of these measures involved an increasing segregation of the Indian and European populations, for 1857 had helped convince the British that proximity to Indians might be both biologically and politically dangerous.

British, and especially British Indian, thinkers about cholera resisted ideas that were gaining acceptance in European thought by the 1860s and 1870s. When a cholera epidemic began in 1867 in the northwestern city of Hardwar, where pilgrims had gathered, the different theories came into conflict. In the previous year an international conference on cholera had called India the "natural home" of the disease, and European delegates had urged that the Indian government impose quarantines and controls on the movements of pilgrims, both within India and from India to other places.[44] And indeed the 1867 epidemic seemed to follow the Hardwar pilgrims home, lending credence to the conference's view. But the government of India hesitated to offend religious pilgrims by interference in their freedom of movement, partly because it feared provoking Indian resistance and partly because mid-nineteenth-century British governments tended to favor freedom of movement and trade anyway. And in any case the Indian Medical Service (IMS) as a whole remained unconvinced that contagionism explained cholera; it was a disease of locality, carried through the air.

The 1867 cholera epidemic hinted at a problem that would magnify in the remainder of the century: that the diffusion of disease throughout India would be greatly facilitated by the improvements in infrastructure and modernization of the economy that British rule (and British investment) brought, especially in the decades after 1857. Pilgrimages had always carried serious disease possibilities, for they brought together large crowds in small spaces, crowds that then dispersed to their home villages. Railroads in India—288 miles of them in 1857, 24,760 miles in 1900[45]—increased the number of pilgrims and the distances they could travel, and created their own noxious disease environments, crowded, dirty, without ventilation or water. In 1927 third-class waiting rooms were still called "universal sources of malarial infection."[46] Railroad construction brought large labor forces together and moved them around the country; railroads were built on embankments (to protect them from flooding) that in turn disrupted natural drainage patterns. Railroads were an important element (though not alone) in increased population mobility and agglomeration, which changed the disease environment of India.

Subsequent cholera epidemics might move very rapidly, but official responses to them replayed the themes of 1867. Renewed cholera in the 1880s led to renewed international calls for quarantines, especially from France (fearful of disease reaching its shores through the Mediterranean) and Turkey (in whose territory the great magnets for Muslim pilgrimage were located). But interfering with the travel of Indian Muslims to Mecca seemed politically dangerous to the British rulers, and Indian business interests (especially the merchant community of Bombay) also resisted quarantines. Hoping to appease international criticism, the Indian government created a medical board for Bombay and proposed more thorough regulation of allowable space for passengers on pilgrim ships. The medical board was to report "whether the trifling cholera usually to be found [in Bombay] had assumed an epidemic form," and so Bombay joined the long list of cities that found euphemisms for epidemics.[47] The prospect of closer regulation of pilgrim ships divided the Muslim community, for the prosperous classes supported a move that would thin out the noisome hoi polloi, while the poorer elements decried the higher fares that would bar them from fulfillment of religious obligation. In all this controversy the British government found itself hamstrung: between the pressure of France and Turkey on the one hand and the desires of its own Indian government on the other; between some groups of Indians (who demanded more public health action by government) and others (for whom public health action contradicted religious, cultural, or economic values).

The Indian Medical Service, holding to its environmentalist and holistic conception of cholera, also resisted both Snow's theory of cholera as a waterborne disease and Koch's arguments about its bacteriological cause. Many Indian doctors found an ally in the great German sanitationist Max von Pettenkofer. And a pure water supply was not an obvious answer. In Calcutta a piped-in water supply was completed in 1869, part of the sanitary enthusiasm to protect the European population that so characterized the 1860s. Death rates in the city indeed declined in the next several years, but the new volume of fresh water soon overwhelmed the city's inadequate drainage system and death rates rose again. By the 1870s the Indian government had entered into a new phase marked by both economy and a desire to create institutions of local self-government for Indians, and neither the central Indian government nor the newly formed municipal governments wanted to spend money on such expensive projects as sewers and storm drainage. Municipal governments, dependent on the votes of local property owners and taxpayers, resisted raising the necessary taxation. And Bombay medical authorities created their first medical laboratory in 1884 explicitly to refute Koch's bacteriological arguments. But by the 1890s Koch's beliefs had made headway even among members of the Indian Medical Service, perhaps because if cholera was really the product of a bacterium then the disruption of a quarantine was unnecessary.

The reluctance of British doctors in India to accept newer currents of thought about cholera may have stemmed from more general weaknesses in their social position, which among Anglo-Indians was not particularly high. Members of the Indian Medical Service occupied less prestigious social rank than military officers and members of the civil service. Partly for that reason, but also owing to the extreme climate, the low scale of rewards, and the slowness of promotion within the service, the IMS had difficulty recruiting able physicians from British schools. In that situation, Mark Harrison reasonably argues, many Anglo-Indian doctors responded conservatively to the challenge of new ideas, especially when those ideas threatened not only their long-held beliefs but also the economic prosperity and political stability of the state they served.[48]

Plague. Plague, unlike cholera, was not a "domestic" Indian disease. It arrived in Bombay in August or September 1896, probably from Hong Kong. A brief period of denial ensued, perhaps furthered by the fact that the first diagnosis came from an Indian physician whose competence the British doubted. But European states insisted that the menace be faced. An international conference in Venice criticized the government of India for its laxness about plague (as earlier meetings had complained in times of cholera), and quarantines against Indian goods were imposed. Stung by this international action (and perhaps, as Rajnarayan Chandavarkar has argued, driven by panic) the British Indian government responded vigorously, especially in afflicted Bombay.[49] A determined search for plague victims began, with mandated house searches. Sufferers were isolated and their families segregated; goods and houses were subject to disinfection or destruction by fire. Working on the theory that plague was somehow conveyed through earthen floors, authorities dug up and disinfected such floors, an especially expensive and time-consuming response, and one that (as Charles Gregg remarks) simply dispersed rats more quickly.[50] Controls on rail travel resulted in much interference with traffic and some degrading physical examinations of passengers. Internal Indian quarantines were proclaimed on goods and people moving from Bombay.

These measures stirred considerable resistance, and by 1898 such aggressive steps had been softened, even though for some their theoretical justifications remained. The government responded to local pressures, coopting local leaders and indigenous health practitioners into its efforts, making more effort to respect the purdah privacy of women and the sensitivity of Hindus previously taken to hospitals in which castes were mingled. In addition to their greater sensitivity, perhaps (as so often) driven by a fear of provoking another 1857, Indian governments lacked the money to implement a comprehensive public health police state. The international pressures for quarantine eased as well. By 1900 two newer approaches received more attention: the application of a preventive vaccine and the attack on the rat as a likely plague vector.

A plague vaccine was the product of Waldemar Haffkine, who had also developed a cholera vaccine. Haffkine, a native of the Russian Empire, began experiments with a plague vaccine in 1897, three years after the apparent causative organism of the disease had been isolated by Shibasaburo Kitasato and Alexandre Yersin. I. J. Catanach suggests that established practitioners in Indian medicine were slow to respond to Haffkine's work, in part because they resented him as an outsider; but by 1901 a considerable population, especially in the Punjab, was receiving Haffkine's plague inoculation. At about the same time the possibility that rats carried the disease won some favor (although P. L. Simond's 1898 experiments had to be repeated in Australia and India before Indian physicians were convinced). Vigorous campaigns to kill rats commenced, but these were unrealistic and were modified by 1908 to control the access enjoyed by rats to human dwellings. Catanach argues that by that date a kind of apathy had overtaken the antiplague effort in India, an apathy borne partly of racist compla-cency; the disease, though it ultimately killed twelve million Indians, was not spreading as the new Black Death to the West.[51]

This appearance of plague in India generated much social and philosophical conflict. The aggressive sanitation responses of 1897 especially stirred opposi-tion. Textile mill owners objected to the steam-sterilization of their goods, a pro-cedure that they said weakened fabrics. Indians feared isolation hospitals, and fled to avoid them. At least initially, patients in isolation hospitals shared wards regardless of caste, a mixing deeply offensive to some Hindus. The abandon-ment of infected property meant its almost certain loss, perhaps to thieves, and so owners resisted demands for its surrender. More generally, merchants resis-ted quarantines, which deeply crippled their export trades; Calcutta was espe-cially hurt by the European embargo on Indian hides and skins, exports particularly shipped from that city. The quarantine seemed especially unjust because Calcutta had no confirmed plague until 1898, and even after that remained relatively lightly affected. Bombay suffered from the plague itself, from the flight of 100,000 of its inhabitants, and from the quarantines imposed by other Indian cities on trade with the city. Railroad companies resisted attempts to control rail traffic in the name of public health; such efforts seemed both inter-ference with free trade and discrimination against some travelers. Muslims opposed restrictions, insisted upon by the Turkish government, on pilgrim traf-fic from Bombay to Arabia. The Indian government, hoping to please both Turks and its own Muslims, suggested that Bombay Muslims sail from Madras or Karachi instead, but that plan stirred the ire of Karachi and especially Madras, whose Hindu citizens did not want pestilential Muslims moving through their midst.

All these different conflicts (coinciding as they did with periods of poor har-vests) led to general and serious social unrest, especially in 1897. A major riot occurred in Calcutta in June of that year, and an Indian Civil Service officer was assassinated in Poona. The mere suspicion that aggressive antiplague measures were to be enforced in Calcutta resulted in 150,000 fleeing that city in 1898.

The new emphases of the years after 1900 also stimulated social controversy. Campaigns against rats encountered the ire of devout Hindus, some of whom sabotaged rat traps. Haffkine's vaccination efforts met opposition both from those who favored a heavy state hand for sanitation and from those who felt that the Russian Jew was socially—if not politically—suspect. Much popular sentiment resisted vaccination as well. Although not all Indians set themselves against the vaccine (and Radhika Ramasubban has even argued that leading elements of indigenous Indian opinion were quicker to support vaccination than were British authorities),[52] as early as 1898 rumors circulated through Calcutta that Haffkine's vaccine was in fact a poison prepared by the government; another report claimed that the vaccine had been prepared in the flesh of pigs and cattle, the same explosive mixture that had ignited the 1857 rebellion by inspiring both the disgust of Muslims and the devotion of Hindus. And when, in the middle of the massive inoculation of about 500,000 Punjabis in 1901–1902, nineteen subjects died of tetanus, anti-Haffkine and antivaccination opinion seized the moment. The government, right up through the viceroy, Lord Curzon, laid the blame on Haffkine.[53]

The conflicts within indigenous Indian groups, and between those groups and the British-led government, therefore often limited public responses to disease emergencies. They also confirmed British critics in their view that India was uncivilized and incapable of self-government, while the persistence of disease in cities joined political fears to make places such as Calcutta the "focus of deep-seated European anxieties."[54]

South Africa

The disease history of South Africa in the nineteenth and early twentieth centuries illustrates additional interactions between the expansive European world and other societies.[55] At the start of the nineteenth century South Africa already had a European population (estimated at about 42,000 in 1819), and as the century went on further migration augmented the European numbers, especially after about 1870 (at which point the Europeans might have numbered about 250,000).[56] The original European settlers, the Afrikaners—an amalgam of French Huguenots and Dutch—had begun creating a pastoral society in the seventeenth century, one whose produce replenished ships calling at the Cape of Good Hope on their transits between Europe and Asia. This initial arrival of Europeans displaced some indigenous Africans; here as in the Americas smallpox played a role, greatly diminishing the number of the indigenous Khoikhoi in the Cape area.[57] As the Afrikaner population grew so too did the area it controlled, for many Afrikaners had little interest in staying close to the seaports and instead preferred an isolated self-sufficiency that drew them further inland. The British seizure of the Cape (first in 1795, then confirmed in 1815) accelerated that Afrikaner movement, as the "Volk" escaped the restrictions and different society of the British. British settlers themselves began arriving in the 1820s. The British and their settlers regarded the Cape as of great strategic importance, supplying and protecting Asian traffic; the Afrikaners regarded its lands as divine gifts wherein they could create a godly pastoral society, excluding unbelievers and enslaving the inferior sons of Ham. In either case the area controlled by Europeans remained basically agricultural.

Remarkable mineral discoveries changed the economy of South Africa dramatically. The first of these occurred at Kimberley, about six hundred miles inland from Cape Town, where diamonds were found in 1869. European fortune hunters and African laborers quickly poured into Kimberley, but events there were overshadowed by the discovery of the tremendous gold fields on the ridge called the Witwatersrand, near the Afrikaner capital of Pretoria, in 1886. Within a few years Johannesburg, on the Witwatersrand, became one of the world's great boom towns. Dense populations of miners, laborers, and entrepreneurs gathered in both Kimberley and Johannesburg; by 1910, 200,000 African miners worked on the Witwatersrand. The populations of coastal towns—Cape Town, Port Elizabeth, Durban—grew as well, as the mineral wealth of South Africa flowed into world trade.

South Africa, therefore, experienced an unusually rapid concentration of population into urban centers. Immigrants poured in from Europe and Asia, and a considerable internal migration of Africans occurred as well. Movements of people distorted the economies of rural areas. Many of the urban workers, as miners, both lived and worked in extremely hazardous conditions. For some of the most powerful people in the society commerce rapidly assumed central importance, which might dictate state policy; yet others remained committed to the maintenance of a white settler society, heedless of commerce and scornful of black Africans. All these elements affected South Africa's disease history.

Shula Marks and Neil Andersson have remarked that "[f]ar from being some tropical inheritance, the diseases of twentieth-century South Africa— malnutrition, tuberculosis, typhus, cholera, typhoid, VD—are the diseases of nineteenth-century industrial Britain."[58] While that statement is true, the South African histories of such diseases reflected some particular and colonial circumstances. Movements of people both to and within South Africa had special significance for disease, for example. In the course of the nineteenth century South Africa received two different streams of European immigrants.[59] By the middle of the century consumptive Europeans, especially British, regarded the magnificent climate of South Africa as ideally restorative. If tuberculosis was not yet endemic in South Africa (and it probably was), middle-class Europeans made it so by creating resorts for the consumptive. The numbers of such migrants may not have been demographically significant, but their epidemiological weight was disproportionately large. Poor eastern Europeans, especially Russian and Polish Jews, made up the later and much larger migration, beginning in the 1880s. They arrived with the full complement of microbes carried by all residents of congested and poverty-stricken European towns and cities, especially (again) tuberculosis. In the burgeoning cities of South Africa they met African laborers and miners, recruited from what had been a rural population (and in fact Transvaal law had barred Africans from living in European towns), arriving in the cities after a difficult journey, perhaps on foot with pauses at overcrowded camps, perhaps on similarly overcrowded trains. After a period of brutally hard mine work some of these Africans would return to their rural homelands.

All these circumstances clearly facilitated the spread of epidemic diseases, and when epidemics arose the sometimes-conflicting economic and social goals of the governing classes added interesting epidemiological complications. The 1882 smallpox epidemic that began in Cape Town displayed the differing pressures of commerce and racial segregration. The mine owners first feared that the disease would reach Kimberley, and to prevent its spread there instituted a rigorous quarantine of traffic from Cape Town. "Hijacking travellers for fumigation at the expense and behest of the mining companies," note Marks and Andersson, would be a "useful precedent" for the future South African state.[60] But the Kimberley diamond lords, with little practical control of routes to town apart from the railroad from Cape Town and with no desire to cut off the movement of African labor to their diggings, could not prevent smallpox from reaching Kimberley. When it did they attempted to deny its presence, fearing that others would not send them labor or food. Edmund Sinclair Stevenson, a Cape Town physician, provided the necessary reassurance. "If it was smallpox, a quarantine would be called, the result being that the comparatively large population, mostly niggers and others, would be thrown out of work. . . . Needless to say we pronounced it chicken-pox, otherwise it might have led to serious trouble."[61] It was more important to keep Africans at work than alive.

But as a rapidly urbanizing society at the end of the nineteenth century, South Africa's greatest epidemic problem was tuberculosis. The combination of European immigrants with a high level of tuberculosis infection and Africans with high susceptibility to the disease set up a dangerous situation, especially when—as was true in the 1890s—those populations often lived and worked in close proximity with each other. Many factors increased the susceptibility of Africans to tuberculosis. The disease was probably not new to the indigenous South Africans in the nineteenth century, but their rural and thinly settled population could not sustain tuberculosis at the epidemic level; relatively few people therefore had hereditary experience with it. The demand for mine labor rapidly outstripped its supply, and recruiters scouring the villages could not be fussy about the health of potential miners. Many of the recruits came from some distance to reach Kimberley or Johannesburg, and the journey itself might be weakening, involving long walks and nights in overcrowded (and disease-ridden) labor camps, or extended trips on similarly overcrowded trains. Many African laborers therefore arrived in the instant cities in imperfect health.[62]

But conditions of life and work in the mine towns played a larger role. Miners worked in close contact in conditions of minimal ventilation. European miners in South Africa sometimes were tubercular, and more often suffered from silicosis, even before they began working in Africa; it was among them that the African miners worked. The introduction of water-fed drills in mines cut down the dust and hence the silicosis, but created a moister atmosphere in which the tuberculosis bacillus moved easily from one person to another. The wages of miners remained low, for mine owners had devoted many of their resources to capital equipment and acquisition and so claimed that little was left for workers' wages; eventually white miners were able to wield political power, but black Africans were shut out by governments committed to maintaining the privileges of a white settler society. African miners were housed in overcrowded barracks; in response to worries about lack of fresh air, such barracks were often opened to drafts, which caused the miners (sometimes migrants from warmer climates) to cluster close together for warmth (and tubercular infection).

In these conditions mortality from tuberculosis soared. Mortality rates from tuberculosis for black Africans reached 1,500 per 100,000 in Port Elizabeth in 1900; although rates were lower in Johannesburg, Randall Packard believes that the policies of mine owners masked the true extent of the disease in mine towns.[63] The mine companies saw certain advantages in a transient work force that worked for a time and then returned to home villages. If nothing else such "seasonal" labor required less "paternalistic" care; mine owners could excuse barracklike housing on the grounds that the workers regarded their places as temporary anyway, and caring for long-term illness might be left to the families in villages. And while some African miners fell victim to the rapidly fatal "fulminating" tuberculosis, many others became more chronically ill away from the mines. This movement of miners also contributed both to further diffusion of tuberculosis back in the villages and to keeping a reservoir of relatively unexposed laborers flowing into the mines.

In this period "South Africa" consisted of several separate political entities. Kimberley lay within the territory of the Cape Colony, in the British Empire but possessing a fair amount of self-government dominated by Europeans; until 1902 the Witwatersrand was in the Transvaal Republic, in some theoretical sense under British suzerainty but in practice ruled by Afrikaners. After that date the Afrikaner states of the Transvaal and the Orange Free State fell directly under British rule, until all the separate British holdings in the area were federated in the Union of South Africa in 1910. Although differences in degree existed among different political authorities, none of them had much interest in political rights for black Africans. Prior to about 1900, political and public health leaders hoped to educate the native workers out of their "bad habits"; they should, for example, give up their inappropriate Western clothing, which they persisted in wearing even when it got cold and wet; they should realize that slums were unhealthy, and not live in them.

Then came another and more frightening disease: plague, which appeared in Cape Town in February 1901. Fear of this disease energized South African governments to the new public health policy of "sanitary segregation." Separate communities should house the dangerous Africans, apart from the European populations of the cities; in 1901 a "location" was hastily constructed outside Cape Town for some 6,000 Africans. Maynard Swanson has shown that this solution emerged from a context in which the segregration of Africans had been proposed as a means by which employers could gain greater social control over their work forces; in 1899 the Cape Colony had passed a "Native Labour Locations Act" with that intent, and another law in 1902 extended government powers to create such "locations." The extent to which concern for sanitation and public health may have been a simple gloss on racial prejudice and social control was suggested by the statement of A. J. Gregory, medical officer for the Cape Colony: "Indeed if only the sanitary condition of the premises is to form the basis of the decision then practically a very large number of Natives could be allowed to reside in Cape Town."[64]

The segregation policy neither worked very well nor helped control disease. At least in the years right after 1902, segregation of the work force met much economic opposition. Employers did not like to see their workers isolated too far from their jobs, and too many black Africans (at least in Cape Town) had become property owners themselves and resisted compulsory resettlement. Native towns could also spring up outside the official locations, over which the authorities had little control; and questions of costs arose between the colonial and municipal governments, mirroring conflicts in India. So many African laborers remained outside the "locations," while for those in them health conditions did not improve.

The South African experience, though it differed in significant ways from the other imperial illustrations in this chapter, confirms some general points. Imperial governments could only partially control public health; private economic interest did not always coincide with proclaimed state policy; medicine could be a justification for stronger social control, but at times that control faltered anyway, and eradication of disease rarely followed. Tuberculosis in South Africa began declining among the European population by 1912–1914, and while Africans and "colored" briefly shared in that decline, World War I brought a more comprehensive industrialization, intensified urban crowding, and for the non-Europeans, increased residential segregation and poverty. With those phenomena tuberculosis rose again, now joined by serious epidemics of typhus in 1917–1924, 1933–1935, and 1944–1946. South Africa was indeed reprising the disease history of an industrializing society.

"Tropical Diseases"

Early European attempts to reach into the interior of the tropics, especially in sub-Saharan Africa, had been repeatedly thwarted by the assaults of malaria, yellow fever, and diseases that assailed European livestock. Tropical disease frustrated occasional Portuguese efforts to reach up the Congo or

Zambezi rivers in the sixteenth and seventeenth centuries, and such troubles persisted into the eighteenth and early nineteenth centuries as well. Willem Bolts, a Dutchman in the service of the English East India Company, put 152 Europeans ashore at Delagoa Bay (Mozambique) in 1777; by 1779 only 20 survived. In Mungo Park's 1805 expedition to the Niger all 44 Europeans died; Macgregor Laird, pushing to the same river in 1833, fared little better, losing 39 of 48.[65] This European frailty in the tropics meant that Western powers maintained their military presence in Africa and the Indies only tenuously, and at considerable human cost to their troops.[66] Philip Curtin's tables of "relocation costs" dramatically illustrate the differences between mortalities in Europe and in the tropics for European military personnel. Whereas deaths per thousand of troops stationed in Britain, France, or the northern United States in the 1820s and 1830s varied between 15 and 20, for French troops in Algeria it was over 78, in Guadeloupe about 107, in Martinique about 113, and in Senegal over 164. British troops fared no better, suffering death rates of 71 in India, 130 in Jamaica, and a dreadful 483 in Sierra Leone. Obviously maintenance of a colonial tropical empire required serious sacrifices of manpower. And sometimes diseases contributed to the collapse of an entire imperial holding, most dramatically in French Saint Domingue (Haiti). In the early 1790s the Haitians had won considerable independence from the French, and retained it despite the complications of an invasion of British troops. When Napoleon Bonaparte, then consul, attempted to regain control in 1802, the French army was overwhelmed by a combination of Haitian resistance and yellow fever, so that by 1803 Bonaparte abandoned the French claim altogether.

Between the 1830s and the first decade of the twentieth century the tropics lost most of their terror for European travelers, and the steep gradient of death rates that European troops or administrators faced when posted to Africa or the Indies fell away. Both preventive environmental measures and therapeutic medical responses contributed to this dramatic demonstration of Western cultural power. And while the germ theory did intercede powerfully at the end of the period, earlier measures had already had important effects.

Europeans in those warmer climates faced several different disease problems. Some were relatively familiar though in some cases intensified: dysentery and diarrhea, and cholera, especially in its endemic Indian home. As was true in Europe, those diseases lost some of their grip with the gradual extension of improved water and sewer systems, improvements first extended to European settlements and military cantonments. Sewer systems that used water to flush wastes out were fairly easily installed in island locations such as the West Indies, where they simply ran into the sea. In India, however, the "dry earth" method (related to the ancient Indian latrine system) persisted. The use of sand filters for water purification also began in the middle of the nineteenth century, although the rationale for their effectiveness was only demonstrated in the 1880s by Robert Koch. The imposition of these new water and sewer systems resulted in declining incidence of the waterborne diseases, although it may have also contributed to a surge in typhoid fever in both Europe and elsewhere; sewage in rivers increased, and unscreened sewage (to which flies had access) remained in dry systems.[67]

Although cholera was in some sense a "tropical disease," the institutes founded for the study of "tropical medicine" in the 1890s concerned themselves more with malaria, yellow fever, schistosomiasis (bilharzia) and other worm problems, and sleeping sickness. Of these malaria and yellow fever were the great barriers to European movement in the tropics. The two posed different problems, although they were often lumped together and diagnoses of them were often imprecise. Malaria is a chronic ailment caused by species of the genus *Plasmodia*. These protozoa are carried from person to person by mosquitoes of the genus *Anopheles*, which includes hundreds of species (although relatively few are important malaria vectors). Several different species of *Plasmodia* produce different forms of malaria, of differing degrees of severity. The disease therefore includes a spectrum of symptoms, made wider by its chronic character; degrees of debility vary widely from time to time in the same individual. Its epidemiology is a complex tangle involving several different causative parasites and a larger number of insect vectors that may flourish in different environments, as well as different levels of human resistance.

Malaria had a long history in parts of Europe and North America, and it was only in the nineteenth century that Europeans began to consider it a "tropical" disease at all. As Randall Packard has argued, that happened, in part, because changes in methods of agricultural production in turn led to ecological changes that affected malarial environments. Those changes themselves were ultimately the outgrowth of Western political and economic power and modernization. With agricultural development, areas in the Western world that had been malarial became less so, while areas of Asia and Africa introduced to systems of Western-controlled plantation agriculture became more so. Many imperial agricultural enterprises involved large labor forces (often seasonal or migratory), little technological investment, deforestation, and haphazard irrigation systems, all of which led to both poverty for the workforce and environmental change that favored malaria.[68]

Eradicating *all* of the relevant *Anopheles* mosquitoes has proved to be extraordinarily difficult. But in the seventeenth century (see Chapter Six) the Western world had learned of an indigenous South American remedy—cinchona bark—that had both curative and preventive powers. In the early nineteenth century quinine, the chemically active component of cinchona bark, was isolated and came into increasing Western use by the 1830s. Daniel Headrick lays great weight on quinine as a prime tool of empire that made the tropics safe for Europeans. Philip Curtin, more cautious, sees quinine use working together with improved drainage in European tropical stations, but both agree that European mortality from malaria in the tropics declined rapidly in the years between 1840 and 1860. Morbidity may have remained higher, since quinine could not entirely prevent *Plasmodia* from entering bodies, and drainage schemes (as we shall see) were often incomplete, especially away from easily managed island environments. The connection between malaria and mosquitoes was made only in the 1890s, so drainage had no precise target; malaria had for centuries been the definitive "miasma" disease, and was then associated with general "filth" by nineteenth-century sanitarians. Alphonse Laveran found the plasmodium in 1880; Patrick Manson began showing the role of insects in filariasis in the late 1870s; Ronald Ross completed his arguments that connected *Plasmodia* and *Anopheles* in 1898.

Yellow fever, an acute viral disease, posed an immediate short-run threat to European lives, for its mortality rate could rival that of plague. But some features of its epidemiology meant that it was both less widespread and easier to escape than malaria, and so its demographic effect was less. Yellow fever—again like plague— exists primarily as an enzootic disease, in its case usually in forest populations of monkeys. It occasionally and endemically reaches humans from the monkey population, through a mosquito vector. Yellow fever becomes epidemic in human populations when mosquitoes carry it from one human to another. Several factors limit its spread. The principal vector, the single mosquito species *Aedes aegypti*, has domestic habits close to human dwellings, a short range of flight, and a constant need for water and warmth. Cool weather or dry conditions will therefore halt an epidemic, and some Europeans and North Americans escaped yellow fever by simple flight, as British troops did in Guyana in 1861. And the acute character of the infection also limited its spread. The symptoms of the disease in fact vary widely, although many cases can be dramatic and the mortality rate may be high; many children in sub-Saharan Africa or the West Indies probably contracted mild cases that conferred subsequent immunity, and thus the disease might run out of unexposed humans and "burn out" fairly quickly, and so either die out or return to the enzootic state in the neighboring forest.

If malaria was a chronically debilitating (and sometimes fatal) problem, yellow fever remained in the nineteenth century an occasional terror. Any Western city maintaining a trade connection with the West Indies was especially vulnerable, if a ship carrying the virus and *Aedes aegypti* arrived in its harbor. Philadelphia suffered in 1793 (see Chapter Six), Barcelona in 1821, New Orleans in 1853, St. Nazaire in 1861, Swansea in 1865, Memphis in 1878. To unexposed Europeans in Africa or the West Indies yellow fever was extremely dangerous, and quinine had no effect. In the earlier nineteenth century the incidence of yellow fever may have been reduced by flight and by some swamp drainage, although the first was more often an intuitive than a reasoned response and the second was undertaken usually as part of a broad-spectrum assault on the general causes of "miasma." Then in the late 1870s the Cuban physician Carlos Finlay y Barres advanced the theory that mosquitoes—specifically *Aedes aegypti*—transmitted yellow fever; apparently Finlay got the idea of the mosquito's role from Patrick Manson, who in 1878 had argued that mosquitoes carried (or "nursed") embryonic filariasis. But Finlay's epidemiological theory was not followed up until 1900. As François Delaporte argues, the intervening decades of the 1880s and 1890s were dominated by zealous bacteriology, which encouraged a search for the causative organism of yellow fever as well as for most of the other ills of humankind.[69] Yellow fever—a viral disease—defeated the bacteriologists, while interest in possible vectors waned.

In 1898 bacteriology enjoyed one of its great triumphs, when Ronald Ross showed that some mosquitoes carry (as intermediate hosts) malaria *Plasmodia*. Two British researchers in Havana, H.E. Durham and Walter Myers, first saw the analogy between Finlay's vector theory of yellow fever and Ross's intermediate hosts in 1900. Havana at that point was effectively under United States control, in the wake of the American war against Spain in 1898; American military physicians, following the lead of Durham and Myers, pursued a possible yellow fever–mosquito link with a series of risky experiments, in the course of which one of them (Jesse Lazear) died of yellow fever after being bitten by an infected *Aedes aegypti* mosquito. Later in 1900 Walter Reed repeated these experiments (and won more historical acclaim), and Reed's work convinced American and Cuban authorities that the answer to yellow fever epidemics lay in the eradication of *Aedes aegypti*. The subsequent assault on possible breeding places and homes of that insect yielded spectacular results, as the incidence of yellow fever (and malaria) in Havana plummeted.[70] More dramatic American military success was to follow, in Panama.

The American conquest of the environment in Panama has often been told as perhaps the greatest "triumph" of Western imperial health. But its historical lessons are not simple, and its consequences for other imperial health policies were mixed. A French company had begun working on a canal across the seductively narrow isthmus in 1881, but it encountered tremendous difficulties, not the least of which were the ravages of malaria and yellow fever on its work force. (The company might have expected this, for the laborers who built a railroad across the isthmus in the 1850s had been similarly decimated.) The canal work was abandoned in 1889, with the company bankrupt and the number of deaths (even then very uncertain) in the thousands. Driven by its experiences in the 1898 war with Spain, the United States government saw the advantages in quickly connecting its naval units in the Pacific and the Atlantic, and so it acquired the French diggings in 1904 and began its own canal, completed in 1914. The eradication of yellow fever and malaria from one of the most malarial places on earth made that success possible.

The eradicator, William Gorgas (an American army physician), had begun a huge and indiscriminate clean-up campaign in Havana in 1899. After the work of Lazear, Reed, and their colleagues had convinced him of the wisdom of focusing his attention on mosquitoes, he had done so. In 1904 he moved to Panama to repeat his methods. Those methods depended on a massive military-style assault on a community, fumigating property, screening houses, and above all attacking mosquito breeding grounds by draining swamps and puddles, clearing vegetation, and lavishly spreading such possible larvicides as carbolic acid and caustic soda. In Panama Gorgas was given a large budget and a substantial work force. The results were startlingly successful: the last yellow fever epidemic was in 1905, while malaria mortality quickly declined (from 40 per thousand in 1906 to 9 per thousand in 1908) and so did morbidity (from a frightening 800 per thousand in 1906 to only 16 per thousand in 1916).[71] But the costs were staggeringly high. George Goethals, the engineer in charge of the American canal construction, told Gorgas that every mosquito he killed cost ten dollars.[72] The wealthy United States might spend that, in a relatively small area of unusual importance for both national security and commerce; but even the vast British Empire had no chance of duplicating such expenses across (for example) the subcontinent of India.

Nevertheless the eradication model, so successful in Panama, drew imitators. At the very least, the same enthusiasm that seized Americans in Cuba and Panama, an enthusiasm for combining the genius of bacteriology with that of engineering, worked elsewhere as well. Across the British Empire different territories began attempts to eradicate mosquitoes. Ronald Ross arrived in Sierra Leone with high hopes, believing that draining about one hundred puddles would eliminate malaria from Freetown. By 1901 he realized that the job was bigger, and he began a more elaborate drainage campaign. But dramatic Havana results were not obtained, perhaps because Sierra Leone was far more malarial than Cuba to begin with. The Royal Society of London's Malaria Commission shied from the prohibitive costs of eradicating mosquitoes in Sierra Leone and instead recommended a system of residential segregation, which would at least isolate the Europeans from the fever-infested natives. A hill town outside Freetown was constructed and the eradication campaign was abandoned. In populous Nigeria the British authorities reached the same conclusion: improving the health of the indigenes simply cost too much. In India, where some local self-government existed by 1900, the size of the problem defeated the willingness of governments to raise money to meet it. An extensive and expensive attempt was made, for example, to drain irrigation canals around the military cantonments of Lahore between 1901 and 1909. It failed, which increased the Indian government's conviction that protecting native quarters was hopeless; all the more so since the indigenously elected local councils proved their incompetence (at least to Europeans) by refusing to raise money for sanitation.[73]

Segregation, as a cheaper "remedy" than a costly Panama-style eradication, was pursued by other European powers as well. In 1910 the German rulers of Cameroon proposed to relocate the entire indigenous population of Douala inland, leaving the coast for European settlement. And in Dakar (Senegal) the French authorities decided that the Africans followed lifestyles that were incompatible with European standards of sanitation. Daniel Headrick points out that some of these unsatisfactory lifestyles in fact grew out of poverty and differential treatment.[74] When the French built up Dakar as a naval station between 1898 and 1908 they lavishly supplied the city with water from newly dug wells, but most of the water was reserved for the harbor and military installations and for European residences; Africans in the rapidly growing town had to husband their water carefully in barrels that became homes for mosquitoes. On such grounds the French justified residential segregation, although they agreed that Africans who obeyed European sanitary rules could live in European quarters. Segregation in Dakar was therefore based on habits, not race, although a racially based decision about water supply helped create the "habits." South African arguments remained more purely racial. As we have seen, a sense of emergency generated by the appearance of plague there in 1900 led to plans for residential segregation, and Maynard Swanson argues that this "sanitation syndrome" became a useful support for social control founded on racial prejudices.[75]

These different African and Indian examples illustrate that other remedies might vie with the wholesale (and prohibitively expensive) eradication of mosquitoes by drainage. Laboratory science also offered other alternatives: therapy (both preventive and curative) and the chemical assault on insects, as opposed to the massive engineering works of Panama drainage. As we have seen, quinine could both deter malaria and contribute to its cure. Angelo Celli, the influential Italian student of malaria, came to believe that widespread quinine treatment was the surest antimalaria path, and Robert Koch agreed. Chemical insecticides gained favor in the years after World War I as another eradication technique. Still another road was not often taken: the improvement of the living conditions of masses of working people. Malaria and yellow fever, like cholera and tuberculosis, might truly have been seen as diseases of poverty, rather than "tropical diseases" that came with the supposedly savage and backward. Before World War I Celli suggested that if people could afford adequate diets and good homes with screens to bar mosquitoes, then mosquito-borne diseases could be overcome. But biomedicine was easier than social reform.

Conclusions

In the nineteenth century Western imperialism both spread diseases and altered the human and natural environments in which diseases existed. In those respects imperialism qualifies more as human disaster than as human triumph.

The West did achieve some limited or mixed successes in the "conquest" of diseases elsewhere in the world. Most dramatic were several campaigns, based largely on mosquito eradication, against yellow fever and malaria. Yellow fever, carried by one fairly domestic species of mosquito, proved easier to attack than malaria, borne by a number of species of varied ranges. Truly effective insecticides came after World War I, and their results—again mixed—will be seen in Chapter Eleven. Cholera, like dysentery and typhoid, was being brought under control by sanitation methods in the West, but those measures only slowly extended to areas under Western control elsewhere. Many Westerners were convinced that the "natives" were hopeless about such amenities and so extending sanitation was futile; Western colonial governments often had little money to spend, or were caught in wrangles about who should bear costs; indigenes sometimes resisted the changes in ways of life or systems of property that sanitation entailed. Plague inspired excited reactions, but until after 1900 those reactions consisted of unfocused "clean-ups"; more effective attacks on rodent vectors only began after World War I. Western-imposed quarantines did help in some cases, but often only after the horse had left the barn; measles in Fiji became less serious largely because the population acquired exposure to it.

If many of the "tropical diseases" (and others) persisted in the Western imperial world, it was largely because economic and social conditions, especially poverty, persisted or were deepened by colonial rule. Plague, typhus, cholera, tuberculosis, malaria, trypanosomiasis, and hookworm diseases all flourished where people lived in close proximity, where houses could be easily invaded by mammal and insect disease vectors, where water supplies could be tainted by sewage, where nutrition was inadequate, where people worked in bare feet. Larger dwellings more solidly constructed, screened windows, iron pipes, adequate reservoirs, varied diets, and shoes were marks of prosperity. Western colonial rule eventually tried to justify itself by claiming to promote economic development, but in the nineteenth century it was most often simply exploitive.

But even with the best will, the Western imperial governments could not impose a clear vision of health on the lands they ruled. Policies could too often inspire internal conflicts between those who wanted to publicize disease (whether in Kimberley or Bombay or, for that matter, in San Francisco) and those who wished to preserve commerce, between those who wanted vigorous action and those who feared indigenous reactions to it, between those who favored the focused attack made possible by bacteriology and those who wished to continue (or revive) a general environmentalism. The ability or even competence of much colonial medicine was not clear even then. Ronald Ross "had no predilection at all for medicine," and only became a physician because that would "allow him leisure for shooting and riding and other such hobbies";[76] William Gorgas only became a physician after he failed to gain admission to a military academy. Western physicians in the imperial world did not all model themselves on the saintly David Livingstone; Leander Starr Jameson and Frederick Rutherfoord Harris took leading roles in the looting of Rhodesia. And even if the rulers could agree among themselves and could employ able and disinterested medical practitioners, it remained true that (as Megan Vaughan puts it) colonialism had a "limited impact on cultures and the identities they created."[77]

Biomedicine's greatest triumph by the end of the nineteenth century was probably over the European mind. Europeans were convinced that they understood the causes of diseases and could take at least preventive action against them, either through immunizing vaccines or through interrupting the vectors that carried microbes. This knowledge elevated them, they believed, above other "lesser breeds" of humanity, whose diseases could be explained perhaps by biology but increasingly as the products of ignorance and hence human failure. The development of this confident biomedicine forms a theme of the next chapter.

Ten

The Scientific View of Disease and the Triumph of Professional Medicine

At the beginning of the nineteenth century physicians occupied an uneasy position in the world of Western healing. Although they still possessed many privileges, in practice the distinctions between them and other healers remained unclear. Thus while physicians belonged to corporate bodies that enjoyed privileges recognized in law, surgeons and apothecaries had begun establishing similar claims; for the most part graduates of universities, physicians enjoyed the status of a learned profession, which elevated them above craftsmen (such as surgeons) and tradesmen (such as apothecaries) in Western social hierarchies, but in at least some places such distinctions were losing their force. Two factors in particular had contributed to fraying the boundaries of the physician's authority. It had proved very difficult—in practice—to enforce the privileges of any one corporate body of healers, particularly in an age when no one group possessed any clear therapeutic advantage over others. Especially in western Europe and North America the eighteenth century was also an age of an increasingly vigorous entrepreneurial economy, which made the maintenance of monopoly hard to sustain; this free market competition had particular force in the health business, where consumers often dictated the terms of service.

Nineteenth-century developments would greatly strengthen the professional position of physicians. In the course of the century increasingly tight connections were drawn between a physician's education and a license to practice awarded by the state, a license that eventually depended on completion of an "appropriate" education or even on an examination administered (or authorized) by the state that confirmed the results of that education. States gradually recognized exclusive rights to practice healing by employing different sanctions against those who fell outside the charmed (that is, the educated and licensed) circle. These changed circumstances were partly the product of political forces and partly the result of pressures from within communities of physicians and other healers, as an examination of several national cases will show. But physicians' changing relationship to science also improved their position, as did changing perceptions of the curative power of the remedies that physicians espoused.

By the second half of the nineteenth century science had come to inspire enormous confidence in its explanatory power. Enthusiasts for science had promoted its virtues in the seventeenth and eighteenth centuries, so by the nineteenth a well-established tradition of scientific faith existed. In the nineteenth century, furthermore, science shared the prestige and evident success of industrial technology, in an age when (for a large complex of reasons, including science's success) religion slowly lost some of its hold on beliefs. Medicine both benefited from and contributed to the perception of the power of science, for not only could technology conquer distance, scientific medicine could conquer disease. Winwood Reade's *The Martyrdom of Man* (1872) may stand as an extreme example of the faith:

> The God of Light, the Spirit of Knowledge, the Divine Intellect, is gradually spreading over the planet and upward to the skies. . . Disease will be extirpated; the causes of decay will be removed; immortality will be invented. And then, the earth being small, mankind will migrate into space, and will cross the airless Saharas which separate planet from planet, and sun from sun. The earth will become a Holy Land which will be visited by pilgrims from all the quarters of the universe. Finally, men will master the forces of Nature; they will become themselves architects of systems, manufacturers of worlds. Man then will be perfect; he will then be a Creator; he will therefore be what the vulgar worship as a God.[1]

Physicians may not have been gods by the end of the nineteenth century, but the triumphs of science (especially the newly articulated germ theory) conferred on them powers that to some seemed little short of miraculous.

Changing Professional Situations

The professional situation of physicians first changed clearly in France. In the 1790s the revolutionary governments scrapped the ancient universities—including the traditional university training of physicians—and created a new national system of higher education. For medical education the new schooling meant a closer relationship between the educations of physicians and of surgeons than had previously obtained. Although (as Chapter Six suggested) the changes may nave been more gradual than revolutionary, the education of physicians now included more first-hand experience of anatomy and physiology and more clinical practice in a hospital setting. Then in 1803 Napoleon Bonaparte's Consulate enacted new laws providing for a uniform licensing system for physicians, surgeons, and "health officers"; a state license depended on completion of a specified number of years in the new state medical universities, followed by a state examination. This uniform, national system (national for the physicians and surgeons at least) replaced the tangle of old regionally based corporate privileges and monopolies that had grown up prior to the Revolution. Those responsible for the legislation intended to draw a much sharper line between licensed and "irregular" medical practitioners than had obtained in the past. Nevertheless the 1803 laws did not change the French medical world overnight. Numerous loopholes remained, through which more irregular practitioners slipped to continue their careers; French physicians only slowly developed institutions that might control professional positions; and university-trained physicians remained the representatives of an elite subculture, not widely trusted by the general population. But the system of state licensing and control imposed a measure of uniformity, and when (later in the century) dramatic new therapeutic science appeared, it could be adopted by a profession that had already been given a shape, defined by a common state-imposed educational, examination, and licensing process.[2]

In the German states a bewildering assortment of privileged bodies existed in the eighteenth century, if only because there existed a bewildering assortment of over three hundred states. After the drastic political rationalizations of the revolutionary and Napoleonic eras, Germany in 1815 still contained thirty-nine sovereign states. In at least some of these the structure for an organized and monopolistic medical profession already existed, for many contained universities that were (and had been for some time) under state control; their medical graduates might be automatically licensed to practice. But would states desire to give physicians privileged powers of monopoly? In the eighteenth-century German states the traditions of enlightened despotism and cameralism had won important adherents, more so than in France or Britain. Those traditions might mandate an active and perhaps intrusive state role to increase a ruler's wealth and power, and thus support state public health regulation. Johann Peter Frank's multivolumed treatise on "medical police," published between 1779 and 1819, urged states to license physicians, to regulate or suppress irregular healers, and to employ physicians as state health officers. Early nineteenth-century German states proved more or less eager to follow Frank's advice, and if they did the prestige and monopoly position of physicians increased. But the issue was never clear, for the rival liberal ideology urged the virtues of free competition, which left much room for irregulars. The ultimate unification of the German states under the aegis of the kingdom of Prussia occurred at a time (1866–1871) when many physicians opposed state restrictions, yet as their numbers increased by the 1880s they pressed for greater power to restrict the market.[3]

In both Great Britain and the United States the legal position of the medical profession was much less clear in the early nineteenth century. In Britain a number of privileged bodies existed for physicians, surgeons, and apothecaries, some of considerable antiquity; the (English) Royal College of Physicians had been chartered in 1518. But their powers were slight. The Royal College of Physicians, the most prestigious, was only empowered to license physicians within a seven-mile radius of London. The college was prone to insist—largely to maintain the gentlemanly aspect of a "profession"—that its members be graduates of Oxford or Cambridge universities, where in fact little serious medical education was pursued; and while possessors of Oxford or Cambridge medical degrees might practice medicine anywhere in the United Kingdom, little or no legal machinery existed to prevent other practitioners from competing for the trade. Among the members of different corporations (physicians, surgeons, apothecaries, from England, Scotland, or Ireland) lively professional rivalries and jealousies persisted. Only in the nineteenth century did these different bodies, with some assistance from changes in the law, begin to demand meaningful qualifications of their members. In the years after 1800 the College of Surgeons began imposing on aspiring members specified terms of apprenticeship, as well as an education that included attendance at a number of lectures. In 1815 the Society of Apothecaries obtained, through a parliamentary statute, powers of licensing that included setting an educational standard and examining candidates for proficiency. But it was not until 1858 that the British government created a legal category of "licensed medical practitioner." The license, it was true, could be granted by any one of a number of corporate bodies, on the model provided for the Society of Apothecaries in 1815; but the registration of the licensed was placed in the collective hands of a "General Medical Council," on which the medical corporations and the universities were represented, and that body had the further power of striking off the registered lists those whom it deemed unqualified. Although British law still did not outlaw irregular medical practice, only registered healers could be employed by government bodies, and after 1858 unlicensed practitioners might be liable for criminal prosecution for assault or manslaughter if their patients wished (and were able) to complain.[4]

The legal powers of physicians in the United States were murkier still. In the colonial period no privileged corporations for the healing professions existed (except those from Britain whom the colonists chose to recognize), and so "doctors" were entirely self-described. In the 1760s some of the colonies began attempting to license physicians, but without any agreement as to uniformity of training. Medical schools in British America also began in the 1760s, but American physicians continued to acquire their credentials by a varying combination of apprenticeship and attendance at lectures at such a college; others simply started practice as "physicians" with no formal training at all. Hostility to the claims of a privileged guild remained strong in the young United States, so much so that by the period between 1820 and 1850 those American states that had previously attempted to license physicians gave up the effort. In the mid-nineteenth century, therefore, American medical practice was entirely unregulated, and a wild variety of healers, expounding different philosophies, competed for the public favor. Then between the 1870s and the 1890s a growing number of American states began conferring increasing powers on physicians, who could be licensed if they earned a diploma from a medical college. The states gradually assumed the power to determine the validity of the diploma and/or to insist that physicians seeking a license pass a state examination that would validate their medical education. As Paul Starr says, those steps evolved "incrementally" in the late nineteenth century, so that by the beginning of the twentieth the American physician occupied roughly the same legal ground as his European colleague.[5]

"Science" and Medical Practice, 1800–1860

Shifts in scientific ideas and technical medical practice may partly account for the emergence of the physicians' professional monopoly. Between 1800 and about 1860 the beliefs of "orthodox" physicians changed considerably, although how those new beliefs affected what physicians did was not so clear. At the beginning of the nineteenth century most physicians were aware that the Galenic paradigms that had dominated their profession for centuries were of doubtful value. Galenic anatomy—and even more Galenic physiology—had been discredited for some ever since the time of Harvey in the seventeenth century. The Galenic humoral theories had likewise come under heavy fire; since the sixteenth century different arguments had been made for the local (as opposed to the systemic) origin of disease, and those localist beliefs had acquired particular force by about 1800, especially in Paris, then the most important center of Western medical ideas.

But the Galenic paradigm had not yet been replaced by another that had won general assent, and the therapies offered by orthodox physicians remained essentially Galenic, in that they aimed at the immediate relief of visible symptoms by manipulation of body fluids. Bleedings and purgings with that end in view remained the order of the day for the early nineteenth-century physician, however much he might have forsworn allegiance to Galenic humors. Thus Broussais, a fervent exponent of the local character of disease, found all disease to be a product of malfunctioning solid tissue, and urged that those malfunctions be relieved by bleeding. Benjamin Rush, the influential American physician, proposed another "unitary" theory of disease, which he believed to be based on "capillary tension." Bleeding ameliorated such tension. The use of the lancet and the prescription of such powerful purgatives as calomel symbolized early nineteenth-century medicine, so much so that an important British medical journal founded in 1823 bore the simple (though politically meaningful) title *The Lancet.*

This view of the importance of local sites for explaining disease, still uncertain at the start of the century, gained much strength between about 1800 and about 1860 as a result of experimental evidence and arguments. That evidence was most important in pathology, where it gained weight incrementally and gradually. Xavier Bichat, one of the most vigorous proponents of a local view of disease, was also an enthusiastic pathologist. Spurred by his belief that disease affected individual tissues, not organs as a whole, Bichat performed a remarkable number of autopsies in a few years of work before his premature death in 1802. In the next fifty years a large body of pathological knowledge accumulated. One of Bichat's Parisian successors, P. C. A. Louis, used his considerable pathological experience to urge the creation of a "numerical" medicine in which conclusions—especially those drawn from pathology—should be formed from statistical evidence. In Britain the availability of corpses for dissection and research was put on a legal footing by the Anatomy Act of 1832. That act had other political causes and consequences that will be discussed presently, but for the moment it may be taken as a symbol of the growing strength and solidity of anatomical research, and of the conviction that medical enlightenment and anatomical science were closely related. In Vienna Karl von Rokitansky accumulated a huge volume of pathological observations, summarized in his writings of the 1840s.

The general pathological interest that these examples represent culminated in the career of Rudolf Virchow, who began to make his name with microscopic pathological studies in the 1840s. Virchow, impressed by the cell theories of Matthias Schleiden and Theodor Schwann, focused his attention on the cell as the heart of the pathological process, while he also came to believe that cells themselves divide and so create other cells. It followed that a "diseased" cell might divide and so by replication, or "mitosis," spread disease. The implications were clear: disease originated in microscopically local sites, and only became "systemic" by spreading over a growing number of such sites. Virchow's reputation as a pathologist became immense, bolstered both by the prestige of his position as a professor at the University of Berlin, the flagship of German *Wissenschaft,* and by his political renown as a leading German liberal, a participant in the Prussian revolution of 1848 and later a deputy in both the Prussian Diet and the imperial Reichstag.

This concern with local organs and local sites of disease also manifested itself in physiological studies, especially in the understanding of the nervous system. The body came to be seen in an increasingly mechanical or chemical light, while human physiological processes were increasingly subjected to deliberate

experimental manipulation. Bichat straddled old and new physiological conceptions, being drawn both to explaining the "vital" properties of organs (as Harvey
had been) and to regarding organs as inert subjects of experiment; surgery
might help him "analyze functional organic dependencies."[6] François Magendie
(1783–1855), in the next generation of Parisian physiologists, employed both
chemistry and surgery experimentally, isolating the chemically active principles
of substances (such as quinine from cinchona bark) and showing their actions
on body organs. A growing body of evidence, accumulated especially by
Johannes Müller in the 1830s, suggested that specific sensory nerves responded
to specific stimuli and thus gave rise to specific sensations. And by the middle of
the century Magendie's successor Claude Bernard had shown that because the
body itself could perform the chemical synthesis of such a complex substance as
sugar, the interruption of chemical processes in the body could artifically bring
about disease. The conclusions of Magendie, Müller, and Bernard argued that
medicine might be a genuinely experimental science: chemically prepared substances could precisely affect human organs, physiologists could experimentally
tamper with nerves, pharmacologists could understand the body's functioning
chemistry and manipulate it in detail.

The local views of disease and of the human body received futher reinforce-
ment from another quarter: the changing tools of diagnosis available to physicians. At the start of the nineteenth century physicians still mainly relied on the
symptoms reported to them by patients, together with visual examination of skin
and excreta. Some thermometers existed to measure body temperature, but they
were awkward and so little used. The same could be said of watches to measure
the pulse. Percussion of the chest, introduced by Leopold Auenbrugger in the
1760s, produced diagnostically useful sounds. Then between 1816 and 1819 René
Laënnec developed the stethoscope (which he "discovered" almost accidentally).
The mercury manometer made possible more accurate readings of blood pressure by the 1820s. Between 1848 and 1854 both the ophthalmoscope and the
laryngoscope came into use, allowing the examination of the eye and the larynx,
while in the 1850s Carl Wunderlich began showing the importance of systematic
records of body temperature, regardless of the clumsy nature of the available
thermometers. The convenient body thermometer, no more than six inches long,
was designed and put into use by Thomas Allbutt in the 1860s. These diagnostic
tools had several immediate effects. They allowed physicians to focus on particular parts, organs, and functions of the body, which may have both confirmed
a "local" view of disease and contributed to the growth of specialization among
physicians; an individual physician might gain a reputation for his special skill in
the interpretation of chest noises, for example. These tools also enabled their
users to pose as detached observers of the body, simply and objectively recording the facts, especially if those facts were quantifiable, as body temperatures,

blood pressures, and pulses might be. Patients thus began the long process of putting themselves in the hands of "scientists" whose judgments depended on "objective" measurement, not on subjective interpretations of the patients' own reports of symptoms, reports necessarily couched in words, always susceptible to shades of meaning. And the new diagnostic tools also increased the assurance of physicians, which may have bolstered their prestige with the general population.

The introduction of new methods of anesthesia conferred further prestige on orthodox healing in the mid-nineteenth century. Medicine here benefited from its de facto alliance with surgery, especially in the United States (where the professional distinctions between surgeons and physicians had never been clear) and in France (where common education and licensing procedures had worn such distinctions away). Between 1845 and 1855 the use of anesthetic gases revolutionized surgical practice. Some forms of anesthesia had been used for centuries, notably different preparations involving opium, mandrake, and/or alcohol, but none of them could do more than moderate the horror of amputations or deep incisions into the viscera. Some surgeons experimented with "compression" of the nerves of a limb during amputation; others hoped to use the trances induced by "mesmerism."

Exciting developments in anesthesia, however, stemmed from the eighteenth-century discovery of gases. By about 1800 one of the pioneers of gas chemistry, Thomas Beddoes, together with his assistant Humphry Davy, had learned the curious properties of nitrous oxide, "laughing gas." In subsequent decades nitrous oxide was first demonstrated by the charismatic Davy in his popular lectures at the Royal Institution in London, and its use then became a party entertainment, as did the use of ethyl ether. A gas evening gave those who attended a chance to be silly, which (as one sarcastic observer noted) may not have been a surprise: "The first subject was a corpulent, middle-aged gentleman, who, after inhaling a sufficient dose, was requested to describe to the company his sensations: 'Why, I only feel stupid.' This intelligence was received amidst a burst of applause, most probably not for the novelty of the information."[7]

By the 1840s experiments had begun on the use of such nepenthe-like substances in surgery, initially by dentists. Horace Wells of Hartford, Connecticut, began using nitrous oxide on patients while he extracted their teeth, but when he performed a public demonstration of the technique in Boston in 1845 the "painless" effect was unconvincing. A Boston surgeon, William Morton, impressed despite the inconclusive result of Wells's trial, used ether in 1846 in the extraction of teeth and, more notably, in the public excision of a tumor. Morton's demonstrations, quickly and widely reported, spread the techniques of gaseous anesthesia to Europe, where by the end of the same year a leg had been amputated in London while the patient lay unconscious from the effects of ether.[8]

In the next year the technique was extended to childbirth, with chloroform becoming especially popular for that purpose. In 1853 anesthesia in childbirth received the highest social blessing when John Snow administered chloroform to Queen Victoria during the birth of her eighth child. Victoria, who did not like the experience of childbirth, referred to "that blessed Chloroform . . . soothing, quieting & delightful beyond measure."[9]

The rapidly spreading use of anesthetics transformed surgical practice. The previous high premium on speed in surgical procedures, requiring of the surgeon considerable strength, gave way to a concern for precision. Since the patient no longer howled and writhed in agony, the surgeon could be meticulous. Both the greater care of the surgeon and the painlessness of the operation gave patients much more confidence in the prospect of surgery, and that confidence redounded to the prestige of the medical profession. This confidence, further strengthened by the gradual adoption of antiseptic methods in surgery (to be discussed shortly), resulted in a considerable increase in the number of surgical procedures performed and in the total of operations in general.[10]

By the mid-nineteenth century, then, medicine and its ally surgery could claim greater diagnostic power and improved (and certainly gentler) surgical remedies. Medicine seemed in some sense more a science, allied with chemistry and even with physics and statistics, while the organs of the body were being seen in a more thoroughly chemical or perhaps electrical light.

The Professionalization of Nursing

In an indirect way, the position of physicians in the eyes of the general public may also have been improved by the changing position of and regard for nurses, a development which ran in tandem with the professionalization of physicians. Certainly the professionalization of nursing made the medicalization of disease and its treatment in hospitals a more appealing prospect, and although conflicts often arose between nurses and physicians over positions of power and authority in the world of the sick, on balance the physicians benefited from the nurses' new dignity.

Nursing had an ancient tradition in the Western world, historically connected with religion. Early Christian communities emphasized the care of the sick as a virtue or an obligation, and in the medieval period religious orders (of both men and women) performed nursing services. The Protestant Reformation, hostile to the religious orders of medieval Catholicism, helped to fracture nursing traditions. In Catholic Europe, at least in some places and cases, religious orders devoted to the nursing of the sick remained strong, as was true, for example, of the Sisters of Charity founded by St. Vincent de Paul in France in the early seventeenth century. But in Protestant states, where religious orders had been discouraged or suppressed, nursing had generally fallen into disrepute by the eighteenth century. Without intangible religious compensations, nursing was a task in which low wages combined with ugly drudgery.

Enlightenment thinkers and governments made several efforts to change that dismal picture. The emphasis on the role of the environment in causing (or preventing) disease obviously suggested the importance of an improved environment for the sick. Some governments, especially in Germany, acted under the influence of a cameralist ideology, perhaps along the lines suggested by Frank's "medical police"; Frank urged the state provision of nursing services that would enforce sanitation standards. In the Rhenish Palatinate the medical reformer Franz May founded a nursing school in connection with a hospital in Mannheim in 1781 (in the same period in which the education of physicians was becoming more associated with hospital experience). May emphasized general deportment together with instruction in dietary routines, bathing, bleeding, and following the orders of physicians. This training, which combined scientific lectures and practical hospital life, was an essential part of May's attempts to create a professional corps of nurses, attempts that also included a careful selection of applicants, the issuance of a certificate on completion of training, and the provision of servants for the nurses. The Mannheim system established a secular model for all future Western nursing; it spread, slowly and unevenly, through other German states in the late eighteenth and early nineteenth centuries.

One of those German nursing centers greatly influenced Florence Nightingale (1820–1910), the most celebrated figure in nursing history. Nightingale, an Englishwoman of some social standing and wealth (and a great deal of intelligence and organizational drive), found in nursing a career that allowed her to break free of her family's conventional assumptions about the proper domestic role of an upper middle-class woman. Residence in the German nursing institution at Kaiserswerth, founded by Theodor Fliedner in 1833, introduced her to disciplined professional nursing. After taking the superintendency of the Institution for the Care of Sick Gentlewomen in London in 1853, Nightingale traveled to the Crimea in 1854 to organize sanitation and nursing for the British army fighting the Russians there. Her career in the Crimea assumed mythic proportions in the English-speaking world, where she was universally revered as the "Lady with the Lamp," caring for the soldiers, although in fact she was more a ruthless sanitary reformer than a compassionate nurse. Her subsequent prestige assisted her establishment of a nursing school on the Mannheim model at St. Thomas's Hospital in London in 1860. She then had a long career as an organizer and agitator for sanitary reform, both in Britain and in India; for many years she was a self-proclaimed invalid, confined to a bed, working (and driving her colleagues) under the pressures of imminent death, although she lived to the age of ninety.

Much of Nightingale's efforts centered on the health of troops, and states seemed particularly willing to take measures in the cause of military efficiency. The British government first moved against prostitution to protect troops from venereal disease, and war spurred others (in addition to Nightingale) toward nursing reform; Jean Henri Dumont's visit to the battlefield of Solferino, in the Austro-French War of 1859, so moved him that he organized what became (with the support of some governments) the International Red Cross, and the same impulse manifested itself in the work of Clara Barton in the Civil War in the United States in the 1860s. Professional nurses, trained in the May model, backed by the prestige of Nightingale who harnessed nursing to a devout sanitationism, made hospital care of the sick a far more palatable prospect by the end of the nineteenth century. The professionalization of nursing, together with developments in surgery, thus reinforced the trends that medicalized disease and isolated the sick in hospitals over which physicians presided.

The Scientific Paradigm and Medical Education

As we have seen, governments in the nineteenth century gradually imposed a measure of uniformity on the qualifications and education of physicians. Those government controls proceeded independently from the implementation of "more science" in a physician's education, and in some cases preceded it as well, but curricular changes and the enforcement of uniformity generally worked together. The resultant model required would-be physicians to devote up to four years to the study of human anatomy, physiology, pharmacology (increasingly dominated by chemistry), and pathology as well as acquiring considerable clinical experience, preferably in a hospital. While the model varied widely, and while generalizations about the "product" are risky, a scientific paradigm of medicine encouraged both specialization and greater impersonality. The increasing complexity of a "scientific" understanding of the body and its functions certainly led to concentration on some organs and functions, for how much could the learner absorb? And science demanded a detached view of patients and their diseases, one in which ailments and those who suffered from them might be subject to experiment in order to place them properly in the system of natural laws. The germ theory added training in microbiology to the scientific mix and, as I shall argue shortly, enormously strengthened the appeal of the scientific paradigm by its apparent success; scientific medicine truly "worked," conferring on its practitioners a powerful therapeutic advantage over their competitors.

In France the Napoleonic legislation of 1803 clearly imposed these ideals on the national system of education and licensing. Other Western countries followed, somewhat raggedly, in the French wake. English universities slowly accepted a more central role for science (in their whole curricula as well as in medicine), although the Scottish system had done so much earlier; but both Oxford and Cambridge remained theoretical, and their graduates had to find clinical experience elsewhere. In the German states the spirit of *Wissenschaft* began to affect the entire university system in the first half of the nineteenth century; medical students tended to be swept up in the notion that their education should bring them in touch with the latest research, and those with more single-minded careerist goals were stigmatized.[11] After 1869 the German medical profession depended for certification on nationwide examinations, first imposed through legislation in the North German Confederation and then extended to the new Empire in 1871; before the end of the century those examinations came to assume eight semesters of medical study, including four semesters of preclinical scientific knowledge. The examinations also gradually emphasized greater medical specialization.[12] American medical schools, private and basically unregulated in their early history, took on greater scientific rigor in the 1870s when Harvard University and the University of Pennsylvania began requiring a longer course of study, more clearly related to science and to hospital experience. The foundation of the Johns Hopkins University medical school in 1893 carried the scientific paradigm further into medicine by emphasizing the relation between ongoing scientific research and medical training.[13] For more and more people of the Western world a "physician" was a person who had completed such a scientific apprenticeship. Those healers who did not accept its presuppositions either had to create a convincingly scientific alternative (as did American osteopathy, which began in the 1870s with the healing career of Andrew Taylor Still) or be relegated to some social margin, however substantial some margins might be.

The Persistence of Alternative Healing Modes

For many reasons, many people in the Western world remained hesitant to take their physical troubles to orthodox physicians. Like their medieval ancestors, patients found that physicians might be geographically remote, socially exclusive, or prohibitively expensive. The habits of people in traditional communities changed only very slowly; those who had always had recourse to midwives, bonesetters, and cunning men continued to patronize them. Orthodox medicine at the start of the nineteenth century certainly offered no clear therapeutic advantage over its irregular rivals, and the acute epidemic crises of the nineteenth century—cholera, yellow fever, typhus, diphtheria—would baffle it. And in any case the ailments that nagged at most people were of a more chronic sort rarely treated by physicians. The variety of respiratory troubles, dysenteries, and tumors as well as such chronic illnesses as malaria and tuberculosis were the special province of the village healer and the itinerant vendor of remedies.

But nineteenth-century orthodox medicine also left itself open to specific criticism. Since the seventeenth century, science had raised expectations that both made patients impatient for results and led to claims from "science" that might have little foundation. On the heels of the germ theory came "Radam's Microbe Killer"; on the heels of Hiroshima came "U-235 Drinking Water." Science seemed to encourage certainty and some irregular treatments cheerfully promised it, even if orthodox physicians were more cautious. In addition, the treatments favored by orthodox physicians in the early nineteenth century were especially daunting, involving as they did unpleasant bleeding and purging; a variety of alternative therapies emerged that all specifically boasted of easier, gentler approaches.

Certainly the alternatives to orthodox medicine remained numerous, and they claimed immense followings. In the United States alternative medicine enjoyed special vigor. Orthodox medicine had little or no legal standing, and lacked the tradition of gentility that accompanied it in the more socially stratified European countries. Much of the American population settled some distance from cities in a culture that encouraged self-healing techniques within families, a circumstance in which both geographic isolation and the ideology of the independent literate free farmer collaborated. The often-frightening remedies of orthodox American medicine, under Rush's influence in its most "heroic" mode, may have simply added fuel to a situation ideally suited to the flourishing of medical alternatives. In nineteenth-century America a rich profusion of "sects" took root, many of which simultaneously contradicted and shared the ideas and approaches of conventional physicians.

Samuel Thomson, a New Hampshire healer without formal education, began his practice in the early years of the nineteenth century, and by 1813 had won a United States patent for a system of "botanic medicine." Thomson believed that the maintenance of body heat was crucial to health, and that a variety of botanic remedies could serve to maintain it. Another (perhaps obvious) Thomsonian remedy was the steam (or hot water) bath, and Thomsonians were thus sometimes dubbed "steamers." Thomson's ideas gained a wide following, especially among those Americans moving west in the second quarter of the century; Thomsonianism had something of the character of religious revivalism, and in fact it followed the same geographic path taken by the religious revivals spreading from the "Burned-Over" district of western New York to the "West." Paul Starr notes that Thomson once claimed that his adherents included half the population of Ohio, and that even his opponents granted him one-third.[14] Thomsonianism included a virulent hatred of physicians, perhaps fired by the fact that a physician had once attempted to prosecute Thomson for murdering a patient. That hatred of physicians also expressed a belief in the virtues of the "common man," who needed no fancy European educational pedigree, and Thomsonianism may be seen as an expression of Jacksonian political culture in America.

At least before about 1850 the anti-elitism to which Thomson appealed had deep European roots as well; doctors, especially doctors supported by the powers of the state, inspired widespread resistance, fear, and even hatred. As we have seen, the seventeenth-century Italian resistance to plague regulations found an echo in the British opposition to measures taken against cholera in 1832. British fear of doctors and their state-related power also stemmed from a measure that seemed, on the surface, a model of scientific enlightenment. Parliament, responding to complaints that anatomical instruction (with its emphasis on the actual experience of human dissection) had created the loathsome trade of grave-robbing, passed an Anatomy Act in 1832 that permitted approved anatomical schools to acquire bodies from parish workhouses. The result was deeply hated by the poor; previously, the only bodies legally available for dissection were those of executed murderers, but now poverty alone could command a fate that struck both at traditional funeral customs and at Christian belief in the physical resurrection of the body.[15] For the medical profession's relations with the poor, the Anatomy Act's coincidence with a cholera epidemic created a disaster, even if it also made a more reliable supply of corpses available for medical education. Popular fear of physicians persisted. In 1847 some Norfolk villagers "believed that the state's encouragement of vaccination formed a plot to kill children under five, and Queen Victoria was a modern Herod."[16] Unwillingness to submit to compulsory smallpox vaccination remained, throughout the century, a point of resistance to both the powers of the state and the pride of scientific medicine.

So while Thomsonianism was in many ways a uniquely American movement, many of the other early nineteenth-century unorthodox therapies had European origins. One such was homeopathy, which originated with the German physician Samuel Hahnemann (1755–1843). Hahnemann first developed his theory in the 1790s and articulated it clearly in his *Organon der Rationellen Heilkunde* (1810). Hahnemann believed that ills could be cured by very small doses of substances that—in themselves—produced the same symptoms as the disease being treated; the phrase "like cures like" became homeopathy's watchword. Hahnemann married a wealthy patient late in his life, and lived in some style in Paris. But in America especially his system gained many adherents in the years after 1840, and before the Civil War homeopathic physicians had rapidly developed as a kind of mirror profession with the "allopaths" (as they called the orthodox physicians). Colleges of homeopathic medicine were founded, their memory preserved in the long-lived Hahnemann University in Philadelphia. Unlike the Thomsonians, the homeopaths did not believe that the healing arts lay within the grasp of the common man or woman; their medicine was complex and sophisticated science, to be practiced by well-educated professionals. But it was also true (as it was true of many contemporary German intellectuals) that

Hahnemann located the ultimate cause of physical phenomena in the realm of the spirit; disease for him was fundamentally a spiritual problem.

Hahnemann's homeopathy, while it trained its practitioners in the disciplines of science, therefore also coincided with other more clearly "religious" alternatives to orthodox medicine, some of which gained wide American followings. Hahnemann's ideas overlapped those of the eighteenth-century Swedish religious philosopher Emmanuel Swedenborg, and many of Swedenborg's nineteenth-century American followers (whether or not they were formal members of the New Church) also subscribed to homeopathy. In turn other Swedenborgians were drawn to mesmerism and the other offshoots of belief in a healing "animal magnetism," such as hypnotism and spiritualism.

Hydropathy, another nineteenth-century medical sect, also had European roots. Beliefs in the curative powers of water are of course very ancient and have taken many forms, including the emphasis on bathing and "lustration" found in Greek temple medicine and the popularity of mineral water cures throughout Europe. Such practices assumed a somewhat different form in the ideas of the Austrian healer Vincenz Priessnitz, who (having suffered severe accidental injuries in his late teens) worked a self-cure with bandages of cold, wet towels. In the 1820s Priessnitz opened a water-cure establishment at Gräfenberg, which in subsequent decades became a mecca for health seekers. Similar facilities began spreading in the United States in the 1840s, where hydropathy merged with a larger and more diffuse movement that promoted "natural" health through the reform of diet and dress. American hydropathy had particular importance for women.[17] Hydropathic theorists believed that their doctrines supported the traditional role of the woman as the caretaker of family health, for they emphasized the maintenance of health with sensible dress, diet, and pure water. Those beliefs also reinforced the conviction that ruggedly individual Americans could take care of themselves without the mediation of fancy European physicians. In addition, the hydropathic doctors regarded pregnancy and parturition as normal human conditions, not abnormal illnesses as did many orthodox physicians; and the hydropathic medical colleges, which appeared (as did some of the homeopathic colleges) in the years before the Civil War, enrolled women among their students.

For many sufferers from disease the claims of medicine (whether orthodox or irregular) were never convincing or became too overbearing. Some old religious traditions persisted or revived; newer ones arose as well. Traditional forms of Western Christianity fought some notable battles with the new scientific paradigms in the second half of the nineteenth century, and some of these battles affected healing practices. In 1864 Pope Pius IX issued his encyclical *Quanta cura*, which asserted that it was erroneous to believe that "[t]he Roman Pontiff can, and ought to reconcile himself, and come to terms with progress, liberalism, and modern civilization"; within Roman Catholicism cults of miraculous healing enjoyed a new popularity, perhaps most notably that at Lourdes, in France, associated with the visions of Marie Bernarde Soubirous (St. Bernadette) in 1858. The development of means of rapid mass transportation, particularly the railroad, aided the appeal of such shrines. Many Protestant groups, meanwhile, had difficulty reconciling their beliefs with those of modern science, especially with the theory of evolution by natural selection propounded by Charles Darwin in 1859. For at least one such group, the Seventh-Day Adventists in America, rejection of Darwin went hand in hand with an entire alternative system of health and medicine, laid out in the writings of the sect's leader, Ellen White (1827–1915). Still another "antimedicine" approach emerged from Christian Science, expounded in Mary Baker Eddy's *Science and Health*, first published in 1875. Eddy argued that disease—like sin—was an illusion, a product of the mind. A "cure" therefore must be sought in the mind as well, and the bodily ministrations of physicians (whether orthodox or irregular) were simply irrelevant.

In their appeal to women the hydropaths may have probed an especially dense vein of those discontented with orthodox medicine. The relation of medicine and the care of women has become a richly complex subject in modern historiography, one in which paradoxes and ironies abound. One point of view—which has been argued with some vigor—holds that in the nineteenth century medical orthodoxy regarded "female" conditions as evidence of pathology; for physicians, menstruation, pregnancy, childbirth, and menopause were all "abnormal" conditions that required medical care and a doctor's intervention. Orthodox physicians thus subjected women to a variety of treatments that began as barbaric and became (as the end of the century approached) increasingly distant, "scientific," "medicalized," removed from ordinary experience, designed to place women under a form of discipline and control. At least down to the middle of the nineteenth century, gynecological problems were treated with such horrific measures as cauterization or insertion of leeches into the uterus; menstrual cramps might be solved by a hysterectomy; and by the end of the century physicians, having gradually pushed midwives to the margin, convinced women that babies could best be born in a hospital.

Against this aggression women responded with several different defenses. Some evidence suggests that nineteenth-century women avoided treatment by orthodox physicians and took their complaints instead to other healers: empirics, midwives, hydropaths, medical botanists, homeopaths. The popularity of Lydia Pinkham's Vegetable Compound makes sense if it was an alternative to a hysterectomy for menstrual cramps.[18] In addition, as more conscious feminism appeared by the middle of the century, some women spoke out against their treatment at the hands of doctors and seized on the opportunities that arose to patronize women healers. Josephine Butler, the English crusader against the

(British) Contagious Diseases Acts of the 1860s (which singled out prostitutes) may have spoken for many other women after her visit to Elizabeth Garrett, a woman physician:

> I was able to tell her so much more than I ever could or would tell to any man. . . . Oh, if men knew what women have to endure and how every good women has prayed for the coming of a change. . . . How would any modest man endure to put himself in the hands of a woman medically as women have to do in the hands of men? . . . I pray to God that many Miss Garrett's may arise.[19]

That view, that male physicians had no understanding of women's problems, receives some further support from the changing attitudes of doctors toward abortion in the nineteenth century. In both Great Britain and the United States laws forbidding abortion either appeared for the first time or became more stringent, first with a British criminal statute in 1803, which was progressively tightened in a series of changes down to 1861, and then with a group of laws passed by individual American states between 1870 and 1900. Doctors in both countries supported the new legal stringency and (especially in the United States) actively promoted the passage of the new laws.[20] In part their loyalty to the Hippocratic oath, taken with special seriousness in the United States where professional status was relatively weak, motivated the opposition to abortion; in part doctors responded to new embryological views; but in part the doctors' politics were stimulated by the professional competition of other sects, against whom the orthodox hoped to call down the power of the law. In France either performing or having an abortion was a crime (as was true in Britain after 1861), although the severity of the code of 1810 had the effect of making convictions difficult to obtain; in Germany the imperial penal code of 1872 also sternly outlawed abortion.[21] For some women, the supposed unwillingness of physicians to perform abortions or offer abortifacient advice gave them still another reason to repair to irregular healers and the purveyors of patent medicines.

But it is not entirely clear that women were in fact the victims of doctors, or that doctors fell out of favor with women. Gynecological problems certainly received harsh treatment in the nineteenth century, but so did many complaints and ailments unrelated to sex or gender. The early nineteenth century was, after all, the age of heroic medicine; as Regina Morantz puts it, "Male genitals were cauterized by the same complacent physicians who cauterized their female patients."[22] Some women understandably avoided heroic orthodoxy and sought alternatives, but so did many men. And the "medicalization" of the treatment of women, especially in pregnancy and childbirth, was often a trend in which the wishes of the women ran ahead of the willingness of physicians. Judith Walzer Leavitt has argued that American women turned from midwives to male obstetricians (starting in the eighteenth century) because obstetricians' tools promised a relief from pain, and the same motives resurfaced when ether and chloroform were introduced in the mid-nineteenth century. Physicians feared that these anesthetics might be dangerous or might mask the signs of progress of labor, but their customers demanded their use, as they did again early in the twentieth century when the "twilight sleep" associated with scopolamine was introduced. Leavitt makes the paradoxical point that many women supported such measures despite the evident "loss of control" that they entailed, while many doctors resisted them despite the same "gains of control" they offered.[23]

The arguments about abortion policy may be muddied by similar crosscurrents. Physicians undoubtedly became alarmed by the rise in abortions which they perceived in the nineteenth century, and attempted to bring the practice of abortion both under the ban of the law and under their control in those exceptional cases that the law allowed. But did the rise in abortions (if it occurred) itself offer evidence of what Daniel Scott Smith has called "domestic feminism," the ability of women to take greater control of their private lives?[24]

And finally, real questions remain about chronology. Surely male fear of (and desire to control) female sexuality was not new in the nineteenth century, and surely doctors treated women clumsily before 1800 as well as after it. And how thoroughly were obstetrical and gynecological events "medicalized" even by 1900? Ann Oakley notes that midwives still attended 70 percent of British births in 1876, and that this proportion was undoubtedly even higher in rural areas.[25] Only in the twentieth century did American births move to hospitals; before then, Leavitt notes, home births remained the rule, and women, with their friends and relations, continued to participate actively in the process.[26]

The ambiguities of the relations of women and orthodox medicine are reflected in the fact that early nineteenth-century medical alternatives, and the orthodox physicians who denounced them so roundly, actually shared substantial common ground. Thomson and Priessnitz took a systemic and single-cause view of disease, but then so too did Benjamin Rush; and while European physicians such as Broussais were moving away from systemic views and toward local ones, many of them—with Broussais a good example—remained convinced that one grand cause produced disease. These "schools" simply disagreed about what the grand cause was, not that it existed. They all also fundamentally believed that medicine and health remained subjects of rational inquiry that was not dependent on magic or divine revelation, although Hahnemann did regard health problems as ultimately spiritual. Homeopaths and hydropaths alike aspired to the trappings of an educated profession, founding schools of medicine to mirror orthodoxy, while all manner of healers, whatever their links with the Jacksonian common man, might assume the airs of a brotherhood in possession of arcane knowledge beyond a layperson's reach. Thomsonianism, the most self-consciously anti-elite of these sects, itself gradually adopted more and more allopathic remedies, transforming itself into another sect altogether under the revealing name of "eclecticism." As Paul Starr has convincingly argued, by the period of (roughly) the American Civil War the sects and the orthodox were in fact, if not yet in theory, blending together; homeopaths and eclectics were not so much stamped out by the regulars as merged into them; as the states created their licensing schemes in the late nineteenth century the irregulars either joined the system or found themselves left out of the public favor that came to value the "scientific" claims of orthodoxy.[27]

By the late nineteenth century the orthodox medical community had succeeded in absorbing some of the alternatives that had competed with it earlier in the century. Its greater professional assurance, strengthened by the appearance of some therapeutic success and by the generally rising prestige of "science," and ratified by its connection with university education and government licensure, made it possible for it to exclude—"marginalize"—other, newer heresies (such as chiropractic) within the realm of healing and to more clearly establish demarcations between itself and the realm of religion.

The same theme—that of convergence of irregular and orthodox—emerged in the world of remedies and medications. The line between homemade remedies and items in an official pharmacopoeia was in any case never clear. Physicians, apothecaries, and the vendors of remedies often (and uneasily) inhabited the worlds of both professional healing and profitable commerce. The eighteenth-century North Atlantic world, especially, was already an aggressively entrepreneurial one. Advertising in newspapers, handbills, and pamphlets spread from England to other British regions, and to northwestern Europe and North America as well. By the nineteenth century techniques of marketing were being perfected, with the advertising of remedies for illness taking a leading or even pioneering role. Vendors of so-called patent medicines developed techniques that would identify their products in the public mind: slogans, pictorial representations, trademarks, distinctive packaging such as bottle shapes, all important because the actual products themselves might either vary little from one to another or because the sellers insisted on the arcane character of the remedy, which forbade them from telling the public their ingredients.

Of course the vending of remedies was hardly new. The itinerant quack was already a stock figure in eighteenth-century Europe; Matthew Ramsey calls him an "immediately recognizable type," and he was clearly a well-established traditional figure when Donizetti created the character of Doctor Dulcamara in *L'Elisir d'Amore* (1832).[28] Nineteenth-century entrepreneurs added an enormous increase in commercial volume and an enthusiastic exploitation of the medium of print. Cheap postage, an important item on the nineteenth-century liberal agenda, was adopted in both Britain and the United States in the 1840s; information—and advertising—thus flowed much more freely. The growth of commercial patent medicine paralleled both the development of efficient postal services and the spread of compulsory state education, which created mass literacy in Western societies.

Did mass literacy mean mass gullibility? The astonishing success of some nineteenth-century patent medicines seemed to argue that case. But the rustic Nemorino did not need to read to be assured by Doctor Dulcamara that cheap wine was in fact an elixir of love, and the arguments in support of nineteenth-century medications appealed on a number of grounds. Remedies, their sellers, and the practitioners of irregular systems of medicine all shared (and benefited from) ambivalent attitudes toward orthodox physicians. Patent medicines frequently advertised endorsements from physicians, and drew many of their materials from the same pharmacopoeias to which physicians might have reference. But at the same time patent medicines set themselves apart from the "bad" aspects of orthodox treatment. Thomas Dyott, an early nineteenth-century American remedy manufacturer, reminded his customers that his medication was "mercury-free," unlike that dreadful orthodox standby calomel. Another Philadelphia entrepreneur, William Swaim, produced medicine flavored with pleasant wintergreen.[29] Irregulars could be both "behind" and "ahead" of official medicine. Some claimed that physicians had strayed from the path of "nature" when they took up chemical and mineral remedies, and so they instead urged a return to herbals and the exploitation of the science of botany. That was the appeal of both the Thomsonians in America and the "medical botanists," such as John Frost, in Britain. But other irregulars gleefully seized the latest scientific ideas, in the manner of Franz Anton Mesmer, claiming that physicians were hopelessly conservative and unwilling to recognize the power of (for example) electricity and magnetism. The heightened expectations of science enabled vendors to feed on fears generated by the well-reported epidemic crises of the nineteenth century (and the twentieth as well). Many of the patent remedies also "tasted good" in other and more controversial ways: they contained substantial proportions of alcohol and/or opium. The widely sold Lydia Pinkham's Vegetable Compound, a remedy for "female complaints," was nearly 20 percent alcohol.[30]

The career of William Radam provides an instructive example of the unclear border between vending and science. Radam, a Texas-born gardener, read about the germ theory being enunciated by Pasteur and Koch and concluded that his body teemed with germs. He would eradicate them the way a gardener would kill pests, with some sweeping poison that left the plant (or himself) unharmed. He obtained a patent for his Microbe Killer in 1886, and within a few years the craze for microbiology had made him prosperous. He owned seventeen factories that produced Microbe Killer, he had published a book full of photographs of "bacteria" (hideous creatures that cried out for elimination), and he had moved from Austin to New York's Fifth Avenue. Attacks on his remedy by physicians, lawsuits for libel and slander, simply gave him more publicity. Never mind that analyses of the Microbe Killer claimed it to be over 99 percent water, to which were added small amounts of red wine, hydrochloric acid, and sulfuric acid; Radam flourished anyway. As James Harvey Young asks, how could ordinary people "differentiate between the credentials of microbe-hunter Pasteur and those of microbe-hunter Radam?"[31] Analytical chemistry had become a formidable science by the end of the nineteenth century, but even it might not precisely sniff out a tiny "secret" ingredient that a Radam might claim made all the difference.

By the end of the nineteenth century "patent" medicines were being produced by large corporations, which might deploy impressive laboratory facilities and employ university-trained scientists. The great German chemical firms especially illustrated that trend. With their products the line between quackery and the pharmacopoeia became murkier still. Physicians, even with a modern scientific education, had trouble keeping up with the pharmacological sophistication of Friedrich Bayer's giant works; aspirin, introduced by Bayer in 1899, was a powerful remedy, an enormous source of profit, and a "patent" medicine all at once. Such successful (and "scientific") medication might—and often did—ensnare physicians in a network of commercial complicity.

Germs, Diseases, and Doctors

The germ theory of disease, when taken together with the extension of the phenomenon of vaccination to a general preventive principle, decisively altered the relations of humans and infectious disease. It also altered, perhaps even more decisively, patterns of etiological thought that in some ways had been undisturbed since the triumph of Christianity in the old Roman Empire. But those changes, while their ultimate significance is beyond doubt, did not immediately sweep the nineteenth-century field, were not quickly accepted as self-evident truth, and had only a gradual impact on disease incidence and mortality. The professional position of physicians as healers of choice was, in the long run, immensely strengthened by the germ theory and by vaccinations, but that result was not a foregone conclusion in the last quarter of the nineteenth century, despite the adulation heaped by their successors on the germ pioneers, especially Louis Pasteur and Robert Koch.

The idea that disease might be caused by microorganisms had enjoyed some currency since the seventeenth century, when the early microscopists had first beheld the stunning world of wee life. But at least before the 1870s such conceptions were usually discounted. We have seen some arguments raised against them in connection with cholera and tuberculosis (in Chapters Seven and Eight), arguments that reflected a more general nineteenth-century conviction that complex interactions between people and environments best explained disease.

By mid-century the British sanitationists and the French party of hygiene commanded influence, allegiance, and growing government support. For them the germ theory was too simple; although Pettenkofer ultimately allowed that germs might have a role, the role was in a drama with a large cast of other actors. More generally, one of the great questions in nineteenth-century attitudes toward nature pitted "mechanical" conceptions against "vitalist" ones, and by the middle of the century the mechanical school predominated and vitalism inspired suspicion. Mechanisms, not spontaneous life, explained organic change. "Germs" did not necessarily mean spontaneous life, but they might imply it. They also represented an exogenous outside force perhaps affecting the entire organism, at a time when mechanical failure might be invoked in the widely accepted etiology that emphasized local tissue, whether in the macroscopic sense of Broussais or in the view of cellular anatomy developed by Virchow.

Despite this prevailing environmentalist and mechanical climate the germ theory won many converts between roughly 1870 and 1885 for a number of different reasons. Evidence that some diseases were related to identifiable microorganisms, including fungi, had begun accumulating in the 1830s, starting with Agostino Bassi's studies of diseases of silkworms; in the 1840s trichinosis was related to microorganisms found in both pork and humans, and a fungus seemed to explain the scalp infection called favus. In the 1850s Casimir Davaine discovered a microorganism in animals suffering from anthrax; "no accident," Ackerknecht comments, "that the first pathogenic organism discovered was one of the largest."[32] But evidence for the causative action of such organisms remained thin, and it required the genius of Louis Pasteur to make that evidence convincing to the scientific and medical communities.

Pasteur, one of the dominant scientific figures of the nineteenth century, was born in a small town in eastern France in 1822, the son of a tanner who had served in Napoleon's army. Pasteur carried throughout his life some of the marks of his origins: conventionally conservative, pious, and intensely patriotic, he was also a pugnacious controversialist with a sensitive regard for his own reputation. But his career was marked by several uninhibited leaps, both from one discipline to another and from shreds of evidence to daring assertions of certainty, that belie a view of Pasteur as a cautious small-town conservative. He practiced what Bruno Latour has called a "Theatre of Proof," in which the successful outcome of dramatic "scientific experiments" made an enormous impression on both professional and lay mentalities.

As a young student Pasteur eventually won a place at the prestigious École Normale in Paris, where he developed his first research specialty, crystallography. When he completed his studies he took positions first at Strasbourg and then at Lille, by which time (1854) his interests had shifted to the study of fermentation. The prevailing mid-century view (that of the eminent German chemist

Justus Liebig) explained that phenomenon as the result of chemical and mechanical changes. Sugar molecules underwent a mechanical rearrangement of their constituents and thus changed to alcohol. But others had argued that the yeast present in such a process consisted of one-celled organisms which directly caused the fermentation. Pasteur took that view, and by the late 1850s had won a European reputation by clearly showing the role of microorganisms in fermentation and putrefaction processes. Pasteur was strongly convinced that he had shown how the "infinitely small" could play an "infinitely great" part.[33] He had also offered practical solutions to problems faced by brewers and wine makers; to prevent products from spoilage as a result of overfermentation, the makers simply had to kill microorganisms at the right point, perhaps by heating (or "pasteurizing").

Pasteur's success, as the man who showed the workings of microorganisms in fermentation, inspired others to extend the idea that "bacteria," everywhere present as Pasteur argued, had other effects, including perhaps disease. One such convert, the British surgeon Joseph Lister (1827–1912), believed that such germs might be responsible for the "sepsis," or infection, that followed wounds and surgical openings. In 1864 he began experimenting with different techniques of "antisepsis" in surgery, and while certain success only developed after a trial-and-error process, Lister's antiseptic methods ultimately ranked with anesthesia in changing both the safety of, and opinions about, surgery. But Pasteur, while generally convinced of the importance of bacteria, was after all a professor of chemistry, not a medical practitioner; by the mid-1860s he had become interested in the silkworm diseases to which Bassi had earlier called attention, and his focus remained on those, as well as on beer and fermentation, until the mid-1870s.

Pasteur's work undoubtedly strengthened the hand of those medical researchers who believed that germs might cause disease. Among them was Robert Koch (1843–1910), the son of a German mining official, who received a medical degree from the University of Göttingen in 1866. One of his teachers there, Jacob Henle, himself espoused the germ theory. Koch practiced medicine in small German towns (first in Hannover, then in Posen) and it was from that rural obscurity that he produced (in 1876) an impressive study of the life cycle of the organism responsible for anthrax. Davaine (and others) had earlier associated a microorganism with that animal disease; Koch isolated the organism from sick animals, grew laboratory cultures of it, and then used those cultures to infect healthy animals with what developed as anthrax. The excited Pasteur, shifting to the study of infectious disease, confirmed Koch's findings (incidentally starting a quarrel over priority), and began extending his reach to other diseases of animals: chicken cholera, swine erysipelas, and rabies.

In the course of his investigations Pasteur learned that some animals could carry massively reproducing colonies of chicken cholera bacteria without themselves showing symptoms of the disease. He also discovered—almost by accident—that some cultures of bacteria lose their lethal character for some reason, becoming "attenuated," and may remain so through subsequent generations. These points recalled human experience with smallpox inoculation and vaccination to Pasteur's mind. In those cases some form of attenuated disease "essence" had been engrafted that prevented the serious symptoms of smallpox from appearing in the subject. Could not the same be done with attenuated "essence"—bacteria—of chicken cholera? If so, "vaccines" for diseases caused by microorganisms might be produced at will, provided that a reliable method of attenuation could be developed. A variety of experiments performed in Pasteur's laboratory (he had returned to the École Normale in Paris in 1857) suggested different methods of attenuating microorganisms: age them, warm them, pass them through a succession of animals.

Pasteur staged his first great "Theatre of Proof" in 1881. Anthrax, the disease that had been early associated with a microorganism and then convincingly shown so by Koch, was also a killer whose depredations of sheep and cattle gave it economic importance. In March 1881, when Pasteur announced that he had produced a workable vaccine for anthrax, French (and other) agricultural interests responded. The Agricultural Society of Melun, under the prodding of Henri Rossignol, a veterinarian skeptical of the germ theory, proposed a test, and Pasteur agreed to its terms. A group of animals at Pouilly-le-Fort (eventually twenty-four sheep, six cows, and a goat) would be "vaccinated" against anthrax by Pasteur. Subsequently they would receive a fully lethal dose of the anthrax organism, as would a comparable control group of animals that had not been vaccinated. Two days after this second treatment, on June 2, before an excited crowd that included representatives of the international press, all the vaccinated animals were alive (although one died shortly afterward), while all the unvaccinated were either already dead or dying of anthrax; two sheep cooperatively expired while the assembly watched. The sensation was immense. "Pouilly-le-Fort, as famous today as all the battlefields," wrote Henri Bouley in 1883.[34] Pasteur had taken a gigantic chance and been justified by the results.

Meanwhile claims had been made for the isolation of the agents of some human diseases. Discoverers had more trouble verifying these claims, for they hesitated to follow all of the steps modeled by Koch's anthrax experiments, especially the infection of healthy animals (in this case humans) with bacteria cultivated in the laboratory. That understandable difficulty limited the acceptance of the "discovery" of the causative organisms of leprosy (by Gerhard Hansen in 1868), of gonorrhea (by Albert Neissner in 1879), and of typhoid fever (by Carl Eberth in 1880). Although Koch was not in Pasteur's class as a showman, he provided his own sensation in 1882 when he announced the discovery of *Mycobacterium tuberculosis*; Paul Ehrlich, who was present, recalled that the "audience was too spellbound to applaud or engage in official discussion."[35] In fact in the 1880s the paths of Koch and Pasteur diverged. Koch and his followers embarked on the isolation and identification of causative microbes, in increasingly well equipped laboratories supplied by the German state and university system. Koch, no longer an obscure country practitioner, had become an advisor to the Imperial Public Health Department in Berlin (in 1880) and a professor at the University of Berlin (in 1885). Pasteur meanwhile focused on the development of vaccines, and a vaccine for a human disease afforded him an even more spectacular "Theatre of Proof."

His target—rabies—was a disease with particularly powerful cultural associations. In the nineteenth century rabies affected relatively few people in the Western world; its victims numbered fewer than one hundred per year in both France and Britain, for instance. But it inspired peculiar horror. A disproportionate number of its victims may have been children, bitten by those most domesticated friends of humanity, dogs. The latency of the disease meant that once bitten by an animal a person endured a month of terrible suspense, wondering whether rabies would strike. And if it developed that the biting animal had been rabid, and the disease took hold in the victim, both horrific symptoms and certain death ensued. The symptoms associated the disease with both bestiality and sexuality; victims raged and attempted to bite others, and they seemed in a constant state of priapic sexual arousal. Kathleen Kete has convincingly argued that the combination of violence and sex brought together the most "dreadful topics" for the nineteenth-century bourgeoisie, and gave rabies its particular cultural significance. People in different times and places created different social constructions of the disease. At least for a time among the middle classes of both France and Britain, rabies seemed a disease originating in the undisciplined dogs of the undisciplined lower orders. But in the years after 1850 French opinion tended to lay the responsibility for rabies on the refinements of urban civilization, which created an unnatural life (especially one that denied sexual outlets) for the domesticated pets of the city bourgeoisie.[36] Did rabies develop spontaneously in such frustrated canines? If so, might rabies be a judgment on the overrefinements of civilization?

Meanwhile in Britain the growing popularity of domestic dogs contributed to a debate about the ways in which the state might control them and hence perhaps control the spread of rabies. A British parliamentary act of 1871 gave local authorities power to muzzle dogs, but arguments about the effects of doing so went on into the 1890s.[37] Similar controversy raged in France, where a Paris city ordinance had compelled the muzzling of dogs as early as 1845, but there—as in Britain later—enforcement was sporadic. In addition to the urgings of those who felt muzzles represented cruelty to animals, both class and etiological opinions intruded; the urban middle classes might say that their little lap dogs never came into contact with the ravening brutes of the poor, so why should they be muzzled, while those who believed in "spontaneous rabies" feared that muzzles might simply build up frustrations in the dog and hence make it more dangerous.

Pasteur began experiments on rabies in the early 1880s, hoping to find a causative organism and attenuate it for a vaccine. Finding the organism proved difficult, for rabies is in fact a viral disease whose organism is too small to have been detected by nineteenth-century microscopes. But Pasteur and his associates worked on "vaccines" anyway, using fluids extracted from the tissues of infected animals, assuming such fluids carried the hypothetical causative organism. (After all, Jenner had never seen the smallpox organism, and Koch and his microbiologists hadn't seen it either.) In that way trial vaccines were prepared, and experiments testing their efficacy on animals begun. The long period of latency (between bite and symptoms) made Pasteur believe that the vaccine might still be effective *after* exposure. Then in 1885 the opportunity for theatre presented itself, or was seized. Joseph Meister, a nine-year-old from Alsace, was brought to Pasteur by his frantic parents; he had been bitten by a dog, and rabies loomed. Pasteur (or more properly a physician allied with him, for Pasteur could not treat humans without fear of legal repercussions) administered a series of inoculations of the attenuated vaccine to the boy, who survived unscathed. From that point Pasteur's position as a benefactor of the human race was assured. By November 1886 Pasteur's Paris laboratory had treated 2,500 people with rabies vaccine.[38] In the 1960s a poll asked a group of French schoolchildren to name who had done the most good for the country. Pasteur was named by 48 percent, far ahead of all others, including St. Louis (20 percent) and the then-living President de Gaulle (9 percent).[39]

But the panegyrics lavished on Pasteur, then and since, should not obscure the uncertainties that surrounded both the rabies vaccine and the more general "germ" theory that it seemingly vindicated. Personal difficulties divided the camp of the microbe hunters; Pasteur and Koch had serious scientific differences and quarreled over priority and the effectiveness of techniques, while national rivalries, felt by both men, exacerbated their relations. Pasteur, after all, had returned the University of Bonn's honorary degree when the Franco-Prussian War started in 1870; according to an American visitor, in 1886 Pasteur said: "The Germans are angry, especially Koch, because France has the merit of this new discovery of protection against rabies. They think that because they conquered our country in '70 that they can be our masters in this field and therefore they spread broadcast their skepticism against me."[40] As Gerald Geison has shown, tensions also existed within Pasteur's own laboratory, where his chief assistant, Emile Roux, had serious doubts about some of the master's decisions. The vaccine used in the great anthrax demonstration was not what Pasteur led the public to believe it was. More serious yet, the Meister rabies test was even riskier than it seemed, for Pasteur's animal experiments had not advanced nearly as far as he hinted they had, and the method of vaccination that he used on Meister had not been tried on an animal at all. Those critics (whether inside the camp of microbiology or outside it) who attacked Pasteur's risk taking were on even firmer ground than they realized.[41]

The effectiveness or epidemiological importance of Pasteur's rabies vaccine also came into question. Were the 2,500 people vaccinated in 1886 really saved from rabies, when fewer than 100 in France ordinarily died of rabies every year? Pasteur argued that the morbidity and mortality statistics of rabies seriously under-reported its true extent, but was mass inoculation of everyone bitten by an animal the best way to attack rabies? Was it possible that laboratory-generated strains of the disease might result in more cases rather than fewer? Was the vigorous policing and muzzling of dogs—what might be called the general public health approach—a surer route to the elimination of the scourge than the microbiological? The success of Great Britain in eliminating rabies from its territory by the second decade of the twentieth century by careful policing and quarantine argued that microbiology and vaccines were hardly needed. And as we have seen with both tuberculosis and cholera, the "discovery" of a causative organism did not result in any immediate breakthrough in the prevention and treatment of either; a vaccine for tuberculosis emerged only slowly, incompletely, and surrounded by controversy, and Koch's attempts to impose his bacteriological model on Hamburg during the 1892 cholera epidemic were widely resisted.

But germ theory and the possibility of preventive vaccination commanded enormous respect regardless. Pasteur's daring experiments had *worked*: twenty-four Melun sheep lived, Joseph Meister lived, and the world's press reported it all. Bruno Latour, in a sensitive discussion of the grounds for acceptance of the germ theory, suggests that Pasteur's theatre won converts partly because it was theatre, but also because germ theory provided the dominant "hygiene" or "sanitationist" approach with a crucial tool. Sanitationism or "hygiene" took a very broad view of disease etiology, unwilling to rule out any conceivable variable. But as Latour says, "[s]ince anything might cause illness, it was necessary to act upon everything at once, but to act everywhere is to act nowhere." Students of public health, the party of hygiene, seized upon Pasteur and germ theory because with them the attack on disease gained sudden and dramatic focus. All the problems that consumed the sanitationists—"overcrowding, quarantine, smells, refuse, dirt"—could be "retranslated or dissipated. Either the microbe gets through and *all precautions are useless*, or hygienists can stop it getting through and *all other precautions are superfluous*."[42] Some dramatic attacks on microbes were made in subsequent decades by sanitationists, attacks that vindicated germ theory more clearly than did controversial vaccines; but the success of Pasteur's theatrical vaccine trials had given the sanitationists a direction that they had lacked.

Germ theory established the "objective," "external" view of disease more firmly than ever. Disease had an independent existence, apart from the healthy animal or human frame. Latour notes that anthrax quickly went from being a "cattle disease" to a "disease of the anthrax bacillus," and that model was to be followed for many others.[43] When Florence Nightingale, a sanitationist who did not like the germ theory, insisted that disease was "an adjective, not a noun substantive," she spoke for an earlier tradition, one that placed "disease" and "health" on a continuum; the body was more or less healthy or diseased, never wholly one or the other except in death. Germs located diseases in their own separate organisms, which invaded an otherwise-healthy body. Germ theory also stood as a logical extreme in trends in nosology, which had—since the eighteenth or even the seventeenth century—been moving slowly and fitfully toward more distinct definitions of separate diseases, understanding that small-pox differed from measles in more than just degree. Germ theory explained those distinctions as the product of different microorganisms.[44]

Concluding Thoughts

By the end of the nineteenth century science had reshaped attitudes toward disease in several ways, not always in agreement with one another. Beyond doubt disease could be conquered, as an external enemy. Several different groups of warriors claimed the central place in the battle line: engineers, if one accepted the preventive powers of sanitation; microbiologists, if one saw germs as the great foe. And in any case, microbiology had also suggested new possibilities of cure as well as prevention. If causative microorganisms could be killed after they invaded the body, or if their actions could in some manner be neutralized, then the physicians who mastered those techniques would stand as undoubted healing geniuses. Of course the healers might not be physicians. Pasteur, a chemist, "cured" rabies; Radam, an entrepreneur, claimed to cure many things. But this therapeutic promise came at a time when physicians in the West had clearly associated themselves with "science," and they had also won increasingly strong legal positions of professional privilege, reflecting the prestige of science and the hopes that it inspired.

And the changing character of Western civilization in the nineteenth century also strengthened the hand of the scientific physician. To the extent that the Western world became more urban, it probably lost touch with much traditional healing and with many traditional healers. In part for the same reason, an increasing proportion of the Western population fell out of touch with the everyday presence and pressure of religion. The oft-cited British census of 1851, which included inquiries about religious observance showing that less than half of the population attended Christian services on a given Sunday, stood as evidence of the decline in religious practice. (The same census also showed that more than half the British population could be defined as urban.) In place of religion and traditional healing would come new forces, many of them commercial, still others professional, which would create and reflect both wants and expectations. Some of those expectations related to the conquest of disease, and physicians—and the vendors of medications—promised that conquest. But did the new science win its war? Did germ theory, combined with sanitation, mean an "End of Epidemics"?

Eleven

The Apparent End
of Epidemics

By the middle of the twentieth century some social and medical observers (including historians) believed that the end of epidemic diseases was in sight. The American magazine *U.S. News and World Report,* reflecting in 1955 on the development of a poliomyelitis vaccine, maintained, "There are diseases that offer threats, but, over all, in the field of infectious ones, most of the killing ones are under control." The same magazine confidently predicted that "[m]an one day may be armed with vaccine shields against every infectious ill that besets him." Richard Harrison Shryock, a distinguished historian of medicine, allowed that Condorcet's remarkable Enlightenment prediction that science would free humanity of old age and death "may yet prove correct."[1] Scientific biomedicine had combined with sanitary engineering, sophisticated political machinery, and widespread public enthusiasm for the dictates of health to bring to apparent fruition the promises of science first made in the seventeenth century. One by one the perils of various infectious epidemic diseases seemed to fade away under the combined assault of enlightened public health and sanitation, the extension of the preventive principle of vaccination, and the curative powers of laboratory products, among which antibiotics created the greatest sensation and held out the most exciting prospects. In many ways twentieth-century scientific medicine changed the relations between humans and disease both decisively and for the better. Although scientific medicine owed most of its earlier success to nonmedical factors, a review of recent Western population history will show its demographic significance in the years after World War I.

Two other phenomena have, however, intruded on that progressive picture: scientific medicine succeeded only by fits and starts, and never completely; and some of its consequences were both unforeseen and unpleasant. Disease,

considered as an objective and biological reality, continues its symbiotic relations with its human hosts despite biomedicine's best efforts; considered as a
human mental construct, twentieth-century disease wears many faces, some of
them molded by the purported end of epidemics, but others with a different,
sometimes long (and not often happy) history.

Disease, Medicine, and Demography

The balance of power between people and certain infectious diseases
shifted decisively (although perhaps temporarily) in the first sixty years of the
twentieth century. Mortality from tuberculosis, syphilis, bacterial pneumonia,
diphtheria, whooping cough, measles, and poliomyelitis (among others) plunged
dramatically, in each case as a direct result of the application of preventive or
curative biomedicine. But the demographic significance of those successes is
harder to assess, for they followed on the heels of other demographic change
mediated by human (not necessarily medical) agency.

Were human responses to disease demographically effective even before the
twentieth century? That question has been among the most widely discussed
issues in modern historiography, and its resolution remains elusive, both
because of the very large number of variables determining mortality (many of
them interrelated if not actually interdependent) and because basic data for the
period before the middle of the nineteenth century are fragmentary at best. Some
review of the variables, and of the present tentative conclusions of scholarship,
may place the impact of triumphant biomedicine in a clearer context.[2]

Modern demographic historians now widely agree that the transition to
today's low mortality in the West occurred in two or perhaps three stages. The
first stage, roughly the eighteenth century (or perhaps the period from about
1730 to about 1820), saw a decline in mortality rates. Although that decline was
halted in the early and mid-nineteenth century, it was not succeeded by notable
upward surges in mortality rates of the kind that had marked the cyclical movements of earlier Western population history. Instead, after a mid-nineteenth-
century pause, the decline in mortality resumed with perhaps greater force in
the last thirty years of the century, and that decline, though staggered by the
appalling experience of early twentieth-century wars and an influenza pandemic,
became steeper by the mid-twentieth century, a period that may constitute a third
and separate stage.

Of these periods the first is at once the simplest and the most difficult: simple
because the number of variables may be fewer, especially those of human
agency; difficult because the data are both sparse and controversial. This book
has already noticed some of its likely elements, one of the most important of
which was the decline in "crisis mortality" that followed the disappearance of
plague from the West. The role of human agency in plague's remission remains

dubious (see Chapter Three), although a case has been made for the efficacy of quarantines in checking plague's diffusion. More serious doubts surround the purported decline of other diseases that may have contributed to "crisis mortality," especially smallpox. If the mortality from smallpox declined (an unproven point), was eighteenth-century inoculation both widespread enough and effective enough to have had a demographic impact? Or might the lethality of smallpox have declined autonomously?

Of course human agency may have been more general and less direct than a straightforward attack on specific diseases. Thomas McKeown, whose ideas on the cause of declining mortality have become both a paradigm and a target, argued that improvements in nutrition should receive credit for most of the reduction in Western mortalities before the twentieth century.[3] Applying McKeown's thesis to the eighteenth century has been frustrated by a lack of data, especially about causes of death. The lethality of plague and smallpox has little or nothing to do with victims' nutritional state, and until we know more precisely what killed eighteenth-century Europeans, "nutrition" will remain a speculative explanation. It is true that new high-calorie crops (notably the potato) spread in some parts of Europe. It is also true that in some places a more "national" grain market developed, which may have reduced local shortages and famines, and that the stronger governments of the Enlightenment made efforts to counter subsistence crises.

More important, however, may have been measures stimulated by Enlightenment ideologies, undertaken by a combination of government and the general public. As James Riley has argued, a belief in the importance of "environment" pervaded the Enlightenment, and led governments and private individuals to undertake environmental changes such as drainage and urban cleansing as part of attacks on general "miasmas."[4] The often-inadvertent result may have interrupted the lives of disease vectors, especially insects. Yet more convincing is the suggestion of Marie-France Morel that Enlightenment ideology began an important change in the care of infants, which in turn led to a reduction in infant mortality (at least in France) by the late eighteenth century.[5] Morel notes the Enlightenment view of infancy as a time of uncorrupted goodness, which joined increasing state concerns with ensuring population growth and hence state power. By the time of the revolution French mothers were urged to breast-feed their children, the practices of unskilled midwives were under attack (as were wet-nurses), and leaders of medical and social opinion demanded new levels of hygiene. Of course these measures could only spread through the population slowly, despite any number of government orders; but Morel's data certainly show a decline in French infant mortality after about 1790.

So improved nutrition, attacks on general environmental "corruption," changes in the care of infants, and the beginnings of preventive measures against smallpox may all have been human-mediated causes of declining mortality rates by the end of the eighteenth century. But the most important clue was the dog that didn't bark—plague—and the human role there remains unproved. Alfred Perrenoud makes the stimulating suggestion that our view of the role of climate may have been misplaced, focusing as it has on the relation between climate and crops. The eighteenth century was the heart of the "Little Ice Age" in the West, and Perrenoud argues that it may have therefore been a difficult age for disease-bearing microorganisms and their vectors.[6]

By the early decades of the nineteenth century the disease environment had changed, as we have seen in Chapters Seven and Eight. The great crisis epidemics, especially plague, had receded, although assertions that they had entirely disappeared depend too much on evidence from a few well-studied northwestern European countries. The new importance of more endemic infections, however, especially those that flourished in the urban conditions of the nineteenth century, offset the gains made against crisis epidemics. Airborne diseases of crowds, especially tuberculosis but also diphtheria, measles, and influenza, had greater opportunity, as did waterborne diarrhea, dysentery, cholera, and typhoid. The likely decline in living standards for many urban dwellers, at least in some period of the century, brought together an array of interconnected variables: poorer nutrition, crowded housing, lack of clean water and sewage removal, and exposure to hazardous work environments that may also have included carcinogens. Infants and children may have been particularly at risk from diseases carried by contaminated foods and impure water. For whatever combination of reasons, the declines in infant mortality seen earlier in France and England came to a halt by the middle of the century.

That mid-century check proved temporary, for strong evidence exists that a decline in mortality resumed in the last decades of the nineteenth century (see Table 11.1). To explain that decline requires a truly multicausal analysis. The greatest contributions to the declines came from reductions in infant and child mortality and from falling death rates from tuberculosis. Both those subjects involved a variety of autonomous, social and economic, public health, nutritional and deliberate medical causes, and so well illustrate the complexities of explaining demographic change and its relation to disease.

Infant and child mortality fell partly because the gradual adoption of different child-rearing practices noticed by Morel in the late eighteenth century gained momentum in the late nineteenth. Concerns with national health generated by political fears of national "degeneracy," common, for example, in France after 1871 and Britain after 1899, manifested themselves in many ways, but they included national intervention in infant and child welfare, inspection of premises by public health nurses, and instruction for and propaganda directed to mothers on the benefits of breast-feeding, timely inoculations, frequent baths, hand washing

_____ Table 11.1_____

Death Rates in Selected Countries: Nineteenth Century and c. 1914

Country	Crude deaths/1,000 population	
	19th century	By about 1914
Austria	Over 26 every year until 1897	20.3 in 1913
England/Wales	Over 20 every year until 1881	13.3 in 1912
France	Over 20 every year until 1897	17.5 in 1912
Germany	Over 23 every year until 1894	15.0 in 1913
Italy	Over 25 every year until 1895	17.9 in 1914
Russia	Over 32 every year until 1897	26.5 in 1912
Spain	Over 26 every year until 1903	21.3 in 1912

Source: Compiled from B. R. Mitchell, *European Historical Statistics, 1750–1970* (New York: Columbia University Press, 1975), 105–119.

before food preparation, and the boiling of water and milk. As Morel admits, the spread of such practices could not be dramatically imposed from above, but surely they had an impact.[7] Those conscious attempts to improve infant and child welfare, regardless of their motivations in the gritty realities of nationalist power, combined with the improving home environments that characterized maturing industrial economies. The size of houses increased, reliable piped water supplies and sewage removal systems reached them, and technological changes made household surfaces easier to clean.[8]

The incidence and/or mortality of specific childhood diseases began falling in the decades after 1870 for a variety of reasons. Diphtheria, a serious childhood scourge by the mid-nineteenth century, retreated partly as a result of reducing crowding in urban housing, thus decreasing the opportunities for airborne transmission. The beginnings of surgical treatment—tracheostomy—may have contributed to a reduction in mortality. But as Anne Hardy notices, the severity of the disease was coincidentally declining autonomously. Hardy also notes that the fall in scarlet fever mortality ran ahead of morbidity decline, suggesting another exogenous decline in severity, although that disease may also have earlier flourished in crowded conditions where the possibility of larger infective doses existed.[9] Whooping cough's decline may have been related to improved nutrition and also to the gradually improving child nursing habits mentioned by Morel. And although mortality from measles declined more slowly before World War I— its morbidity was kept especially high by the spread of compulsory education in Western states—it too responded to improvements in nutrition, housing, and parental nursing habits. These reductions in childhood infectious disease occurred at different rates in different places. Graziella Caselli's comparative study of England and Italy suggests that by the middle of the nineteenth century England had already achieved some such reduction (as apparently had France), perhaps owing to greater social and economic change, perhaps to Enlightenment-inspired changes in parental customs.[10] Italian rates (and perhaps also German) remained higher until the late nineteenth century, but they then fell dramatically in the face of rapid economic change and state pressure for healthier children.

The case of tuberculosis was especially important for late nineteenth-century mortality, and its complexities have already been discussed (see Chapter Eight). Its severity may have declined autonomously, or Westerners may have gained more resistance to tuberculosis through a grim process of natural selection by the end of the nineteenth century. Improvements in nutrition, if and when they occurred, certainly strengthened the ability of individuals to resist the serious manifestations of a tuberculosis infection. A whole range of "standard of living" improvements in the late nineteenth century may have been relevant, especially reductions in overcrowded dwellings and the provision of fresh air access in workplaces and schools. Reduced residential density, related both to rising per capita incomes and to the developing technology of commuter transportation, generally lessened the likelihood of airborne infection. The isolation of victims in sanatoria, hospitals, and workhouses reduced the chances of contagion. Again, rates varied from place to place (see Chapter Eight), with more dramatic reductions in the areas of greatest economic development. In some cases, but not all, high initial rates also accompanied proportions of urban concentration; England's tuberculosis rate, considerably above Italy's in 1871, fell to approximate the latter's by 1901.[11]

While tuberculosis and childhood infections receded due to a variety of human responses and exogenous changes, the water- or foodborne diseases— cholera, typhoid, diarrhea, dysentery—clearly fell to improved sanitary regimens, including water purification, sewage and refuse removal, and changes in food preparation and personal habits. Regional differences in those diseases remained striking through World War I, depending clearly on the impact of the sanitary gospel. Death rates from diarrhea and enteritis in Italy were three or four times their English equivalents in 1881, and actually increased in the next twenty years. By the end of the century typhus was largely eradicated from countries such as the United States and Britain where sanitation had entered the national ethos (although the disease's specific etiology remained a mystery); in other places it persisted and enjoyed a powerful revival in the filthy (and often lousy) horror of World War I.

Thus while curative medical intervention played almost no demographic role in the late nineteenth and early twentieth centuries, it does not follow that demographic decline occurred solely for inadvertent or exogenous reasons. Deliberate preventive actions—those of sanitation, urban and workplace regulation, housing codes, infant health propaganda—played an important role, joining other more consciously medical preventives such as smallpox vaccination and the growing insistence on antiseptic conditions, the last-named probably important in declining infant (and maternal) mortality. And perhaps most important of all for health, many fully industrial societies achieved a dramatic decline in birth rates. Smaller families had many benefits for the health of their members, including (but not limited to) the mothers of children.

A combination of factors therefore marks the period between (roughly) 1880 and the beginning of World War I as crucial in Western demography. Two other features about disease and demography in the late nineteenth century should be noted. First, if mortality rates for the Western world as a whole declined more dramatically in those years than they had earlier in the century, regional differences might have been partially responsible. Infant mortality and childhood infections, whose decline was a major component of the overall improvement, had apparently been falling more gradually and continuously in Britain, France, Sweden, and the Netherlands; in the last decades of the century Germany, Italy, Spain, and even Russia may have begun to catch up, and their joining the parade clearly swelled its momentum. Second, the late nineteenth century saw an important shift in the death rates of the two sexes. Women's mortality rates had long reflected the consequences of differential nutrition (men got more to eat) and the ravages of pregnancy and childbirth. In the late nineteenth century women benefited from the medicalizing/sanitizing of childbirth, from declining birth rates that reduced pregnancy-related deaths regardless of medical intervention, and from improvements in the home environment. Men, at the same time, faced a greater variety of accidental dangers, and (more important) increasingly weakened their health and resistance to disease by the consumption of alcohol and tobacco. The gulf between male and female mortality would continue to widen in the twentieth century, to the disadvantage of the males. But regardless of differences by region or gender, by the end of the nineteenth century scientific biomedicine was poised to make its own clear contributions to declining Western mortality.

Triumphant Biomedicine
Prevention

By the early twentieth century the aims of public health had acquired a sharper focus. Thanks to the germ theory, attacks on specific microorganisms and their vectors could replace the much more difficult attempt to purge an entire ecosystem. Yet the old broad-gauge approach to public health did not immediately disappear, in part because the associations of dirt and disease still afforded strong resonances with social class. Conscious public health now included both the precise attack on the vectors of disease and the continuing general concerns with clean water, the disposal of human wastes, regulations about the handling of foods, and increasing public and legal pressure on the personal habits of individuals.

Insects suddenly seemed both a menace and an answer to questions about disease transmission. After 1897 *Anopheles* mosquitoes were believed to carry malaria; yellow fever was convincingly traced to *Aedes aegypti* in 1900; in the years between 1895 and 1914 the rat flea accounted for plague; in 1909 and 1910 Charles Nicolle and Howard Ricketts established the links between typhus and lice; the tsetse fly was associated with African trypanosomiasis in 1895. As we have seen in Chapter Nine such knowledge conferred great power on preventive medicine. The American campaigns against mosquitoes, malaria, and yellow fever in Cuba and Panama inspired confidence and understandably fed a desire to find and eradicate other insect vectors. The rapid rise of poliomyelitis in the early twentieth century baffled epidemiological opinion, which wanted to call it a disease of filth carried by the unwashed lower orders. But it occurred with disturbing frequency in the well-scrubbed middle classes. Insect transmission of a poliomyelitis bacterium or virus might explain its appearance in both slums and suburbs, and so health reformers held the fly accountable for the serious 1916 poliomyelitis epidemic in the United States.

Beliefs in insect vectors led logically to extensive campaigns to eliminate the pests, or at least remove them from contact with humans. Breeding pools were drained; attractive sites for insects were cleaned, and when the automobile ousted the horse from city streets in the first quarter of the century the fly lost its beloved horse manure; screens barred flies and mosquitoes from homes and shops; chemical attacks commenced on the insect world, culminating with the employment of dichlorodiphenyltrichloroethane (DDT) as a lethal insecticide in World War II.

Rat eradication became part of a gradually evolving set of responses to the menace of plague, a disease that might have resulted in as many as 13 million deaths (largely in Asia) between 1894 and 1914. In the early stages of that pandemic—for example in British-controlled Hong Kong and Bombay, and in American Honolulu and San Francisco—governments attempted draconian disinfection and isolation of "filthy" populations of Asians. But as awareness of the role of rats grew, such sweeping and indiscriminate sanitation policies took on a narrower focus. The contrasts between the responses of San Francisco authorities in 1900 and in 1907, when plague returned in the wake of the 1906 earthquake, illustrated the evolution. The rat, not Chinatown, became the target.[12] Rat eradication was subsequently pursued, although at times fitfully, in regions of plague epidemics (especially India and Manchuria). A little later the development of the anticoagulant substance called warfarin (between 1939 and 1948) had particular importance in the control of rats and hence in halting the spread of plague.[13]

Such attempts to interrupt the relation of humans and disease vectors were not always simple, and consent for them was not always unanimous. In India, for example, Hindus sometimes objected to the killing of rats; more generally, massive attempts to eradicate mosquitoes might become very costly and hence arouse taxpayer resistance, especially when (as was true of *Anopheles* mosquitoes) their complete elimination meant huge environmental changes to neighboring unsettled areas. DDT eventually had disastrous effects on other species of life. Window screens and the solid housing construction (including roofing) that would separate humans from insects and rodents too often depended on a respectable family income, which meant that the poor often continued to bear the brunt of disease spread by animal vectors. Animals (both wild mammals and domestic creatures, especially dogs) also spread rabies; by the end of the nineteenth century some authorities demanded that dogs be muzzled, while other states—notably Great Britain, favored by its insular position—instituted rigorous animal quarantines, successfully in the British case, for rabies disappeared from that country by the 1920s.[14]

These preventive measures and their apparent precision grew out of the germ theory and the association of specific diseases with specific microscopic (or submicroscopic) agents. Something of the same theory could be applied to more general sanitation. The provision of "clean water" meant water free of certain microorganisms. Sewage should be removed and treated not because it offended tender sensibilities but because the organisms of cholera, typhoid fever, and dysentery made their homes in it. It is also worth recalling how much the successful supply of clean water and the removal of sewage depended on cultural as well as technical factors. Water-and-sewer system construction represented a heavy capital expense that required a consensus of the taxpayers; it might also require a state with considerable powers of coercion to override powerful private property rights. Human behavior itself might have to change if the systems were to be effective; toilet bowls had to be cleaned regularly, and wastes had to actually reach the bowls, to suggest only two actions that should not be taken for granted. The effectiveness of plumbing systems also depended, Anne Hardy reminds us, on the skill with which they were installed; the professionalization of the plumbing trade in the late nineteenth and early twentieth centuries is a relevant subject in the history of preventive public health.[15]

Other public health measures demanded other reformations of personal habits. The preparation, preservation, and handling of foods came under new scrutiny, when it was realized that microorganisms reached the body through the mouth. The social discipline of washing hands, especially after excretion, acquired a new and more urgent rationale. Some foods, it was argued, required special treatment: notably milk, after bovine tuberculosis was linked to infected milk. The "pasteurization" of milk itself meant a challenge to cultural norms of taste. More general social habits also came under censure. Assailed were spitting as a vehicle for the spread of tuberculosis; smoking tobacco (especially in the years after 1960) as a diffuser of lung cancer and emphysema; and—a habit that long had been under public health scrutiny—sex (especially the casual commercial sort) as the transmitter of syphilis, gonorrhea, herpes, and (toward the end of the twentieth century) AIDS. (Further discussion of public health concerns with sex will follow in both this chapter and the next.)

Epidemiology emerged, by the end of the nineteenth century, as a conscious and separate branch of medical science. Its principles entered into the matrix of preventive public health, and in doing so created more social tension and conflict over the proper extent of state power organized against the rights of the individual. Epidemiologists insisted first on the accurate collection of data, which meant the identification of all sufferers from a disease. That required cooperation from physicians (and other providers of care), whose notification to authorities might breach the confidentiality of the healer-patient relationship. Of course "identification" of a disease became much clearer with the acceptance of the germ theory; when disease was defined by the presence of certain microorganisms in the body (which could be discovered by microscopic examination of blood, other fluids, or cells) rather than by external symptoms observed by a physician or described by a patient, "certainty" and "objectivity" asserted themselves. Once a victim was identified he or she could be hospitalized or otherwise isolated, and the process of "contact epidemiology" could begin; tracing the personal contacts of the bearer of a contagion could help to further isolate the disease and contribute to understanding the mechanism of its diffusion, but the procedure also threatened individual privacy and community regard alike. Diseases whose construction carried moral and/or class freight posed particularly hard choices for such contact epidemiology, as we shall see.

The realization that some diseases might be spread by "carriers," who harbored causative microorganisms without themselves manifesting physical symptoms, created some poignant cases. Perhaps the best-known was Mary Mallon, New York's "Typhoid Mary." Mallon, a cook, was employed in some typhoid-stricken houses between 1900 and 1907. Confined after a struggle in 1907, she was found to be "continuously discharging" typhoid bacteria. But by then still-widely-held standards, she was not "sick"; if illness depended on the observation of symptoms she was perfectly healthy. No wonder that she resisted confinement, both physically and with legal appeals. A prolonged period of alternating confinements and releases ensued, as authorities wrestled with the conflicting imperatives of individual liberty and public health. She was eventually isolated on an island in New York's East River. By the time of her death in 1938 New York alone had registered hundreds of chronic "carriers" of typhoid; for reasons having as much to do with gender, class, and ethnicity as with microbiology, Mallon alone was isolated.[16]

Much, though not all, of the public health machinery that contributed to twentieth-century prevention of diseases was inherited from the nineteenth (or earlier) centuries. The late nineteenth-century germ theory contributed the identification of some specific vectors and a rationale for long-standing attempts to purge environments of "filth." What was newer at the beginning of the twentieth century was the extension of the practice of vaccination (against smallpox) into a general preventive principle. The preparation of vaccines (apart from smallpox) began in the 1880s with those which prevented animal diseases (as we saw in Chapter Ten); the great age of human vaccines began after the turn of the century, when an expanding number of preventive specifics joined smallpox vaccine and the use of quinine as a preventive of malaria. A vaccine for typhoid appeared in the 1890s, although its effective use began in World War I. The 1920s brought a number of vaccines, including those for diphtheria, tetanus, and tuberculosis (the so-called BCG, for which see Chapter Eight). In the next decade vaccines appeared for typhus, whooping cough, and yellow fever; the first of those found extensive use in World War II, as did vaccines for influenza (for which unsuccessful vaccines had appeared as early as the 1890s). The dramatic creation of a vaccine for poliomyelitis in 1955 (about which more shortly) was followed in the 1960s by vaccines for measles, mumps, and rubella. The effects of some of these on disease incidence were sensational, at least in the short run.

Nor did preventive medicine limit itself to vaccines against specific infections. During World War II sulfonamides, developed primarily as curatives, also found widespread preventive application against streptococcal and meningococcal infections, especially scarlet fever. The science of pharmacology created a host of substances that chemically readjusted physiology, in the hope of preventing diseases of degeneration (thus remedies for hypertension) or of psychiatric distress (thus a great variety of antidepressants). Even mechanical or electrical devices (such as heart pacemakers) could interfere with errant physiology.

Cure

In the twentieth century, biomedicine apparently gained enormous ground in its ability to diagnose and cure diseases, especially infectious epidemics that had previously been beyond control. Quinine had given humans some power to cure malaria; mercury compounds had some effect on syphilis. Otherwise—before the twentieth century—medical intervention had usually been futile. After 1900 laboratory scientists discovered specific remedies for more diseases, developed the general technique of serum therapy, and then moved to more general curative substances, notably bacteriostatic agents, which halted the spread of microorganisms, and antibiotics, which killed them. And just as mechanical and electrical technologies were employed in prevention, so too they entered into cure, although with less success than that of bacteriostatic and antibiotic substances.

The first new specific—against syphilis—was developed by the German bacteriologist Paul Ehrlich, a disciple of Robert Koch. Ehrlich sought a "magic bullet" that would be specifically toxic for a particular organism and harmless to the organism's host. Ehrlich experimented with aniline dyes, which had had a central place in German industrial chemistry since the 1860s. He tested their effects on malaria and the protozoan diseases caused by the trypanosomes, including syphilis. In 1909, on his 606th trial, he produced a compound called Salvarsan (or "606") that proved effective against the syphilis trypanosome. By 1912 he had produced Neosalvarsan, which had less serious side effects. As we shall see, a number of social and "moral" problems accompanied the use of these specifics; while they were effective against syphilis (though not against its neurological symptoms) their use was not universal. Neosalvarsan did not eradicate syphilis.

More exciting than specific magic bullets, because more general, was the principle of serum therapy. In the late 1880s bacteriologists discovered that the microorganism responsible for diphtheria produced "toxins," and that these toxins had pathological effects. Soon afterward Emil von Behring and Shibasaburo Kitasato, colleagues of Koch, showed that animals could be treated by doses of such toxins in increasing strength, that such animals then had blood serum (that is, the fluid that separates from a blood clot) which could counteract subsequent toxins, and that such serums might be transferred to the blood of other animals to serve as an "antitoxin."

Von Behring and Kitasato had originally worked with the disease tetanus, which also fed toxins into the bloodstream. Tetanus, a disease most often carried into the body from wounds, may have been declining by the late nineteenth century because of economic and social change. Tetanus especially flourished in rural areas where cuts and punctures were common among populations that worked with agricultural tools. The decline of the proportion of the work force in agriculture affected the incidence of tetanus. But the same forces made diphtheria, an airborne disease, increasingly common. Diphtheria obviously flourished in urban settings, especially those of overcrowding, and most especially among children. The spread of systems of universal state education, common in most of the Western world between 1840 and 1900, created more opportunities for such a crowd disease of childhood. Von Behring and Kitasato turned their attention from tetanus to diphtheria, and when von Behring dramatically treated a sick child with diphtheria antitoxin—on Christmas Day 1891—he joined Pasteur and Koch in the bacteriological pantheon. Other serum experiments and developments were less successful. Attempts to produce serums to treat typhoid and erysipelas simply failed. Serums for pneumonia, which evolved with the realization (after about 1910) that "pneumonia" included several types, required sophisticated diagnosis and equipment to administer the correct type of serum. Serums for scarlet fever appeared by about 1930, but their value was never clearly established. The success of serum therapy for tetanus and diphtheria kept alive interest in the extension of the antitoxin principle, however.

More exciting yet were the sulfonamides, or "sulfa drugs," the first of which was produced by Gerhard Domagk in 1935. Like Ehrlich, Domagk experimented with chemical dyestuffs. While in the employ of the German chemical firm I. G. Farben, he learned that a certain dye, "prontosil red," protected mice from streptococci. The dye was converted in the body to sulphaniamide, which had a bacteriostatic effect on parasitic microorganisms, inhibiting their multiplication and thus giving the body's antibody defenses a chance. Several other sulfonamides were developed between 1935 and 1940, and until about 1950 medical practitioners and biomedical researchers responded enthusiastically to them. They often had dramatic effects on the streptococcal diseases, erysipelas, puerperal sepsis, some forms of pneumonia and meningitis, gonorrhea, and dysentery. Between 1935 and 1950 over 5,400 articles about sulfa drugs appeared in medical journals, and as early as 1941 physicians administered 1,700 tons of sulfa compounds in the United States alone.[17]

The excitement over sulfa drugs, while intense, was relatively short-lived largely because of the nearly contemporary development of antibiotics. Sulfonamides inhibited evil bacteria; antibiotics annihilated them, much more satisfactory in the century of total war. The first antibiotic seemed in some ways to be a serendipitous discovery, although in fact the theory of antibiotics had been established in the late nineteenth century. William Radam's Microbe Killer now seemed to come to life. In 1928 Alexander Fleming, of St. Mary's Hospital, London, observed that a mold grew (accidentally) on a plate where he was cultivating staphylococci organisms, and that the staphylococci subsequently dissolved. The mold was of the species *Penicillium notatum,*and from it Fleming extracted the active substance penicillin. Attempts to concentrate this substance in quantities sufficient to allow testing failed until the late 1930s, as attention shifted to the sulfa compounds. But in 1940 Howard Florey and Ernst Chain of the University of Oxford produced enough penicillin to allow a test on a mouse infected with streptococci. The successful result led to a human trial in April 1941, briefly successful until the penicillin ran out and the patient died.

Frustrated by his inability to interest pharmaceutical companies in war-torn Britain, Florey took his arguments to the United States. Partly through the mediation of Alfred Richards of the American government's Office of Scientific

Research and Development (itself organized in 1941 to relate science to war activities), several American companies became interested in manufacturing penicillin. By the spring of 1943 enough tests had been performed to convince American officials that the substance had an important future in preventing war wound infections, especially those involving staphylococci that had proved resistant to sulfonamides. By the end of that year American production of penicillin had become massive; although most penicillin was intended for military use, word of its miraculous powers reached the general public and pressure for its release to the civilian world increased. By the end of the war, extravagant possibilities for the antibiotic were foreseen: as a household salve, in eyewash and mouthwash, in toothpaste, in contraceptive jellies, in throat lozenges.[18]

For penicillin had in fact displayed powerful curative powers against a wide range of infections: forms of pneumonia and meningitis, staphylococcal infections, such streptococcal problems as puerperal sepsis, erysipelas, and scarlet fever, gonorrhea, and (perhaps most exciting) syphilis. Although sulfonamides had also been employed against many of those, penicillin seemed both more effective and more benign. Could other active substances be similarly isolated from living things to create more "antibiotics"? Selman Waksman, a cell biologist at Rutgers University in the United States, discovered an active (but lethal) antibiotic in 1940 which he called actinomycin; then he obtained streptomycin from a fungus, and reported its antibiotic properties in early 1944. By 1950 streptomycin was shown to be an effective cure for tuberculosis, although the chronic and sometimes latent character of the disease made evaluation difficult and the proper dosage of streptomycin proved elusive. When the antibiotic was combined with para-aminosalicylic acid (PASA), an even more successful treatment for tuberculosis resulted. In the next decade other antibiotics joined the fray, notably isoniazid (effective against tuberculosis, and also used in preventive doses for that disease), the "broad spectrum" antibiotics, aureomycin and terramycin (whose range was even wider than penicillin), and chloramphenicol (which attacked rickettsial diseases such as typhus). This armory of antibiotics expanded under the twin urgings of competitive academic research (Fleming, Florey, Chain, and Waksman had all won Nobel Prizes by 1952) and the gigantic profits foreseen by pharmaceutical manufacturers.

Antibiotics seemed to free humanity from the grip of bacterial diseases and bacterial infection. When combined with the spreading systems of preventive vaccines and the widespread acceptance in the West of the gospel of sanitation, they made the belief in the "End of Epidemics" plausible by the third quarter of the twentieth century. Did that in fact occur?

Mortality figures suggest that the application of biomedical methods of cure and prevention indeed had some effect, but that they basically strengthened trends that had begun in the late nineteenth century. A dramatic decline in

_____ Table 11.2 _____

Deaths per 100,000 Population, 1871–1960: Diarrheal and Digestive Diseases

Year	England/Wales	France	Italy	U.S.A.
1871	136			
1881	75		290	
1901	119		330	
1910				118
1920				54
1926		49		
1930				26
1940	15			10
1950/1	6	5	42	5
1960	5	1	12	5

Sources: This table, and Tables 11.3, 11.4, 11.5, and 11.6, have been abstracted from Samuel H. Preston, Nathan Keyfitz, and Robert Schoen, *Causes of Death: Life Tables for National Populations* (New York: Seminar Press, 1972), 261–267, 284–287, 296–303,408–411, 728–731, 752–755, and 764–767; and from Graziella Caselli, "Health Transition and Cause-Specific Mortality," in R. Schofield et al., eds., *The Decline of Mortality in Europe* (Oxford: Clarendon Press, 1991), 74, 76, 80–81, and 89–90.

_____ Table 11.3 _____

Deaths per 100,000 Population, 1871–1960: Pneumonia, Bronchitis, Influenza

Year	England/Wales	France	Italy	U.S.A.
1871	317			
1881	313		400	
1901	272		449	
1910				184
1920				219
1926		95		
1930				106
1940	233			73
1950/1	201	105	106	33
1960	114	67	77	39

Sources: See Table 11.2.

deaths from waterborne diseases marked a "second stage" in mortality transition, between 1870 and 1920, although Italy trailed other major Western states (see Table 11.2). Public health and sanitation apparently needed little biomedical help in their defense of the digestive system. Social changes had a powerful effect on mortality from respiratory ailments (see Table 11.3), but the toll from such

_____ Table 11.4 _____

Deaths per 100,000 Population, 1871–1960: All Infections

Year	England/Wales	France	Italy	U.S.A.
1871	556			
1881	415		551	
1901	297		276	
1910				265
1920				196
1926		194		
1930				124
1940	116			76
1950/1	54	78	64	34
1960	12	30	28	12

Sources: See Table 11.2.

_____ Table 11.5 _____

Deaths per 100,000 Population, 1871–1960: Diseases of the Circulatory System

Year	England/Wales	France	Italy	U.S.A.
1871	247			
1881	255		275	
1901	254		307	
1910				284
1920				281
1926		234		
1930				325
1940	495			406
1950/1	603	414	360	492
1960	599	386	414	514

Sources: See Table 11.2.

diseases remained relatively high in 1940, especially in England. The declining respiratory death rates of the 1940s and 1950s may reflect antibiotic treatment of bacterial pneumonia. The pattern of infections (see Table 11.4) is similar: considerable reductions in late nineteenth- and early twentieth-century mortalities, thanks to social changes and improvements in public health, and then a *coup de grace* administered by mid-twentieth-century biomedicine.

Disease pressures remained, however, modified by new circumstances. Mortality from neoplasms and diseases of the circulatory system surged (see Tables 11.5 and 11.6). Perhaps the fruits of the end of epidemics allowed people

_____ *Table 11.6* _____
Deaths per 100,000 Population, 1871–1960: Malignant Neoplasms

Year	England/Wales	France	Italy	U.S.A.
1871	44			
1881	56	41		
1901	92	55		
1910	81			
1920	88			
1926	84			
1930	106			
1940	175	129		
1950/1	214	186	127	142
1960	219	206	151	152

Sources: See Table 11.2.

to reach the age of physical degeneration; perhaps industrial success produced affluent diets, extravagant habits, and a toxic environment. But several examples will illustrate that the "End of Epidemics" also remained ambiguous even on its own chosen ground, the conquest of infections.

Diseases under Modern Attack
Syphilis

Syphilis had been a subject of Western discussion and concern since the late fifteenth century, but in the late nineteenth worry about the "pox" had become more urgent.[19] This heightened consciousness grew in part from the increased stress placed in many Western states on the "national health" of the people, a stress related in part to perceived military necessities and in part to economic ones. The late nineteenth century saw both the development of mass conscription armies and the increasing economic competition between industrial national states, and both required a healthy national population. To these concerns were added a greater consciousness of the role of "race," and of the importance of maintaining the health of the family as the central social unit that must be preserved against the dilution of the national stock by alien races or inferior social orders.

Syphilis menaced the health of those families and populations, especially since by the late nineteenth century Western conceptions of syphilis had become grimmer. Alfred Fournier (1832–1914) established a clearer understanding of the frightening tertiary symptoms of the disease, which unequivocally related madness and paralysis to an initial infection that many rakes had taken lightly for centuries. Fournier also emphasized the hereditary character of syphilis, which doomed future generations to the same appalling symptoms. The hereditary grip of syphilis drove the plot of Ibsen's *Ghosts* (1881), a play called by one London critic "an open drain, a loathsome sore unbandaged."[20] By the end of the century syphilis had become the subject of a volume of propaganda designed to frighten people into behavior that would halt its spread, and this view of syphilis—as a terrible menace to be avoided by sexual continence—persisted far into the twentieth century.

Behind this excitement about syphilis lay a long history, as well as particularly modern concerns. Syphilis—or as it was long known, the "great pox"—had been associated with sexual transmission almost from the start. By the seventeenth century (at the latest) venereal disease seemed evidence of disobedience to the laws of religion and morality, and those who suffered from it got their just deserts. Treatments for syphilis had emerged early in the disease's Western history (see Chapter Four), and mercury and guaiacum continued to be offered for centuries. But since sufferers could easily be seen as sinners the possibility of long-term care often gave way to ostracism, which was certainly cheaper than the provision of a charitable lazaretto. The spiritual ambiguities that surrounded medieval lepers did not extend to victims of the pox. And even in the sixteenth century, says Claude Quétel, "the tendency was to avoid giving advice regarding individual prophylaxis on the grounds that it was not wise to encourage sexual excesses by guaranteeing those who performed them impunity [*sic*] from venereal disease."[21] In these circumstances it was logical that remedies might enjoy popularity if they were discreet. "Van Swieten's liquor," an eighteenth-century mercuric compound in alcohol solution, could be self-administered and so (although physicians approved it) patients could keep their secrets. Not surprisingly syphilis presented a fertile field for the charlatan and the concocter of patent remedies, who offered relief without a potentially compromising call on a physician. In the nineteenth century respectable bourgeois seized on the possibility that syphilis might have a nonvenereal cause, including the long-popular toilet seat; that hope was not new either, for the sixteenth-century anatomist Fallopio satirized women who claimed to have caught the pox from Holy Water.[22]

With the association of syphilis and sex came its linkage, again quite old, with prostitution, and in the nineteenth century more elaborate attempts were made to regulate that trade. Earlier attempts to do so had generally foundered on the incorrigible combination of sexual appetites and economic needs, but nineteenth-century states mobilized more regulatory resources. In a series of measures between 1800 and 1804 the Napoleonic regime in France compelled prostitutes to register with the police and set up a system of officially recognized brothels. A hospital in Paris was set aside for the care (and confinement) of pox-ridden prostitutes. Britain compelled medical inspection of suspected prostitutes between 1864 and 1883, but only in certain enumerated garrison and port towns;

London, the Great Wen, remained unregulated. The nineteenth-century debates about prostitution prefigured many of the issues that surrounded twentieth-century attempts to combat syphilis.[23] Those favoring regulation—which might involve medical examinations, isolation or quarantine, and state licensure of prostitutes—began with moral or religious convictions that prostitution was an evil, but then added public health arguments. Syphilis was a great epidemic threat, disseminated by prostitutes; prostitutes lived in quarters seen as the main foci of venereal infection. The sexual urges of males could not reasonably be restrained, and so better to recognize that fact and provide healthy sex with clean, registered prostitutes, especially for the troops on whom the security of the nation depended.

Against these seemingly reasonable and scientific propositions a storm of objections arose. Some were functional: regulation of such a trade would not work. Inspectors could make mistakes, could miss hidden or small chancres, or could be easily corrupted. Many prostitutes—perhaps most—could escape regulation and inspection altogether, as certainly happened in France all through the nineteenth century and as happened in the United States in the midst of World War I attempts to close brothels near army garrisons. Regulation might lead to a false sense of security. And while some medical or public health arguments supported such regulation, other physicians asked why only women were being regulated; were not the bees, going from flower to flower, the true propagators of epidemic? Principled objections appeared as well. Did not regulation of an evil amount to tacit recognition of it? Proto-feminist opinion, especially in Britain, objected to the singling out of women for regulation. More generally, regulation in the name of public health raised fundamental questions about the power of a state over individuals. On what grounds could a policeman detain a woman and order her to undergo medical inspection? Civil libertarians defended individual freedom from arbitrary detention; socialists saw regulations aimed at particular social classes (or ethnic groups, or races) as excuses for an elite exercise of police repression. The experiences of "respectable" British women mistaken for prostitutes showed how class expectations could conflict with the letter of the law. Advocates of medical inspection and regulation could only respond that the greater social good outweighed individual rights, or that wrongdoers (especially prostitutes) had placed themselves outside the bounds of civil society and its rights. Disease—syphilis—menaced society; prostitutes spread syphilis; therefore prostitutes must be controlled.

These arguments, both about the regulation of prostitution and (by extension) about the powers of the state to attack syphilis with an intrusive machinery of public health, were further sharpened in the early twentieth century by two new circumstances. New and powerful therapies against the disease came on the scene, and Western states became involved in wars on a new and total scale.

Ehrlich's "magic bullets," arsphenamine and neoarsphenamine (Salvarsan and Neosalvarsan), appeared in 1909 and 1912. The Wassermann test (1906) made possible a more precise (but not infallible) definition of the disease in individuals. Although mercury compounds continued to command some favor, Ehrlich's arsenicals became the treatment of choice for those defined by a Wassermann test as syphilitic; in a Paris hospital in 1920, 33,480 neoarsphenamine treatments were administered, and only 49 of mercury.[24]

Medical science had other weapons in its armory. In addition to Ehrlich's arsenicals, some bismuth compounds were employed. The discovery that the syphilis trypanosome could be killed by heat led to another radical therapy in which doses of malaria were induced in syphilitic patients, and the resulting fever "cured" syphilis. Trading syphilis for malaria was thought a gain. But penicillin overshadowed and supplanted all these remedies. Between the mid-1940s (when that antibiotic was first employed) and the mid- to late 1950s the number of primary and secondary syphilis infections in the Western world tumbled dramatically, falling below 5 cases per 100,000 inhabitants in most countries; in the United States, for example, from 70.9 in 1946 to 3.9 in 1956.[25]

These biomedical approaches coincided with unusual social stresses. World War I made huge demands on the manpower and materials of the states that took part in it; governments struggled to maintain the health of the soldiers whom they sent to be slaughtered, while the experiences of the war may have significantly changed popular attitudes toward sexual morality. "If these young men, alive today and dead tomorrow, if these young women who, as they read the casualty lists, did not seize experience at once, they knew that for many of them it would elude them forever," recalled a British observer in 1936.[26] To the social disruptions of the war, which certainly also contributed to changing the economic positions of women in Western societies, were added the interactions of technology, popular culture, and changes in sexual habits and standards. The automobile represented a new locale for sexual experience, away from the compromises of a parental home. The radio and the phonograph, not to speak of the cinema, presented new experiences to the senses, and contributed to changing standards of behavior more rapidly than older generations could accept. World War II repeated World War I's demands on populations on an even grander scale.

Those events and their accompanying stresses created the social matrix within which the new chemotherapies of syphilis treatment were employed. Dominating responses in the United States and France, as Allan Brandt and Claude Quétel have shown, was a barrage of propaganda and education aimed at establishing abstinence from sex outside marriage as the goal of both public morality and public health. The successful chemotherapy was a dangerous ally precisely because easy cure removed the morally useful punitive function of syphilis. The stage and screen were enlisted. Eugene Brieux's play *Les Avariés* was first read in Paris in 1901; performed the next year in Belgium, it received permission from censors for a Paris production in 1905, and reached the United States as *Damaged Goods* in 1913. In it the rakish protagonist ignores his doctor's warnings and marries despite his disease, which then devastates his family life. Although its discussion of syphilis (more explicit than the oblique references in Ibsen's *Ghosts*) was a daring airing of issues usually left in the dark, its message certainly reinforced the lesson that syphilis should be prevented by the moral actions of individuals, who should keep themselves clean for marriage. The same theme informed the American military training film of World War I, *Fit to Fight*.

After the war such openness (justified at the time by the need to maintain the health of the troops) was attacked in American society; *Fit to Fight*, with a highly moral message that endorsed sexual abstinence, was judged an obscene film by the New York State Board of Censors in 1919.[27] Both Brandt and Quétel agree that in the years between the world wars American and French societies, while obsessed with syphilis and its dangers, concentrated on preaching abstinence and otherwise retreating in shame before sexual openness. The chief of police in Lansing, Michigan, laid down clear rules for dancing:

> Right hand of gentleman must not be placed below the waist nor over the shoulder nor around the lady's neck, nor lady's left arm around gentleman's neck. Lady's right hand and gentleman's left hand clasped and extended at least six inches from the body, and must not be folded and lay across the chest of dancers.[28]

Maurice Bernay, a French physician, allowed that some sexual encounters might still occur, but urged men so involved to be careful:

> Those who have remained unwounded should carefully inspect the terrain as they march into battle. They should put on their most fetching smile and caress the lady's neck, feeling at the same time for swollen glands under her skin. They should express enthusiastic admiration of her mouth and tongue, but take particular care to glance at the lips, gums and tongue. They should praise the bosom, but examine the skin for possible suspicious blotches.[29]

During World War I objections had been raised to treating soldiers with prophylactic doses of mercury or arsenicals, on the grounds that the terrors of syphilis should be maintained for the sake of morality. The return of peace strengthened such arguments, for no longer could military necessity excuse the treatment of the syphilitic warrior. "Contamination"—infecting someone with syphilis—became a crime in Denmark, Sweden, Czechoslovakia, and the Soviet Union.[30]

While possible therapy was entangled in a moral quagmire, preventive public health encountered other political obstacles. The Wassermann test had opened the possibility of tracing the disease through a population, if its use could be combined with a careful contact epidemiology. Those infected by the spirochete could then be identified, warned of their condition, perhaps forbidden to marry, perhaps confined until treatment cured them. But such a program had first to overcome the reluctance of doctors to break confidentiality by identifying their patients, the reluctance of lovers to betray their contacts, even the reluctance of individuals to admit to themselves that they had a disease. And the greater the weight of moral stigma the disease carried, the greater became those obstacles. The Wassermann test was not foolproof; should happy marriages, or the maintenance of employment, depend on its results? Could the state compel its administration? What grounds justified "suspicion"? Different writers were clearly willing to consign different groups to the social margins as likely carriers. Léon Legendre assured a French agricultural college in 1928:

> It is particularly prevalent in intellectuals, the state of whose blood plasma serum, and even of the nervous tissue itself, differs from (1) that of the peasant who lives in the open air and uses his muscles much more than his brain; (2) that of the Arab who drinks nothing but water, eats nothing but couscous, fruit, dates and bananas, and who has nothing to do but bask in the sun.[31]

But prostitutes, the poor, and (in the United States) emigrants and blacks were much more likely to be singled out than were intellectuals. When black American troops arrived in St. Nazaire in World War I, the panicky mayor insisted that black women be brought from the United States for them. The United States army was prone to assume that all black troops were syphilitic and so all should be required to undergo chemical prophylaxis. The image of African Americans as a "syphilis-soaked" race persisted in the United States; the considerably higher rates of syphilis infection among African Americans were explained as a product of moral failure (perhaps hereditary), with little regard for alternative social or economic explanations. Economic conditions (and cultural barriers) meant that blacks were much less likely to be able to seek treatment, and so their infections persisted; when African Americans did seek treatment they were much more likely to repair to a public clinic, not a private physician who might hide their disease from the national statistics.[32]

The conjunction of biomedicine's zeal for experiment and American racial conceptions about syphilis led to a particularly disturbing moral and political example, when the Tuskegee Study (beginning in 1932) deliberately left over four hundred poor African-American males untreated after they had been tested as positively infected with latent syphilis. The goal was the tracing of the tertiary symptoms of the disease through their entire course, and the experiment continued long after penicillin had made possible the cure of the subjects; the study ended only in 1972, by which time a public outcry had arisen against the persistence of racial assumptions and the imposition of medical power on the marginal members of society.[33]

Penicillin dramatically affected the incidence of syphilis, but it did not eliminate it. The precipitous decline in syphilis rates ended in the late 1950s in most Western countries; since that time syphilis has tended to hold its own, with occasional upward spikes in incidence, for example in the United States in the late 1980s and early 1990s. By the 1970s primary and secondary stages of syphilis infected 11 or 12 people per 100,000 in the United States. Social and political factors largely explain this revival of the old pox. As long as a disease is allowed to stigmatize its victims, contact epidemiology will remain incomplete; some will not seek treatment, others will respect the confidentiality of their sexual partners. Some have argued that the easy treatment of venereal disease afforded by penicillin, combined with the birth control pill, opened the door for the moralists' worst fears; an age of permissive and promiscuous sex ensued. But did promiscuity—if it occurred—correlate with venereal disease? Allan Brandt is not so sure, and argues instead (or in addition) that the persistence of the moral approach must bear some responsibility. Attitudes toward sex education and venereal disease remained highly moralist in the United States even when syphilis (or pregnancy) could no longer threaten those who disobeyed chastity's injunctions; as a result, conspiracies of silence about sex and sexually transmitted diseases continued, and youth remained ignorant of preventive methods that would protect them from venereal disease. The apparent disappearance of a public health problem enabled uncomfortable discussions of sex to be conveniently forgotten. And although the syphilis-causing spirochete showed no signs of adapting to better resist the onslaught of penicillin, gonococci did so evolve, leading to an increase in gonorrhea for biological reasons as well as social.

Still a further twist on the public discussion of venereal diseases came with the growing awareness of AIDS in the 1980s. Its effects on the position of syphilis have been mixed. The sense of crisis accompanying AIDS (see Chapter Twelve) has certainly led to a much franker acceptance of discussion of and education in preventive techniques; condoms may be advertised on television. But the impact of such discussion may be greater in some socioeconomic groups than others, leading to class differences and stigmas; the very openness of preventive talk has stirred moral backlashes; AIDS itself has been thoroughly configured as a disease affecting only marginal groups of society, and such discussion has given new strength to the general notion of disease as sin; and finally, as Quétel suggests, syphilis may lurk hidden behind the greater terror of AIDS, if only as an opportunistic infection assailing weakened immune systems.

Poliomyelitis in the United States

Poliomyelitis had a peculiarly twentieth-century history.[34] It apparently appeared in epidemic form for the first time in the late nineteenth century, and for a time it shook the public confidence in biomedicine. Ultimately it afforded a triumphant reaffirmation of that confidence, but not before certain old themes had been replayed, some with decidedly twentieth-century twists. As the epidemic increased in severity so too did public clamor and even hysteria. That public pressure was channeled into support for research which sought a "cure" for this modern scourge, and in the process various new determinants of scientific behavior manifested themselves.

Poliomyelitis—which at different times has had a variety of names, the best-known ones polio and infantile paralysis—is triggered by a virus, called simply poliovirus. Although poliomyelitis epidemics are relatively new, the poliovirus has very probably been a companion of humanity for many centuries. Its effects on the human body range over a wide spectrum of severity; many people can be invaded by the virus and show no symptoms at all, while others suffer an attack on their central nervous system that can lead to paralysis. The disease is rapidly contagious, moving from person to person most often through the mouth. Apparently before the late nineteenth century poliomyelitis was a common "disease" of infancy and young childhood (though not recognized as such), one in which the vast majority of "cases" either displayed no symptoms or revealed themselves only in a brief mild fever. Occasionally the central nervous system was affected, perhaps resulting in a period of stiff neck and back muscles, or more serious muscle weakness, or even a paralysis that lamed the victim. But no connection was made between common mild fevers and the occasional cripple. Most children experienced the disease while still quite young and enjoyed subsequent immunity from later attacks.

This picture began changing in the late nineteenth century, perhaps because of the very success of the gospel of sanitation. The growing thoroughness of sanitary practices, and attention to personal hygiene, may have increasingly isolated American and European infants from early exposure to the poliovirus. Perhaps as a result larger communities of unexposed older children and young adults existed in some places by the end of the century, when the first epidemic reports began accumulating. Some of these early epidemics occurred in relatively isolated small towns in thinly settled districts. Thus 24 cases were described in Modums (Norway) in 1868; a further 13 cases in Umeo (Sweden) in 1881, 25 cases in Sainte-Foy-l'Argentière (France) in 1885, and 132 cases in Rutland County, Vermont (United States) in 1894. By that time an urban epidemic had occurred as well, with 44 cases in Stockholm in 1887. That experience, together with the Rutland epidemic, subsequent Stockholm episodes in 1899 and 1903, and, dramatically, over 1,000 cases in Sweden in 1905, established poliomyelitis as an epidemic disease in the West.

These outbreaks of the disease differed from the occasional paralytic cases of previous centuries, and they stimulated new understandings of it. By the twentieth century greater numbers of older children or even young adults were involved; in the 1894 Rutland epidemic over 25 percent of the victims were over the age of six, and in the large 1905 Swedish epidemic over 61 percent of them were. Two Swedish investigators—Karl Oskar Medin and Ivar Wickman—put forward the idea that paralysis (and other involvement of the central nervous system) was a later manifestation of the same disease that might only appear as a mild fever. Wickman also argued (on the basis of the 1905 experience) that the disease should be regarded as highly contagious, traveling to remote villages along the lines of ordinary human traffic. Wickman's views of the disease's spread did not gain universal assent, however, and in subsequent years the epidemic mechanism of poliomyelitis remained a bone of contention that confused some community responses.

Poliomyelitis's epidemic appearance in the United States coincided with a period of great faith in the importance of sanitation, a faith that awkwardly coexisted with the emergence of the germ theory model. Belief that "dirt" produced disease was hard to expunge, as responses to poliomyelitis illustrated. The first major American urban epidemic of poliomyelitis occurred in 1907, when between 750 and 1,200 were afflicted in New York. The disease struck Cincinnati and New York in 1911, and Buffalo in 1912. But the most dramatic early epidemic came to New York and other northeastern American cities in 1916. In that year 8,900 New Yorkers contracted poliomyelitis, and 2,400 deaths resulted; the United States as a whole suffered 27,000 cases and 6,000 deaths.[35] American medical and popular opinion still believed dirt to be the home of disease, although the germ theory had shifted attention from generally unsanitary conditions to the particular dirty habits of individuals. In 1916 those individuals were the poor and especially the immigrant poor, of whom New York had a vast population. As the epidemic took hold, regulations were applied to them: the activities of immigrants were restricted, their children were forbidden to attend charitably sponsored summer camps (for fear of their infecting others), their neighborhood festivals were carefully monitored. A New York city regulation compelled the hospitalization of sick children if their homes lacked a private toilet, dining space, and nurse for the sick. This ukase in effect forced poor children into hospitals, for (as Naomi Rogers notes) such conditions could be met only by the well-to-do.[36]

Such vigorous government public health measures stirred political controversy and resistance, as they had done so many times in the past. Guenter Risse's study of the reactions of Oyster Bay, New York, in 1916 shows divisions along ethnic and class lines, and also over the validity of medical approaches. Wealthy summer residents attacked the Polish and Irish ethnic communities as harboring the disease; both local authorities and businesses argued about the imposition of quarantines that might close down the vital summer tourist trade;

permanent residents resisted tax increases to provide the public health machinery demanded by the wealthy summer visitors. The medical profession in Oyster Bay was held in generally "low esteem."[37] Oyster Bay, a summer resort community, illustrated what would become one of the major impacts of poliomyelitis on American popular culture; the disease spread in the summer, and as its contagious character was recognized, middle-class American parents became terrified for their children in summer crowds, most notably on beaches, at pools, and at other swimming places.

But the facts of epidemiology did not support a "filthy immigrants" theory, for poliomyelitis was hardly confined to poor immigrant quarters. Nor could a clear pattern of contagion be traced from poor immigrants to prosperous suburbanites. The disease seemed to leap over space; not every sick suburban child lived in a house served by a slum-dwelling immigrant cook or housemaid. Those circumstances justified the popularity of insects as an epidemiological explanation: insects, especially flies, were thought to carry the disease from poor to rich. American medicine and sanitation had after all recently triumphed over insects in Cuba and Panama; the fly, like the mosquito, could be dealt with; the fly had already been implicated in the spread of typhoid fever, so it was an enemy anyway. Settling on the fly enabled authorities to convince the public that the epidemic could be mastered.

The assault on the fly began, a campaign that could involve the population at large. But the disease did not cooperatively vanish, and it (together with the influenza pandemic of 1918–19) became a symbol of the persistent weakness of modern scientific medicine. Polio's apparent cause, a virus, had been "discovered" in 1909 by Karl Landsteiner of Vienna, who isolated *something* that passed through filters that could trap bacteria. The "something" (the individual constituents of which could not be seen with available microscopes) could be blamed for the disease, but how was it transmitted? Did it reach the human body through the nasal passages, as Simon Flexner, the leading American authority, believed? Once in the body, did it primarily affect the nervous system (another Flexner argument), or did it first lodge in the digestive tract? Physicians were also at a loss for therapies. In the prevailing uncertainty the public seized on a wide variety of etiological ideas and therapeutic nostrums. Contaminated milk, spitting (both already blamed for the spread of tuberculosis), domestic animals, unusual foods (especially those of immigrant groups), and contacts with the poor were all suspicious. And as the disease's rates increased in subsequent decades, popular fears and searches for causes and cures intensified. By the time of the 1934 outbreak in Los Angeles public hysteria had become serious and had even affected hospital personnel. At the railway station an anxious crowd awaited the arrival of a team of experts from Yale University and the Rockefeller Institute who presumably would find answers, and their appearance threatened to become a media event. In this atmosphere 2,500 "cases" (in six months) were treated at the Los Angeles County Hospital alone, but only about 1,300 actually proved to be poliomyelitis.[38]

Popular fears of the disease were certainly magnified by the images presented by the therapy prevalent in the years between the world wars. Serum therapy, a great hope in the first decades of the century, had been disappointing. Its failure left most therapy in the realm of orthopedics, which attempted to minimize or reverse the effects of paralysis. To that end orthopedic fashions shifted between exercise of the afflicted limbs and immobility; in the 1920s and especially in the 1930s the advocates of immobility held the field and carried their practices to a zealous excess. Treatment for paralytic poliomyelitis involved the imposition of rigid plaster casts on limbs and the confinement of patients in hospital beds that had the appearance of mechanical monsters. This vision of a crippled youth in the grip of pulleys, casts, and iron framework was reinforced by the appearance of the Drinker respirator, commonly called the "iron lung." Developed in the late 1920s to assist (or even make possible) breathing for those poliomyelitis victims whose paralysis affected such muscles as the diaphragm, the device—an encasing cabinet in which air pressures alternated on the body—was another horrific symbol of the ravages of the disease, although it undoubtedly helped some severely paralytic patients to survive.

Those symbols—the iron lung, the heavy casts and braces enforcing immobility—contributed to shifting the public view of poliomyelitis from fear and loathing toward pity and compassion. The disease still terrified, but by the 1920s and 1930s realization grew that social class conferred no immunity from it. The case of Franklin D. Roosevelt had particular importance in the United States, even before his election to the presidency in 1932. Roosevelt, a member of a prominent American family, had served in Woodrow Wilson's World War I government; he was stricken by paralytic poliomyelitis in 1921, when he was thirty-nine. Although the images of his subsequent political career downplayed his disability—he was most often photographed sitting down or standing behind a podium—his experiences received wide publicity and contributed to the social "respectability" of the disease. Roosevelt's struggles with poliomyelitis joined, and in part inspired, the activities of the massive fund-raising efforts of the National Foundation for Infantile Paralysis, begun in 1937 with Roosevelt's direct blessing. Its activities overwhelmed other earlier philanthropy, including the foundation that supported treatments at Warm Springs, a spa in Georgia favored by Roosevelt (who purchased the property and established the foundation). The National Foundation carried fund-raising against a disease to new heights, in the process posing new questions about the interrelationship of popular philanthropy, scientific research, the allocations of resources, and the cultural configurations of disease.

In its early years the foundation showed most interest in a quick "cure" for the scourge of poliomyelitis, but (especially after the failure of some vaccine trials in the 1930s) it began to shift its emphasis in the direction of basic research. The gradual weakening of Flexner's view of the disease encouraged the shift. Flexner had seen poliomyelitis as first and foremost an attack on the central nervous system. If he was correct the hopes for a vaccine were faint, for any antigen (however attenuated) that first settled in the nervous system was obviously dangerous to the subjects; even experimental trials would carry fearful risks. But by the years of World War II Flexner's view had lost favor to one that saw the digestive tract as the primary site. If that were true, perhaps a vaccine could be prepared that would in some way replicate the mild symptoms (or no symptoms at all) of most earlier poliomyelitis infections. The foundation began pouring its collected resources into virology, in the hope of finding such a vaccine. Private philanthropic support for biomedical research was a relatively new phenomenon in the Western world, one that would be widely copied later in the twentieth century.

Of course philanthropy had long been directed at therapy—witness the thousands of medieval leprosaria—and the foundation undertook that more traditional role as well. It remained at least for a time wedded to the "immobility" approach. This meant that the foundation scorned the arguments of the Australian nurse Elizabeth Kenny, who advocated stimulation and exercise of the afflicted limbs; Kenny gained other American support and began an institute in Minneapolis that practiced her methods. Tensions between the National Foundation and Kenny's followers remained an underlying political issue in the history of poliomyelitis in the United States. Meanwhile the foundation also supported the use of the "iron lung," using its resources to purchase the machines and thus entering the complicated picture of allocation of such expensive therapy. If a limited number of the Drinker respirators was available, on what basis did patients gain access to them? Ability to pay or to travel to their locations? With money raised from the public by a heart-rending appeal?

The foundation's appeals for money from the American public were both highly organized and highly emotional. The annual "poster children" chosen by the foundation combined pathos and plucky determination as they displayed the braces supporting their crippled limbs. A particular stroke of genius was the "March of Dimes," fund-raising that encouraged even the smallest contributions and could thus involve the mass of the population, even children whose dimes could succor other children. When the possibility of a successful vaccine seemed brighter in the years after World War II, the foundation was in a powerful position to direct research with its funds, while at the same time it had become something of a prisoner of the publicity and hopes it had generated. The millions who gave to it demanded a "cure" as soon as possible.

In the years after 1945 two main vaccine possibilities were explored: attenuated (or "live") and inactivated (or "killed") virus. Jonas Salk of the University of Pittsburgh, one of those working on inactivated viruses, boldly presented the foundation with a *fait accompli*. In 1952 he performed experimental trials with such a vaccine; some of his subjects had already suffered from paralytic poliomyelitis: others were mentally retarded children and adults at a state residential school in Pennsylvania. Salk published an account of the successful result of these trials, which involved something over one hundred subjects, in early 1953. The foundation (or at least its administrators), which had created a Committee on Immunization (including leading researchers in the field) in 1951, seized on Salk's report and actively supported his approach, working through a smaller committee of enthusiasts. By the end of 1953 the foundation had set in motion a field trial of Salk's vaccine that was unprecedented in its scale. In the spring of 1954 the foundation enlisted in trials over 1.8 million American children, for the most part between the ages of six and nine, the first fruits of the remarkable "baby boom" in the American population. Some received vaccine, some a placebo; others remained untreated. The investigators then awaited the arrival of the summer poliomyleitis season, and at its end the results could be analyzed. The steady advance of the epidemic, which had reached a peak in 1953, had lent real weight to the emotional appeals of the foundation; American public opinion on the subject was in a frenzy.

The results of the 1954 trials were announced to a huge crowd of news representatives gathered in Ann Arbor, Michigan, on April 12, 1955, which was also the tenth anniversary of Franklin Roosevelt's death. The successful outcome of the trials—over 200,000 children vaccinated with no serious health problems as a result—generated a media circus. In that atmosphere the National Institutes of Health had asked an ad hoc committee to decide whether Salk's vaccine should be licensed for general use in the population. As John Paul says, it was "far past the appropriate time for a deliberative body to have been brought on the scene"; in the superheated atmosphere of Ann Arbor in April 1955 the committee could do little but approve the vaccine for general use, which it did.[39] A disaster followed almost immediately. Within two weeks reports spread of newly-vaccinated children in California and Idaho being stricken by paralysis. For two months in 1955 the huge hopes apparently satisfied by the April 12 announcement were at least suspended, if not dashed, while investigators probed what became known as the Cutter Incident. Vaccine manufactured by one firm—the Cutter Laboratories, in California—apparently resulted in 164 cases of severe paralysis and ten deaths among the children inoculated with it.[40]

But the Cutter Incident was eventually overshadowed by the immense success of the vaccination program that began after April 12, 1955. In the first three weeks after that date four million Americans received doses of Salk vaccine, and by the middle of that year massive vaccination was also under way in Canada, Denmark, France, and Germany. The results in the next several years were stunning. Rates for paralytic poliomyelitis in the United States fell from 13.9 per 100,000 in 1954 to 0.5 per 100,000 in 1961. While the decline was not as dramatic in other Western countries—in part because the initial American incidence was higher, perhaps in turn because American sanitary success had created the most favorable conditions for the disease—poliomyelitis retreated rapidly everywhere vaccines were applied. British and Australian incidence in the early 1960s was 7 percent of their early 1950s figure, while Sweden (another zealously sanitary country with high poliomyelitis rates until the mid-1950s) experienced a decline nearly as steep as that in America.

Although the inactivated vaccine had thus been pushed to the fore in the United States, attenuated forms had received more attention elsewhere. The World Health Organization had encouraged trials of such vaccines, and they began in the then Belgian African colonies of Congo, Rwanda, and Burundi in 1957. Shortly afterward trials of other attenuated vaccines started in Latin America and in the Soviet Union. Meetings in Washington, D.C., in 1959 and 1960 (organized with the help of the Kenny Foundation, which illustrated that rivalry was still an issue) heard of the success of these vaccines, especially that developed by Albert Sabin of the University of Cincinnati. Attenuated vaccines had real advantages, particularly the permanence of the immunity they offered. Like the original Jenner smallpox vaccine, the Salk vaccine needed to be repeatedly reinforced by further inoculations, which would require a sophisticated public health network in a population disciplined to regular treatments. In rural areas, places without such a public health system, and especially among poor populations not in ordinary contact with professional health care, such conditions might not exist. The attenuated "Sabin" vaccine thus became the first choice in much of the world in (and since) the 1960s.

The circumstances of the dramatic National Foundation–Salk triumph in the 1950s raised some disturbing and difficult questions. The public had demanded a quick "cure," and it had been led to a belief that such was possible by a constellation of factors. The relentless publicity of the foundation had itself contributed to that belief, but so too had three centuries of gradually increasing trust in science, and the recent experiences of World War II, which had convinced Americans in particular that science could be mobilized to make quick and successful war on anything: Nazi pests, Japanese pests, bacterial pests, insect pests. Penicillin, DDT, and the atomic bomb all testified to the vast power of science aroused. In demanding a speedy solution the foundation threw its resources into a narrow salient, hoping for success as soon as possible, instead of supporting research on a broad front. Questions—perhaps unanswerable, or answerable only by individual moral choice—surrounded much of the resulting narrative.

At what point in an experimental procedure are trials on humans justified? What degree of safety is "enough"? Could the Cutter Incident have been avoided with more deliberate care in the process? Or would "more deliberate care" have exposed millions of American children to another epidemic season of poliomyelitis in the summer of 1955? Questions about the use of human subjects had already been raised by the experiences of World War II, both because military necessity had been a justification for the rapid introduction of new therapies, and because of the dreadful experiments performed in the name of racial science in Nazi Germany. The 1953–54 trials of poliomyelitis vaccines suggested the difficulties of simple answers.

The autonomy of science, never clearly established at any time, was now challenged from another quarter: the demands of a mass public, fed by the self-interested bureaucracy of philanthropy. One poliomyelitis researcher complained that he and his colleagues were "beginning to look like a troupe of trained seals."[41] The National Foundation certainly diverted resources toward inactivated vaccine research and away from attenuated vaccine research; what motivated it to do so? And while "public opinion" has always at least contributed to the configuration of a "disease," the publicity afforded by mass communication techniques perhaps sped and intensified such cultural configurations. Was the "most diseased" victim (that is, the one to whom resources would be diverted) the one for whom the most pathetic case could be made over television broadcasts?

Influenza, 1918–19

The influenza pandemic of 1918–19 ranks as the greatest disease event of the twentieth century, and as one of the most sweeping in the world's history.[42] According to a recent estimate, perhaps fifty million fatalities resulted from the pandemic and "even that vast figure may be substantially lower than the real toll, perhaps as much as 100 percent understated."[43] In recent years this tremendous episode has attracted renewed historical attention, in part because contemporary fears of "Asian bird flu" or "SARS" have stimulated interest in their predecessor, and in part owing to the exciting 2005 identification of the virus responsible for the 1918 pandemic. Yet Alfred Crosby's term—the "forgotten pandemic"—remains appropriate. A study of its course suggests some reasons why that has been so, and also illustrates other aspects of the strengths and limitations of scientific medicine in the twentieth century.

Influenza, a widespread viral disease, has been almost continuously present somewhere in the world for at least the last several centuries. Its familiar symptoms share much ground with the common cold: sore throat, cough, nasal discharge, fever, general aches and pains, weakness. All these symptoms may vary widely in severity, and most often (even in epidemic or pandemic times) victims recover; frequent high morbidity rates and relatively low mortality characterize influenza epidemics. Influenza is caused by one of several related viruses, the most important sometimes called influenza type A, which passes rapidly from person to person via the respiratory system. Influenza is extremely contagious. It is also extremely mutable, for its unstable virus changes frequently, and the modified forms may present constantly changing puzzles for human immune systems. A case of this year's influenza may not ensure immunity from next year's.

We do not know how long influenza has been epidemic in human populations. But it was clearly so by the early modern period, and a series of pandemics, more or less worldwide, began in the eighteenth century and has continued to the present.[44] These pandemics had certain common characteristics. They probably began when a new subtype of the virus appeared that met little or no resistance from human antibodies. Human traffic carried them from one community to another; they seem, according to David Patterson, usually to have begun in central Asia and moved from east to west, most often in cold weather. Domestic animals, a number of which may be infected by the viruses, may have played a role in transmission as well. Morbidity in these pandemics (in, for example, 1781–82 and 1873) was very high, so that even with low mortality rates the death toll might be considerable. Especially at risk were the vulnerable very young and very old; death might often result from a combination of the effects of influenza and something else, especially pneumonia.

Perhaps the most serious of these pre-twentieth-century pandemics occurred in 1889–90. By that time the Western-centered system of steam transportation had greatly increased the speed of human traffic by sea and land, and (as we saw in Chapter Nine) diseases—among them plague, cholera, and measles—moved more rapidly as well. The swift diffusion of influenza in 1889 created a tremendous morbidity and hence a total mortality that (according to Patterson) certainly exceeded the nineteenth-century ravages of cholera, which attracted much more attention then and since. But although influenza affected millions, most "individual sufferers had little reason to fear death. It quietly killed old people by the thousands" without interrupting the rhythms of society.[45] The 1889 pandemic gave an illustration of the speed with which influenza could spread; if a more dangerous subtype should appear, awesome effects might follow.

In 1918 that more dangerous subtype appeared. It differed from earlier influenzas in several respects, two of them crucial. Earlier versions of the disease had killed mostly the generally vulnerable, those at opposite ends of the age spectrum. The 1918–19 pandemic, however, for reasons still not entirely clear, proved particularly dangerous to young adults. And more than earlier influenzas this one seriously compromised the lungs, resulting in many deaths from respiratory complications. It also began not in the heart of the Old World but in the heart of the New; its first cases apparently occurred in Kansas, in the central United States, and it rapidly spread from there to most (though not all) corners of the world.

It diffused in three waves. The first was noticed in Kansas in March 1918 and within a month had spread widely across the United States. That country had been a belligerent in World War I since 1917, and across the Atlantic moved a stream of troopships carrying influenza to France by the end of April 1918. Sea traffic carried it to the Iberian peninsula and to India in May; by June other western and northern European states were affected, as were far-off Australia and the East Indies. Influenza then seemed to flicker, diminishing through the summer months, only to revive in a more virulent second wave beginning in August. This new outburst began in France, perhaps after undergoing a mutation or recombination there.[46] Sea transport carried the second wave back to the United States (first to Boston) and to Freetown in West African Sierra Leone, and from those initial nodes influenza spread across North America and Africa. By September and October many places in the world were experiencing peak weeks of morbidity and mortality, although the second wave's intensity varied from place to place. But in general the months between September and December 1918 saw devastating influenza tolls throughout the world. The third wave, in large part a fainter echo of the second, spread in the first six months of 1919; it did, however, fall heavily on Australia, which had largely escaped the second wave.

The epidemic vividly illustrated the ways in which modern transportation could facilitate disease diffusion. In addition to the first wave's rapid movement from the central United States to France and to India (a ship carried it to Bombay on May 29), the distant islands of the Pacific were not immune. The second wave reached Guam on October 26, Western Samoa on November 7, and Tahiti on November 16. The second wave in India, while moving generally from Bombay eastward, arrived in Assam and Burma before it affected Bengal and Bihar, probably because it gained a separate port foothold at Rangoon. Ships rapidly moved influenza along the west coast of Africa, and from the east coast of the United States to the gulf and west coasts as well. Certainly the volume of human traffic in troopships in 1918 was an exacerbating factor in the rapid spread of influenza.

Away from the coasts, railroads assumed an important diffusing role. The different experiences of India and China illustrate their power. India, with its extensive British-built railroad network, may have lost 18 million people to influenza. Although Chinese statistics have been less thoroughly explored, estimates of influenza deaths there range from about one million to nine million, in a population substantially larger than India's. One author suggests that China's relatively primitive internal transportation system may have slowed or stopped influenza's course.[47] And within the interior of Africa influenza clearly followed railroad lines.

Although we should not claim that World War I caused influenza, the social, economic, and political circumstances of the war certainly contributed to influenza's severity. The war brought together masses of young men in crowded camps and ships and assembled civilian masses in patriotic rallies and parades. Its demands for doctors and nurses left civilian sectors short of health professionals. In some places war and revolution created social chaos and with it poor nutrition, stress, and the greater likelihood of bacterial infection interacting with influenza. But while war and pandemic acted symbiotically in some areas of the world, the greatest ravages of influenza occurred in places far removed from the stress of fighting, especially India. As the demographic impact of the disease makes clear, the social conditions of poverty played a much greater role in influenza's mortality, although war may have made its spread (and hence high morbidity) more likely.

Influenza stirred a number of responses from both medical professionals and the general public. Physicians, whose confidence rode high on the successes of previous decades, willingly tried "scientific" remedies and preventives. According to Martha Hildreth, physicians in France, acting on the possibility that influenza was either bacterial or related to a specific miasma, urged the antiseptic cleansing of both individual bodies and public places.[48] A variety of antitoxins and vaccines were produced and applied; chemotherapeutic agents successful against other diseases, such as Ehrlich's arsphenamines, were prescribed for influenza as well. Public health authorities likewise applied those measures that they had developed to combat other disease problems: they ordered schools, churches, and theatres closed; they attempted quarantines, for example in colonial territories along the west coast of Africa (which failed) and in Australia (which did fend off the second wave for a time).[49] A widespread belief in the airborne character of the disease led to a number of ingenious attempts to make breathing safe. In the United States some authorities ordered the population to wear gauze masks, which (in San Francisco, for example) resulted in both perceived interference with individual rights and scenes of low social comedy. French doctors urged the benefits of steam vapor mixed with eucalyptus, a measure also adopted by the white settlers of Nigeria, where the black population substituted camphor for eucalyptus.[50]

None of these remedies had a noticeable effect. Influenza's morbidity reached staggering proportions, although figures for it are not reliable owing to widespread underreporting and the difficulties of differentiating influenza from other complaints. Alfred Crosby estimates that 28 percent of the population of the United States suffered from influenza between fall 1918 and spring 1919. Although physicians' remedies were of little avail, the disease's impact was surprisingly fleeting, at least in the developed world. Perhaps thirty million Americans had been ill, but the peaks of epidemic moved quickly through individual communities. Influenza moved on before a siege mentality could set in, although the elaborate public health reactions of San Francisco and Philadelphia described by Crosby suggest that a sense of siege was imminent. The disease came in the midst of the greatest war the Western world had known, a war that provided bigger news, accustomed opinion to the deaths of the young, and imposed censorship on such discouraging news as influenza deaths. (The fact that news *did* come from neutral Spain led to the epidemic's misleading name: "Spanish influenza.") And, as Crosby says, influenza neither crippled nor scarred its victims, nor did it create chronic ill-health.[51]

But Crosby's "forgotten pandemic" also courted oblivion partly because its most dreadful effects were outside the Western world, in places from which Europeans and Americans could hide their eyes. Niall Johnson and Juergen Mueller's recent estimate of fifty million worldwide deaths include about three million in Europe and North America, where mortality rates varied between about 3 and 12 per 1,000 population. (In the United States, for instance, the figure was about 6 per 1,000.) Mortality rates in some Latin American countries (Mexico, for instance) may have been about 20. African rates were huge: 44 in South Africa, 58 in Kenya. Asian tolls were comparable or even higher. I. D. Mills estimates seventeen or eighteen million deaths in India, a figure that would mean a mortality rate of about 60 per 1,000. And—a point that illustrates the invisibility of the pandemic in Africa—in Senegal perhaps 47,000 people died of influenza in 1918, but the 3,000 Senegalese plague deaths in the same year monopolized the attention of French colonial authorities.[52]

Results in isolated communities could be frightful. In Tahiti 10 percent of the population died in twenty-five days after an influenza-bearing ship called on November 16, 1918; similar mortality occurred in Tonga, and in Western Samoa 7,500 people (of a total population of 38,800) died within two months, nearly 20 percent. In the Alaskan village of Wales 170 of a total population of 310 died when influenza appeared there.[53]

Relatively high mortality rates from influenza often related to the involvement of other infections that struck the weakened influenza victim. Many of the deaths due to "influenza" undoubtedly resulted from the combined effects of influenza and subsequent pneumonia. Patterson and Pyle also suggest, with good reason, that influenza contributed to many other deaths attributed to heart and kidney problems and to diabetes.[54] The poverty of Asia, Africa, and Latin America aggravated such complications in many ways. So while Crosby saw little evidence of differential mortality along class or ethnic lines in the United States, Mills finds sharp differences among Indian castes and classes, and Patterson and Pyle see obvious correlations with worldwide poverty.[55] Ethnicity and race clearly mattered in Asia and Africa. Maoris in New Zealand had an influenza mortality rate seven times higher than New Zealand whites.[56] Poor nutrition, poor housing, a slimmer chance of supportive care, all opened the door for bacterial infections that could worsen influenza's effects. Mills also points to correlations between high mortality and damage to crops from unusually severe monsoon rains, and suggests that regions which experienced a wider range of daily temperature fluctuations might be more prone to pneumonia, especially among the poorly housed and clothed. Indian women suffered disproportionally, perhaps because influenza added to the physical stresses of pregnancy, perhaps because as primary care-givers themselves they lacked nursing care when they fell ill. In the European colonies of West Africa, the demands of the war created serious shortages of doctors and nurses, made worse by the persistent poverty of the colonial governments themselves.[57]

Although Western medicine approached influenza with confidence, it offered different etiological explanations, and some aspects of the 1918 pandemic are still mysterious. No consensus was reached about a causative bacterium, although the germ theory was at its most seductive. "Pfeiffer's bacillus" for a time was a likely collaborator with some "virus," but more widespread was a belief in general contagionism, perhaps stirred up by the war and its poison gases and rotting flesh. Wartime xenophobes could readily call influenza an enemy plot, and apparently the idea that influenza came to Europe from Allied-imported Chinese labor began its career as German propaganda. Influenza viruses were eventually identified in 1933. Much more recently (in 2005) samples recovered from frozen corpses in Alaska (and from pathology material preserved in American and British military archives) led to the identification of the particular 1918 virus. But its geographic origins are still in doubt, as is its "newness" in 1918. And why the 1918 variety pounced on young adults remains in the realm of conjecture. Did those born before the 1889–90 pandemic enjoy some immunity? If so the magic age in 1918 would have been twenty-eight or twenty-nine, and the high death rates of "young adults" straddle those years. Were the military generations subject to greater stress? Undoubtedly, but influenza affected young adults all over the world, in places as far removed as possible (both physically and psychologically) from Flanders fields.

The pandemic had serious demographic effects, at least outside Europe and North America. Patterson calls the 100,000 deaths in six months in the Gold Coast (modern Ghana) "the worst short-term demographic disaster in the history of Ghana," while Howard Phillips calls the pandemic "the single most devastating episode in South Africa's demographic history," one that resulted in a "lost generation." Mills makes clear the ways in which the pandemic disturbed Indian demographic patterns.[58] Births in India plunged sharply by the middle of 1919; high morbidity in late 1918 probably meant lower coital frequency, many women of childbearing age had died, marriages were postponed during the pandemic, and many families were broken apart by the death of a marriage partner.

And even in the United States, some evidence suggests that influenza may have changed differential mortalities for men and women for up to fifteen subsequent years, as the gaps between overall male and female mortality rates narrowed.[59] So while the influenza may have been forgotten in Europe and North America (except of course by those families in which death had occurred), the worldwide social and economic effects reverberated through succeeding generations.

The memory of the pandemic now stands in the West as a cautionary tale of the dangers of new influenza strains. The discovery of influenza viruses presented the possibility of preventive vaccines, but their development raised practical and political problems. Could adequate supplies of a vaccine be produced when rapidly mutating viruses gave very short notice of their changes? Or should broader-gauged vaccines be prepared in the hope that they would cover new subtypes of virus? And if something went wrong with vaccine preparation or with delivery systems, would populations again be vulnerable to a pandemic on the scale of 1918? If nothing else, influenza (assisted by poliomyelitis) showed that scientific biomedicine in the age of World War I (and later) had no remedy for a viral illness once it took hold in the body. Regardless of the confidence in the "therapeutic perspective" documented by Hildreth, the possibility of defining disease in terms other than the biomedical persisted.

Unresolved General Issues

For all the confident optimism of biomedical practitioners before 1960, it was becoming increasingly apparent that several issues lay outside their control and might remain so for some time to come. Of those the social issues seemed more complex and intractable, but even if an optimal social situation for the promise of biomedicine could exist, some biological phenomena were still beyond the reach of the physicians.

The elusive character of viruses loomed largest among those biological problems. Viruses could now be identified, and in some cases preventive vaccines could be prepared; but therapy, on the hugely successful model of the antibiotics that conquered bacterial ailments, eluded biomedicine. Bacterial problems emerged as well, for natural selection operated in the microbiological world, as resistant strains of tuberculosis, gonorrhea, and streptococcal and staphylococcal infections developed. The very success of biomedicine cast other "failures" in a harsh light. The promise of serum therapy remained partially unfulfilled, with the outright failure of some serums and the persistent problems that accompanied others: the slow action of tetanus serum was only overcome when curare was added as a relaxant, early diphtheria serums wore off, meningitis serums varied wildly in their effectiveness. Anaphylactic reactions to diphtheria serum foretold the later allergic reactions, some serious, to penicillin.

More blatant human error sometimes crippled biomedicine as well. Twentieth-century healing annals were punctuated by the Lübeck BCG disaster (see Chapter Eight), the Cutter Incident with poliomyelitis vaccine, and other examples of biomedicine's human frailties. Science proposed therapies that later seemed simply odd, if not dangerous: gold salts for tuberculosis; the induction of malaria in syphilis patients in the attempt to kill spirochetes with high temperatures. In fact some diseases had such complex etiologies that they resisted the best efforts of scientific medicine at every stage; tuberculosis remained especially elusive, for evaluation of a "cure" remained difficult, as did the judgment of proper doses of the antibiotic that supposedly could end the scourge. Contact epidemiology could produce remarkable results, but diseases transmitted through the respiratory system remained almost impossible to trace, while some diseases might have a disheartening number of "carriers" who manifested no symptoms.

Most of the problems that rose up in the path before the apparently triumphant scientific paradigm in fact originated in society itself, for the entire biomedical agenda depended on human beings for its implementation. "Disease" persisted, or its social construction shifted, in part for that reason, as well as because of autonomous biological developments. Human cultural behavior changed slowly; issues of cost sometimes dominated medical response or effectiveness; disease incidence continued to reflect socioeconomic differences within populations.

Much of the effect of twentieth-century biomedicine depended on the acceptance of a variety of cultural assumptions and habits by masses of the population.[60] People had to be convinced that taking an ailment to a physician was wise; medical culture urged not only regular visits to physicians but a variety of self-monitorial practices (breast examinations for women, for example) that would make such visits timely. A physician's proposed treatment might require a regimen that patients could easily neglect, especially if doses of medication became complicated or if the point of continuing medication was lost when the overt symptoms disappeared. Thus many patients did not complete sulfa treatments of gonorrhea because they were not convinced of their necessity. The very success of some therapies, especially antibiotics, led patients to demand (and physicians to accede to) overprescription; penicillin seemed to be thrown at every sore throat in the United States. This success also led to relaxation of the vigilance that the biomedical culture demanded of individual habits; the apparent easy conquest of syphilis by penicillin certainly contributed to a more casual attitude to sexual hygiene, and silver nitrate treatments for gonococcal conjunctivitis in newborns lapsed for a time. The demands of contact epidemiology met strong cultural resistance, especially inquiries into sex lives, where the "necessary" openness was hard to achieve. And the tendency of epidemiologists to make political assumptions about subgroups simply increased resistance; syphilis investigations in the United States made assumptions about African Americans on the sole basis of race, for example.

The success of biomedicine hinged on changing broader cultural habits as well. Could parents be persuaded that doctors and nurses should take a hand in the rearing of children? Would they accept hectoring visits from public health authorities, or the trumpeted necessity—sometimes enforced by law—that their children receive vaccines? A variety of personal habits came under scrutiny; public health opinion attacked alcohol consumption almost continuously, and by the second half of the century stigmatized tobacco use even more heavily, especially in the United States. The extent to which habits of personal hygiene were "reformed" remains an interesting subject for social and cultural historians; why and when did washing hands (especially after excretory functions) and foods and scrubbing plumbing fixtures become accepted behavior? And among what social groups?

Those issues of change in cultural habits might affect rich and poor alike. But modern scientific medicine sometimes entailed frighteningly high costs: of treatments, of medicinal products, of the infrastructures of public health and sanitation. Commercial pressures could dictate the development of therapies; Howard Florey and Ernst Chain, finding no British pharmaceutical makers willing to commit to penicillin production in the midst of a desperate war, took their processes to the United States. Such powerful political forces as war also disrupted the efforts of biomedicine, as (again) the case of penicillin in World War II illustrates; military priorities governed its allocation, while the civilian sector clamored for its miracle cures. Costs of individual treatments led to degrading spectacles in which parents appealed to the public, perhaps through the medium of television "entertainment," for funds to allow their poliomyelitis-stricken child access to a respirator.

For wealth and poverty continued to matter. Despite whatever real improvements the maturation of industrial economies brought to living standards, some dwellings remained more congested than others, with more houses per hectare or more people per room; the quality and maintenance of plumbing and sewers depended in part on income; some homes resisted the invasions of disease vectors better than others. Access to physicians depended not solely on acculturation, but on income as well; poverty might mean greater resistance to medical culture, but it might also simply shut a physician's door. The late twentieth-century revival of tuberculosis clearly illustrates the continuing—or reviving—links between the poor and the diseased.

By the late twentieth century two broad social possibilities had emerged that called the triumph of biomedicine into question. One was in a sense new: did industrial maturation, or the evolution of a postindustrial society, mean the continuing improvement in standards of living that the "second industrial revolution" had promised late in the nineteenth century and early in the twentieth? Or had continuing economic development around the world led to a declining per capita income for a large number or even a majority? If so the implications for the maintenance of health were serious. The second possibility was a much older theme, revived and strengthened by the complexities of a shrinking world: the likelihood that societies would continue to regard their marginal members as unworthy of care, that the conflation of the "diseased" with the poor or the aberrant would persist. Thus the social construction of disease lends support to its biological and epidemiological reality.

Twelve

Disease and Power

In two important ways the twenty-first-century West confronts disease
more vigorously than did past societies. The biomedical model has conferred on
its practitioners exceptional power, and the modern Western state has used a
combination of ideology and technology to exert a new level of control over its
populations, their behaviors, and the ailments that beset them. Yet these apparent discontinuities in Western disease history, marked by the undoubted successes of modern medicine and state-sponsored public health, may simply mask
important unchanging realities. The powerful still configure disease as the product and bane of the powerless. Practical limits remain on the extent of biomedical or political power over the incidence of disease, if not over its configuration.
The contemporary epidemic of AIDS has brought both the new powers of biomedicine and the old habits of mind that relate disease to marginal groups and
their supposed behavior into newly sharp focus. AIDS also suggests other continuing dilemmas, especially those stemming from the gulf between the growing
powers of scientific medicine and continuing inequalities in the sharing of world
resources.

The Ambiguities of State Power

States have long had an interest in the health of their populations,
although their motives have not always been clearly expressed or even understood. Early modern European states gradually came to recognize connections
between the size of their populations and both military power and economic prosperity; ambitious absolutists such as the eighteenth-century kings of Prussia
encouraged immigration; enlightened despots of the same period embarked on
programs of "medical police," particularly attending to the control of epidemics

through isolation and quarantines and, in some cases, to the public provision of nursing care and the training of nurses. The concern that eighteenth-century states manifested for the health of their soldiers and sailors suggests the importance of the military motive for such benevolent behavior. By the middle of the eighteenth century some governments had also begun attempts to number their inhabitants, and much late Enlightenment opinion persisted in associating a large population with progress. At the end of the century the English author Robert Malthus cast serious doubts on that equation, doubts that may have coincided with the tendency (in liberal states at least) to leave the health of populations to individuals. As we have seen, however, laissez-faire health policies never became absolute, as a dialectical struggle characterized the nineteenth-century state's attempts to superintend the health of its citizens. Within most states arguments raged over (for example) the registration of physicians, the enforcement of quarantines, and the provision of sewer systems, as well as attacks on particular diseases.

Vaccination

As we saw in Chapter Three, late medieval governments had evolved public health machinery to deal with the specific threat of plague, but its goal was containment rather than eradication. In the nineteenth century Jenner's smallpox vaccine seemed a new and powerful tool, and some governments quickly announced policies to apply it. Bavaria made smallpox vaccination compulsory as early as 1807, and Denmark (1810), Russia (1812), and Sweden (1816) followed.[1] Government compulsion did not, unfortunately, mean effective administration, and the rapid elimination of smallpox certainly did not result. The practical, political, and theoretical barriers that interfered with governmental will illustrate the gaps between intentions and results that have bothered governments since.

National administration of a vaccine faced daunting practical problems in the nineteenth century. For much of the period adequate supplies of vaccine could not be relied on, and their quality varied widely. Even after the serious epidemics of the early 1870s (which prodded several European states toward tighter compulsion) quality and quantity could not be assumed. In the German Empire, where an 1874 law required national vaccination, physicians continued to supply most of their own vaccine by cultivating it in the arms of their patients and transferring it from arm to arm.[2] The skill of vaccinators was unpredictable. Vaccination might therefore be accompanied by considerable pain, expense, and (at the least) inconvenience, so a passive resistance to the procedure was probably widespread everywhere in the Western world.[3] That passive resistance might be more easily overcome in times of severe epidemic, but those distant in time or place from such outbreaks might be more likely to forget vaccination; while if vaccination had some success in reducing smallpox incidence, that very success might lead to popular complacency. Other practical difficulties arose from the too-slow realization that one vaccination did not confer lifetime immunity; compulsory state rules in the early nineteenth century required only a single vaccination, presumably in infancy, and the development of smallpox cases later in life seemed to prove that the technique did not work. And while government might "compel," obedience to government might depend on local leaders of opinion—teachers, clergy, landowners, healers—and their ability to persuade others.

Both political and theoretical issues might drive such passive resistance to more active opposition. Many healers insisted, all through the century, that vaccination was unproved at best, and perhaps positively dangerous. Could the procedure spread other diseases? Syphilis especially was blamed on it, and the dirty practices and instruments of some vaccinators lent credence to such beliefs. As earlier chapters of this book (especially Chapters Seven and Ten) have shown, the notion of disease as a discrete entity made only gradual headway in the nineteenth century, while many thinkers continued to insist on a miasmatic or environmental explanation that they applied to smallpox as well as to more obvious candidates. Based on the "contagion" theory, vaccination was by those lights inadequate to halt disease.

These theoretical medical objections overlapped with, or were overshadowed by, more general political and cultural arguments. The religious or moral view of disease—as punishment sent to sinners by God—continued to sway some opinion; vaccination was thus an impious interference with God's will.[4] Others objected generally to the extension of state power that compulsory vaccination represented, especially because it brought the state into the family, interfering with parental (and particularly paternal) rights in the care of children. In Great Britain the objections of the antivaccination movement of the 1870s and 1880s coincided with the campaigns waged against another salient of state health regulation: the Contagious Diseases Acts of the 1860s, which licensed and controlled prostitution in an attempt to preserve the health of the military. Those measures and vaccination were alike seen as intolerable intrusions of state power into the lives of individuals. In some other cases resistance to vaccination may have grown out of ethnic conflict, as in Quebec in the 1870s; sometimes state enforcement mechanisms touched raw nerves of class, as was true in England after 1840.[5] In that year the government began to provide free vaccination to the poor, made available through the local administrators of the Poor Law. But this seemingly benign policy came on the heels of a reform of the system of poor relief that had created a widely hated bureaucracy. Many of the poor shunned vaccination simply because it brought them to the workhouse. When vaccination was made compulsory for all infants in 1853, the procedure remained in the hands of Poor Law guardians, guaranteeing its continued unpopularity.

In the face of political and cultural resistance (which took an increasingly organized form in many states by the 1870s and 1880s) governments responded in several ways, not always consistently. In some countries compulsion was a last resort; France adopted compulsory vaccination only in 1902. Others attempted to sweeten the prospect, hoping to induce compliance with the carrot rather than the stick. Thus Prussia (in 1835) urged schoolmasters to accept only vaccinated pupils in their schools, and made possession of a vaccination certificate a prerequisite for receipt of state benefits. Prussia simultaneously threatened parents with arrest if their children became sources of smallpox infection. Such methods produced vaccination rates roughly equal to those achieved by German states (such as Bavaria) that employed outright compulsion.[6] Some evidence even suggests little correlation between legal penalties and rates of compliance. According to Naomi Williams's studies of British policy in the 1870s, some regions (for example, Buckinghamshire) had high rates of both prosecutions and compliance, others (including London) had low rates of both, while Leicestershire— much higher in compliance than London, lower than Buckinghamshire—had a much higher prosecution rate than either.[7]

Compulsion, therefore, clearly needed popular conviction as well as the iron fist of the law. R. J. Lambert (1962) certainly exaggerated when he called the 1867 British provision of repeated penalties for evading parents a "savage, cat-and-mouse provision totally unprecedented in health legislation" (remember Florentine torture in the seventeenth century), but wider compliance everywhere probably followed not Draconian penalties but a careful government monitoring of the vaccination process that reassured the population about its safety.[8] The German government began such a policy in the 1880s, one involving detailed codes of instruction for vaccinators, parents, and policing authorities alike. Compliance rates soared as a result. Vaccination illustrated that state medical power functioned more successfully when a population accepted its own "medicalization."

Despite the varied difficulties, some states achieved the eradication of smallpox. Sweden was apparently the first, declaring itself smallpox-free in 1895; in the first half of the twentieth century a growing number of Western (and some non-Western) states joined this list. As Donald Hopkins says, this result was a "byproduct of attempts to vaccinate entire populations" rather than the achievement of a deliberately announced national goal of eradication.[9] Compulsion played an inconsistent role. At about the time when France belatedly made vaccination compulsory (1902), Britain (between 1898 and 1907) backed away from strict compulsion by allowing parents to refuse vaccination on grounds of conscience; a number of American states, beginning with California in 1911, adopted a similar policy, and by the 1930s four American states actually forbade local authorities from requiring vaccination for schoolchildren. Only ten American states compelled vaccination. Yet despite that apparent laxity Britain was free of smallpox in 1939 and the United States in 1949. Popular acceptance of vaccination, helped along by such indirect "compulsions" as requiring international travelers to prove vaccination, apparently eliminated smallpox from Europe and North America by 1950. These efforts also received help from an autonomous source: the rapid spread of the mild *Variola minor* form of smallpox in different areas of the world in the twentieth century. That disease in effect inoculated millions of people from the effects of *Variola major* without any human intervention.

In parts of Asia and Africa, however, smallpox remained a serious killer. Its eradication by 1977 resulted from a combination of new medical technologies, a new epidemiological approach, and the first effective stirrings of international cooperation. The preparation of a freeze-dried vaccine, in use in 1949 and in full commercial production in 1954, made available a vaccine that retained its potency for months without being refrigerated; the warm and poor regions of the world could thus be vaccinated reliably. Many doubts about the possibility of eradicating smallpox in poor countries were overcome between 1966 and 1970 when, after a World Health Assembly meeting vowed to eliminate smallpox in ten years, a number of contiguous West and Central African states succeeded in rapidly stamping it out. In the process of that campaign the attempts to vaccinate whole populations were abandoned, and the strategy of "surveillance-containment" adopted, one that concentrated on the immediate loci of the disease. That proved dramatically successful. Only six countries reported smallpox in 1972, and by 1977 the last natural case of the disease in the world (in Somalia) occurred.

Nations in Peril

Vaccination also gave states experience in the attack on specific disease entities. Those attacks became much more frequent in the twentieth century, in part because of the growing strength of biomedicine, but also because several circumstances pointed states toward more active concern with health. In the years between the Franco-Prussian War of 1870–71 (and the resultant unification of the German Empire) and World War I the major Western states fell into a rivalrous set of military alliances, struggled with one another for world economic and colonial supremacy, and developed a far higher level of bureaucratic activity and efficiency involving many facets of life from tax collection to economic promotion and mass education. Universal military conscription became the rule for the European continental powers, so a direct correlation existed between numbers in the population and in the armed forces. In those contexts Western political and military leaders invoked not so much Malthus as Darwin, for by the end of the century Malthus was apparently being proved wrong, while the ideas of social Darwinism supplied a language in which states could give voice to their national hopes and fears.

The specter of Malthusian overpopulation receded in the most industrially advanced states, which (at different dates) began experiencing a demographic transition. Their death rates fell, but so too did their birth rates, and the explosive population growth that had characterized most of nineteenth-century Europe leveled off. Was France—the great early exception with its slow growth—really the model for the rest? French leaders, with a population outnumbered by rival Germany in the ratio of eight to five, wanted to reverse the trend by promoting population growth; Germans held up degenerate France as an awful example, and urged their people to remain healthy and fruitful.[10] And while the apparent failure of the Malthusian prediction threatened the quantity of the nation, other forces imperiled its quality. Could the breeding of inferior stock overwhelm the health and vigor of a "native" race? Both environmental and genetic hazards loomed. British leaders, hoping to retain their country's imperial and economic primacy, recoiled in horror from the evidence of the effect of urban slums on the health, fitness, and physical stature of the Britons resident in them. According to one report, 565 of every 1,000 recruits for the army in 1900 (during the Anglo-Boer War) failed to meet the minimum height of 5'6", and such data stimulated a "nation in peril" alarm.[11] At the same time Americans faced a deluge of immigrants from southern and eastern Europe, who seemed to concentrate in the large cities rather than diffusing to the healthy "natural" countryside as had their German and Scandinavian predecessors. In ideology that thoroughly confused nature and nurture, both British and Americans regarded their "race" as threatened by the new human situation, and some of them proposed extreme state action to counter the dangers.

Nationalists (and governments) perceived both general and specific threats to the health of the people, and they responded to each in a variety of ways. In their general approaches to the health of the nation, states could rely on the well-established environmental theories of disease causation that had so attracted nineteenth-century sanitationists and miasmists. Policing the environment had become, as we have seen, an important early justification for state activity that continued into the twentieth century. But other possibilities presented themselves as well. "Nations are built of babies," proclaimed an Ontario Board of Health pamphlet in 1913, and many Western governments agreed, attempting to provide clean milk, promote breast-feeding, educate mothers in child care, and encourage routine medical care of infants.[12] The purity of foods and drugs became a state concern. In initially modest ways governments began investment in medical research, funding that by the mid-twentieth century had become enormous. Governments had also begun acting against disease by insuring their citizens' medical costs, a policy begun in Germany in 1883 and subsequently adopted (in different forms) in many Western states. Such actions certainly aided in the "medicalization" of the population (and of views of disease), for state insurance might only be paid to those healers recognized by the state, and the state insurance schemes arose coincidentally with the most vigorous period of professional assertion by physicians. States also expressed more indirect interest in health, which might take the form of official promotion of healthy diets (through such diverse mechanisms as state-subsidized colleges of agriculture and instruction in "health" and "home economics") and of physical culture (through physical training in state schools and the insistence on universal military training).

More sinister possibilities lurked in this panoply of largely benign state initiatives. Could the health of the nation be improved by a more careful—or regulated—attention to its breeding stock? Darwinism certainly carved the "survival of the fittest" on many late nineteenth-century walls and minds; Darwin left little doubt that inherited variations related to survival, but he left considerable doubt about the mechanism of inheritance. By the end of the century two different concepts seemed to strengthen the role of "nature" as opposed to "nurture," of genetics as opposed to environment, in the determination of inheritance. Gregor Mendel (when his arguments were belatedly accepted) seemed to establish inheritance on a clear footing as the transmittal of particulate traits, without blending and certainly without environmental interference; red and yellow parents produced red and yellow offspring, not orange. The mathematical precision of Mendelian genetics lent strength to the certainty of "heredity" as a determinant. Meanwhile August Weismann's arguments convinced many that the "germ plasm" alone carried the principles of inheritance, that changes in the "soma" were not reflected in the next generation. Weismann seemed to dismiss any role for "acquired characteristics" in evolution.

In the prevailing climate of nationalist fears, magnified by the apparent failure of Malthus's population predictions, the rampant forces of industrially driven social change, and the movement of peoples, the ideas of eugenics gained widespread and influential currency.[13] The study of breeding a fitter humanity by identifying desirable traits and encouraging their possessors to be fruitful was first consciously advanced by Francis Galton in the 1860s and 1870s; he coined the word "eugenics" in his *Inquiries into Human Faculty and Its Development* (1883). The ideas of Weismann and Mendel seemed to add weight to its assumptions. Thefollowers of eugenics believed not only that desirable traits should be encouraged, but that the propagation of *undesirable* traits should be discouraged. If human weaknesses or "degeneracies" were inherited, then breed them out. Eugenicists quickly agreed that a number of such weaknesses were inheritable, including various levels of "feeble-mindedness", epilepsy, insanity, alcoholism, a propensity to crime and prostitution, and a susceptibility to tuberculosis.

That list coincided with many of the most widely perceived threats to national health in the late nineteenth and early twentieth centuries, and those almost invariably included (or were headed by) tuberculosis, venereal disease, and alcoholism. The social costs of such "disease," especially if the plastic category of "feeble-mindedness" were included, were reckoned as appalling. State expenditure could be reduced, and more important, the health and fitness of the nation could be strengthened, if such "disease" could be stamped out. Vaccination suggested that disease could be extirpated, at least in theory. The eugenic idea—the use of inheritance to breed out degeneracies and their "disease"—gained such wide favor that Jean Webster's *Dear Enemy* (1915), a popular American girls' story, could blithely tell fifteen-year-olds:

> It seems that feeble-mindedness is a very hereditary quality, and science isn't able to overcome it. No operation has been discovered for introducing brains into the head of a child who didn't start with them. . . . Our prisons are one-third full of feeble-minded convicts. Society ought to segregate them on feeble-minded farms, where they can earn their livings in peaceful menial pursuits, and not have children. Then in a generation or so we might be able to wipe them out.[14]

The stories of the "Jukes" and the "Kallikaks" entered into American figures of speech, and the "degenerates" were indeed segregated on "feeble-minded farms." As early as 1879 the state of New York had created an institution for the housing of supposedly feeble-minded women of child-bearing age, and other states copied this initiative. Eugenically based government restrictions on marriage spread. The American state of Washington, for example, prohibited marriage for the feebleminded, the insane, habitual criminals (all disturbingly fluid categories), epileptics, and those with venereal disease or advanced tuberculosis.[15] The evolving biomedical definitions of the latter "degeneracies" made their detection easier, for the Wassermann test for syphilis and the tuberculin test for tuberculosis both appeared in the first decade of the twentieth century.

Bureaucracy might also literally cut lines of inheritance. In 1902 an Indiana physician, H. C. Sharp, urged vasectomy as a eugenic solution, claiming that he had already performed it on forty-two Indiana state prison inmates. Between 1907 and 1918 fifteen American states passed laws allowing the sterilization of criminals and the feeble-minded in state institutions, and while these laws were applied only irregularly and inconsistently, they enjoyed widespread popularity. By 1941 over 38,000 institutionalized Americans had been sterilized by the power and with the blessings of the state. Many European countries as well as Mexico and Japan approved similar laws; only Great Britain had explicitly rejected such legislation.[16] The obvious cultural component in the definitions of "degeneracy" or "disease" conferred disturbing legitimacy on the eugenic practices of Nazi-ruled Germany; when Winston Churchill (in 1940) memorably foresaw the "abyss of a new dark age made more sinister, and perhaps more prolonged, by the lights of perverted science," the lights may have been closer than he realized.

As Paul Weindling says, although "eugenics was authoritarian in that it offered the state and professions unlimited powers to eradicate disease and improve the health of future generations," it was not necessarily related to racism and it was not "inherently Nazi."[17] Adolf Hitler and his National Socialist party came to power in Germany in 1933 espousing an explicitly racist ideology, and they found eugenics (or some of its points at least) congruent with their theories. As racists they believed in the supreme importance of inheritance; as nationalists they wished to improve the health of the German people; they shared with Italian fascists the conviction that struggle was natural and desirable. Some of their beliefs (or the emotions to which they gave voice) found support among members of the German medical community. Many German physicians had developed a hatred of socialism, which they associated with the German state's health insurance schemes, while at the same time some felt threatened by a free-enterprise world that imperiled the corporate privileges of professions. Naziism promised attacks on the evils of both socialism and unrestrained capitalism. Anti-Semitism was widespread among German physicians, many of whom believed that Jews monopolized valuable places in the profession: places that—if Jews were removed—would open to them. More specifically, some German physicians saw that the implementation of eugenic principles would increase the activities and standing of their calling. If the state made eugenics a central point of its policies, physicians would find themselves in the high councils of government; physicians would take the lead in the breeding of a new and higher German race.

Of course Nazi ideology and practice did not completely harmonize with the science of eugenics or—for that matter—with scientific biomedicine as it had emerged in the early twentieth century. In many ways the Nazis were hostile to the intellect, and certainly hostile to open inquiry. The position of highly trained elites was problematic in the Nazi world, suffused as it was with anti-intellectualism and appeals to mass violence. Much Nazi sentiment was consciously anti-modern, appealing to older German mythology, folk art and craft, a preindustrial society of peasants and elves. Alternative healing modes such as homeopathy attracted some Nazis; others extolled the ideas of Paracelsus as an expression of peculiarly German genius.[18] As Nazi policy moved from support for eugenic sterilization toward euthanasia and then toward the medicalization of anti-Semitism, many doctors found themselves with deep internal contradictions.

In 1933 a German Sterilization Law singled out nine "diseases" as genetic problems meriting sterilization: epilepsy, Huntington's chorea, schizophrenia, manic depression, severe alcoholism, and "hereditary" feeble-mindedness, blindness, deafness, and malformations. As had been true of the earlier American state legislation (with which considerable overlap existed) most of these categories were largely culturally determined, but in 1933 at least the German law had no explicit racial component. Between that date and the end of the Nazi regime (1945) perhaps 360,000 sterilizations occurred in Germany, but the numbers declined—as did interest in the sterilization approach—after about 1937. The greatest number of the sterilized suffered from either schizophrenia or "feeble-mindedness."[19]

Interest in sterilization declined as the goal of eugenically benefiting the population, or benefiting individual families, became confused with the Nazi goal of racial purification. The issue of race clearly appeared in the German marriage laws of 1935. Those laws forbade marriages between the healthy and the hereditarily ill, a notion consistent with the attempts of American states to compel Wassermann tests before marriage licenses could be issued; but the 1935 German laws also prohibited marriages between Jews and non-Jews and spelled out a careful set of genetic rules defining a "Jew" by ancestry. Thus the definition of "disease" underwent a new expansion.

This slippery eugenic slope led to further state measures, including euthanasia, apparently under way with the German government's quiet blessing by 1938. Just as earlier economic arguments had supported sterilization, the proponents of euthanasia urged that the costs of maintaining the feeble-minded and their like could not be justified. (These arguments had been voiced for decades. In 1877 Richard Dugdale had calculated that by that date the family called the "Jukes" had cost New York $1.3 million, for which better uses could surely have been found.)[20] In October 1939, after the outbreak of World War II in Europe, the German government began taking a direct hand in the "processing" of patients for "wartime economic purposes."[21] Central direction of euthanasia emanated from the vaguely named "Reich Association of Mental Hospitals," also sometimes called the "T-4" program from its office in Berlin. At its beginning the T-4 program set a target of 70,000 psychiatric patients to euthanize by the end of 1941; when that goal was met and the medical and political criteria for the "useless" were increasingly conflated, the program apparently became both more loosely organized and more widespread. Among those singled out were the tubercular, the homeless, those unwilling or unable to work, and criminals of many sorts. Götz Aly cites the example of a seventeen-year-old girl, with some mental and physical handicaps but able to work, who was judged "impudent, disobedient, no longer listens at all . . . has already had sex with several men." This stereotypical rebellious teenager was ripe for euthanasia, and so died in a "Special Treatment Ward."[22] These euthanasia activities provided alarming precedents: the disappearance of patients was blamed on convenient outbreaks of "epidemic disease"; plausible explanations were offered for the transfer of patients to "new facilities"; euthanasia centers disguised gas chambers as shower stalls.

Michael Kater argues that "[f]rom the beginning to the end, the Nazi solution to the Jewish question was a medical one, in which German physicians played a key part."[23] Aly agrees, but also sees the euthanizing actions of doctors as part of what they maintained was a total program of medical reform, in which more rational and intensive care and therapy could be offered to those worth saving, those not condemned by heredity. The crucial step was the definition of socially established criteria as hereditary disease. The Jew was "disease incarnate," a hereditarily diseased race from its origins and/or suffering from a higher rate of disease as a product of the "miscegenation" that according to much eugenic opinion (not only German) produced inferior stock. Public hygiene demanded that such a population be—at the least—isolated in quarantine, in ghettos; as Robert Proctor says, such isolation in crowded and ill-served ghettos made the Jew as "disease incarnate" into a "self-fulfilling prophecy."[24] The first commandants of the extermination camps of Sobibor, Belzec, and Treblinka all came to their positions from the T-4 program.[25] Aly makes the disturbingly suggestive point that the euthanasia program of 1939–1941 showed that both German government administrators and the general populace would accept state-sponsored killing in the name of public hygiene.[26] Thus, as Kater says, Auschwitz was the "logical extension" of earlier German marriage, sterilization, and euthanasia policies.[27]

Diseases as Cultural Constructs

The world's experience with the Nazi regime should have stilled any surviving doubts that disease may be a cultural construct. Defining "race" as "disease" stands as the limiting case of such cultural determinations, but it is hardly a unique one. Yet paradoxically the modern world has also witnessed the most energetic assertions that disease is a purely autonomous biological entity. In the course of the twentieth century different configurations of disease, some maintained both simultaneously and inconsistently, wrestled for attention. Much of the inconsistency stemmed from the prevalence of the biomedical model, which internally denied that disease could have any cultural meaning, but was employed in concert with such cultural constructions.

Some contemporary disease formulations, furthermore, have grown out of earlier relations of disease to social power and weakness. When poliomyelitis first emerged as a serious American scourge, it was immediately associated with poor urban immigrant populations; later, the first subjects for poliomyelitis vaccine tests came from orphanages and state institutions. Dominant American opinion, including medical opinion, located the "disease" drug addiction in different marginal groups: opium in Chinese immigrants, cocaine in African Americans, heroin in the subclass of "criminals"; in each case "war" (as the appropriate response to an "epidemic") was declared on the drug use, which might also have been war on the social customs of a subpopulation. Venereal disease continued to be associated with race and behavior, or in some cases (as in early twentieth-century Russia) with general poverty and backwardness, despite its apparently clear biomedical explanation; did a spirochete cause syphilis, and/or was it inevitably linked to race or habits? Tuberculosis remained shameful because of its inferred causal connection with poverty as well.[28]

The biomedical model also served to break down traditional cultural constructions. Germs and viruses respected no class or racial lines. The tubercle bacillus might be found in (or travel to) anyone; even if the social and economic conditions of urban poverty made its spread more likely, poverty itself was no longer sufficient cause. Ideas about the strictly moral or social cause of a disease were quickly contested, often successfully.

But biomedicine imposed constructs of its own. An increasing number of human complaints and conditions have been "medicalized," that is, called "disease," and hence have been assumed to be amenable to biomedical treatment. Some of these have also involved the long-standing imposition of practices and ideas by the powerful on the weak. The medicalization of pregnancy, menstruation, menopause, and (now) "premenstrual syndrome" has been extensively documented by modern historians, who have shown that physicians thus extended their professional power, sometimes with the enthusiastic cooperation of women and sometimes not (see Chapter Ten).[29] Many of the complaints suffered by women, whether explicitly related to the female reproductive system or not, were also interpreted by the (largely male) physicians as "hysteria" or its modern descendants. Joan Jacobs Brumberg has shown that the problem now called anorexia nervosa grew out of a complex tangle of social causes, medical perceptions, and the successful pressures of capitalist enterprise, yet its treatment fell firmly in the hands of biomedicine.[30]

In some ways the very success of the biomedical model has generated a new target for stigmatization: the disease itself, seen as an exogenous force, operating independently of the body, the product of (and perhaps essentially consisting of) germs, viruses, or malign occurrences. Victims of disease have been shunned without belonging to any marginalized social group; being a cancer sufferer was by itself shameful, and a remarkable pattern of circumlocutions and euphemisms developed to avoid the word "cancer."[31] Campaigns against cancer—and against many other diseases and problems, including drug addictions—were usually called "wars," as though declared on some sovereign foreign power. For the understanding of the totality of disease this trend has been a mixed blessing. Biomedical understanding of diseases has weakened much of the rationale behind those moral judgments that allowed some groups to bear the blame for epidemics. But at the same time biomedical reductionism also has weakened attempts to take social contexts such as poverty into account when constructing defenses against such epidemics. It has consistently been easier and cheaper to make war on an organism than on underlying social problems.

The epidemic with which this book must end—that of a disease called, in true contemporary style, by an acronym—illustrates many of the ways in which cultural and biological meanings of disease have come to intersect in the modern world. Social, economic, and political pressures still have great power to define a disease and associate it with marginal groups in a population. The biomedical model shapes much of our response to an epidemic, limits our ability to respond to the social issues it raises, yet may also limit the prejudicial power of moral judgments. State power over disease, while actively asserted and pursued, remains uncertain in its efficacy. The disease itself remains an enemy, outside us.

AIDS

Between 1979 and 1981 a number of anomalous and not yet clearly connected disease events occurred in the Western world, events that shortly thereafter began to be knit together as a new epidemic.[32] A Los Angeles physician noted an increase in serious cases of cytomegalovirus; a few cases of Kaposi's sarcoma, a relatively rare cancer, appeared in an atypical population of young New York men; a Copenhagen man died of *Pneumocystis carinii* pneumonia; another Los Angeles physician wondered why cases of cytomegalovirus seemed to involve serious immunosuppressive effects, including the appearance of *Pneumocystis carinii*. In January 1981 a New York man died of toxoplasmosis, a disease usually associated with cats, after his immune system collapsed. In the spring of that year the Centers for Disease Control, an agency of the American government, took notice of a surge in orders for drugs prescribed for *Pneumocystis carinii* coming from New York physicians, and a Kaposi's sarcoma patient appeared in San Francisco, one whose immune system had started to fail as early as 1978. In June 1981 the Centers for Disease Control's *Morbidity and Mortality Weekly Report* carried an account of five severe cases of *Pneumocystis carinii* pneumonia in young Los Angeles male homosexuals, a report that subsequently seemed the first sounding of a tocsin.

Within a month the Centers for Disease Control had issued another report, on the appearance of Kaposi's sarcoma (26 cases) and *Pneumocystis carinii* among homosexual men in New York and California. By late August the number of such patients had climbed to 108; by November it was 159, with others suspected. *Pneumocystis carinii* cases developed in Europe as well, in Paris, Barcelona, London, and Switzerland. Between 1981 and 1984 the number of cases grew rapidly, while biomedical research wrestled with the causes of the "disease." By the end of 1982 the Centers for Disease Control had enumerated over 750 cases in the United States, while the World Health Organization found over 1,500 cases worldwide; by the end of 1984 the respective numbers were over 8,000 and over 12,000. Victims seemed to share some common characteristics, in addition to an alarming collapse of their immune systems and the development of unusual infections and carcinomas. Male homosexuals—at least for a time—seemed to predominate, and so as early as 1981 the name Gay-Related Immune Deficiency ("GRID") was proposed for the disease. But other at-risk populations appeared as well: Haitians, sufferers from hemophilia, heroin addicts, Europeans who had contacts in the United States, and other Europeans who had contacts with Africa. As will be seen shortly, the occurrence of the disease in different subgroups of the Western population quickly led to a complex pattern of stigmatization.

Meanwhile researchers sought a causative organism, perhaps one whose action was triggered by some characteristic of homosexual life. Agreement about the causative virus was not reached until after the disease received its name: "AIDS," "acquired immune deficiency syndrome." This term began to be used in 1982, when it simply (as Mirko Grmek puts it) "suggested a clinical, not a pathologic, concept."[33] In the course of 1983 two research centers dominated the search for a cause: the Pasteur Institute in Paris, and the National Cancer Institute, a division of the National Institutes of Health, near Washington, D.C. A Paris team led by Luc Montagnier discovered a likely culprit in January and February of that year, which they called lymphadenopathy associated virus (LAV); in May, about the time that Montagnier's discovery became known, Robert Gallo and his NCI colleagues argued that their discovery, human T-cell leukemia virus-I (HTLV-I), was the likely agent. An unseemly wrangle ensued, involving disputes over priority and allegations of academic dishonesty as well as uncertainty about the "right answer." Gallo described another candidate (HTLV-III) in 1984; several months later it was shown that Montagnier's LAV and Gallo's HTLV-III were identical, and seemed to be the "cause." In 1986 an international commission suggested another name, thus avoiding the priority battle, and that term gained general acceptance: human immunodeficiency virus, or "HIV."

HIV was a representative of a recently discovered class of viruses, the retroviruses, so-called because their RNA material had the power to reverse the usual biological sequence and transcribe itself into DNA. The particular effect of HIV was that of an apparently inevitable weakening of the body's immune system, the result of an attack on the lymphocytes which are vital components of that system. An acute infection by HIV first manifests itself as a brief mild illness, which might be mistaken for influenza. A period of latency then ensues, of still-indeterminate length—perhaps many years, perhaps much shorter—but eventually the damage to the immune system becomes clear and the victim suffers from a wide range of possible "opportunistic" infections, against which the body can muster no effective defense. The victim at that point passes from being "HIV positive" to suffering from AIDS.

Although many possible modes of transmission of HIV have been discussed, and many more feared by the public, medical researchers generally agree that it passes from one person to another only through the exchange of body fluids, especially blood and semen. Such exchange occurs most obviously in the course of sex, when both blood and semen may be involved in either vaginal or anal penetration, particularly if either vaginal or anal ulcers facilitate the passage of blood or semen into the recipient's circulatory system. The other important method of exchange is through injections that carry another's body fluids, perhaps blood being supplied in a transfusion or blood carried incidentally on a reused needle injecting drugs. The late twentieth century world afforded those methods ample opportunities. But panic about other possible means of contact has remained strong; many public washrooms in the 1980s began featuring electric-eye sensors to flush toilets and operate faucets, so that users' hands did not touch plumbing fixtures.

By the early 1990s the epidemic of AIDS had spread over most of the world, and it had claimed impressive numbers. The World Health Organization estimated in early 1992 that between 9 and 11 million people had been infected with the virus, and that perhaps 1.5 million cases of AIDS had developed, of whom about 90 percent had died. Of those infected, 6.5 million lived in sub-Saharan Africa. By late 1996 the number of infected had climbed to 22.6 million, 90 percent of them in "developing" countries. It was clearly increasingly difficult to configure AIDS as a disease of homosexuals. The U.S. Centers for Disease Control reported that the percentage of AIDS cases traced to male-to-male sexual contact fell from 66.5 percent in 1985 to 46.6 percent in 1993.[34] Although male-to-male sexual contact remained the most common vehicle for AIDS transmission among white American males, African-American and Hispanic-American males were roughly equally likely to have contracted the virus through injected drug use as through homosexual contact, and women were increasingly subject to infection through heterosexual contact. Reports from Africa—where statistics were far less precise—placed overwhelming emphasis on heterosexual contact as the prime mode of transmission.

The worldwide AIDS epidemic had its origins in Africa.[35] At some point, perhaps in the fairly recent past, two different forms of the virus called HIV were transmitted to humans from apes that had been infected with an allied "SIV" (simian immunodeficiency virus). The earliest clear evidence of an HIV infection comes from Kinshasa, Congo, in 1959; other cases probably existed in the 1950s in western equatorial Africa. It is likely, moreover, that by the 1970s AIDS might have become epidemic in Kinshasa (and perhaps elsewhere), well before Western eyes had focused on it, or even before the very concept of a retrovirus had been articulated. Two important circumstances, the products of the virus's epidemiological pattern, contributed to hiding the epidemic's presence. What we now know to be its very long incubation period (an indeterminate number of years between infection and the manifestation of symptoms) made the dating of its "first" appearance almost impossible. And the "symptoms," when they emerged, were in fact those of other infections, most of which were clearly identifiable as "other" ailments.

But it is important to understand the significance both of the African origin of the epidemic, and of the long period of the 1970s and early 1980s when it spread largely unrecognized through populations in sub-Saharan Africa. As John Iliffe insists, Africa has been most ravaged by the disease primarily "because it had the first epidemic established in the general population before anyone knew the disease existed."[36] The epidemic in effect gained a huge head start on the African population, and that circumstance lay behind the scale of the subsequent disaster.

To be sure, particular conditions in Africa contributed to the initial appearance and spread of the epidemic. Some of the initial contacts with the virus probably were made more likely by the aggressive imperial economic penetration of equatorial African forests by European colonizers, especially French and Belgians. With different goals in view—the expansion of land under cultivation, the extraction of rubber, logging, even hunting—that penetration brought African laborers into closer contact with wildlife (including apes) and insect parasites. Opportunities for human contact with a mutant simian immunodeficiency virus thus multiplied. Diseases formerly restricted to narrow ecological niches ultimately appeared, sometimes inspiring the frissons of horror that accompanied the first appearances of the Marburg and Ebola viruses in (respectively) 1967 and 1976.

Rapid social and economic changes occurred in Africa that aided the spread of an epidemic. Although cities all over the world grew quickly in the twentieth century, some of the most breathtaking urban growth was African. Kinshasa—Leopoldville under Belgian rule—was a sleepy colonial capital of about 40,000 people in 1940. By 1960, as Congo gained its independence, Kinshasa's population had reached 400,000, and by 1990 it had swollen to 3.8 million. As late as 1960 no sub-Saharan African city had one million inhabitants. By the early twenty-first century, twenty-seven cities had surpassed that number.[37] Medical and sanitary changes facilitated reductions in death rates, while birth rates remained high. The resulting surge in the population of the young had ominous significance for an epidemic transmitted by sexual contact.

Much of Africa remained very poor, despite urbanization and greater integration into the world economy. Peasant farmers lacked the capital to take advantage of new agricultural methods, and that contributed to the economic necessity driving migrants (especially the young) to cities. And as Chapter Nine has suggested, the social and economic changes that accompanied Western colonial rule disrupted traditional social systems and frayed traditional social controls. Those changes often deepened after World War II despite the demise of Western colonial power.

A particularly dangerous social situation developed in many African cities and towns. Spouses were often left behind as people (more often males) moved to cities. Poverty especially affected women, forcing them into dependent relationships with (often older and at least marginally more prosperous) men. For some women the "escape" from poverty might be the sex trade; some men took advantage of the opportunity for multiple concurrent sexual encounters, and it was that very situation that fed into the peculiar epidemiology of HIV. That virus is apparently most infective in people who themselves have been recently infected. As a result, societies in which multiple sexual encounters are concurrent, rather than sequential, are ones in which the virus can spread most rapidly. Some of the tragedy of the African AIDS epidemic emerged from that circumstance.

And African political turmoil exacerbated the situation. Repeated civil wars followed the collapse of the Western imperial regimes. The newly independent states often occupied areas that had been defined (with some level of ignorant abstraction) by European powers and that did not necessarily coincide with traditional tribal or language groups. The new states therefore often contained populations that shared only a common European occupying power, and which—when that power left—fell to fighting among themselves. As this book has repeatedly shown, war and civil turmoil often create optimal conditions for the spread of disease. In mid- and late-twentieth century Africa such conditions certainly existed, magnified by the movement of soldiers within the continent and of mercenaries into it. Rape committed by a rampant soldiery, hardly unique to Africa, constituted another grimmer version of multiple concurrent sexual contact. Periods of peace brought greatly increased volumes of international business travelers and tourists, as well as easier transit for migrants.

At least some of these trends were relevant to developed North America and Europe as well, including urbanization, the rapid movement of peoples, and disruptions of traditional social mores. Particularly relevant in the West was the assertion of new and much freer notions of sexual behavior, in part related to biomedical technology in the 1950s and early 1960s. Freed by penicillin from the fear of venereal disease and by contraceptive pills from the fear of unwanted pregnancy, young people in Western countries proclaimed a new era of sexual liberalization. Some expressions of that liberalization overlapped with another Western trend of the 1960s: the assertion of the civil rights of those subgroups that had previously suffered legal sanction or social discrimation. Western homosexuals combined the civil rights and sexual liberty movements, demanding both an end to discrimination and (more serious) a recognition of the social legitimacy of their practices. Many (though hardly all) homosexuals reveled in newly asserted freedoms in the 1970s; some subcultures of homosexuals in cities such as New York and San Francisco saw a remarkable spread of promiscuity as overdue public self-affirmation. The bathhouses of such subcultures became nearly ideal diffusion environments for sexually transmitted diseases. European homosexuals traveled to the American cities to enjoy the new dispensation.

Modern medical technology also played a role in the diffusion of AIDS. The idea of blood transfusions was an old one, tried by the zestful experimenters of the scientific revolution. Their transfusions from sheep to people did not work well, and the practice lapsed until the early nineteenth century. But its successful practice depended on techniques to prevent blood from clotting while in transit, and on the realization that different blood groups existed that were incompatible. Beginning about 1900 Karl Landsteiner of Vienna discovered the so-called ABO blood groups, and continued to work on different blood types; eventually, in 1940, he discovered the Rhesus-factors as well. Some transfusions were performed in the battle heat of World War I, but their true coming of age was World War II, when combatant nations began storing blood in "banks" for transfusion into the wounded. The subsequent frequency of recourse to surgery was symbiotically related to a booming (and sometimes international) blood trade; more surgery demanded more replacement blood which in turn made possible more surgery. Transfusions of blood and plasma made hemophilia a more manageable condition; transfusions reduced the risks of Rhesus-factor incompatibility between mother and fetus. Transfusions, dependent on the "gift relationship" of blood donation (in Richard Titmuss's phrase), became important elements in the maintenance of late twentieth-century health. And the "strange virus of unknown origin" entered into stocks of blood in the 1970s and early 1980s, from donors who had as yet manifested no symptoms of illness and whose virus was not then recognized, let alone screened, by blood collection agencies. Especially significant was the surge in transfusions in sub-Saharan Africa, which rose from 600,000 in 1950 to 6.8 million in 1985, when the transfusion rate approached that of the cities of Europe and North America.[38] The worldwide character of the blood business ensured worldwide dissemination.

Another piece of modern medical technology played a role in the diffusion of AIDS: the plastic syringe, in theory disposable, and far cheaper than the earlier nineteenth-century metal and glass versions. Its low cost made possible its wide distribution. In the developing world (for instance in Africa) inexpensive syringes entered a culture that already saw the needle as the prestigious symbol of successful Western biomedicine. The most obvious triumphs of the Western doctors—vaccinations and the administration of antibiotics—both gave the needle talismanic status and assured its continuing use. The poverty of developing nations, however, increased the likelihood that the disposable plastic syringe would be reused. The plastic syringe entered into Western epidemiology as well, for it facilitated the intravenous use of narcotics. The narcotics user received a more powerful and immediate sensation from injecting heroin than from smoking an opium pipe. The narcotics user was also much less likely to discard a used syringe, whether for reasons of poverty or indifference or ignorance. So reused and unsterilized needles spread infected blood throughout Africa and the West alike.

Western biomedicine contributed to the emergence of AIDS in still another, albeit indirect, way. It eliminated much of the competition. To some unknown extent AIDS may have existed in populations where people died of tuberculosis or smallpox or some other infection that the West set out to abolish. In another of the coincidences noticed by Grmek, the last confirmed case of smallpox in the world occurred in 1977, just as AIDS, or at least HIV infection, began to surface. Medicine's success against infectious disease has opened the door for much higher mortality rates from neoplasms and cardiovascular and cerebrovascular ailments. As we now understand, AIDS too should be regarded as a chronic condition, more nearly akin to cancer or to tuberculosis than to acute plague, smallpox, or cholera.

That understanding evolved with our construction of the disease. By the late 1990s, the AIDS epidemic had proceeded through several stages, both in its effects and in the ways in which societies configured it. In its first few years (between 1981 and perhaps 1986) AIDS seemed a new killer epidemic, the Black Death of the twentieth century, and a disease of unknown cause. The latter fact gave rise to a variety of explanations of it, associated (in the manner of many past confrontations with the unknown) with social issues, personal behavior, and personal and societal morality. By 1986, as agreement approached on the essential role of a virus, and agreement (very symbolically) was reached about that virus's name, thinking about AIDS became more "scientific," or "bio-medical," or "reductionist"; the emphasis on social-context explanations diminished. But the construction of AIDS as a new violent Black Death faded more slowly. In 1988 Elizabeth Fee and Daniel Fox edited a collection of essays intended to bring AIDS into the context of past acute epidemics and social responses to them; only in 1992 did the same scholars produce *AIDS: The Making of a Chronic Disease,* in which the historical parallels were no longer plague, cholera, smallpox, and yellow fever, but tuberculosis and leprosy.

Initial reactions to the new disease followed some well-established historical precedents, especially in their stigmatization of marginal groups. Leprosy came from fornicators, plague from the Jews or from sinners in general, cholera from the poor, the irreligious, or the immigrants. AIDS in its early history came from the "4-H" group (a particularly ironic reference in the United States, where the 4-H Clubs, a long-established rural youth association, are symbols of virtuous country life), three of which were easy targets for blame: homosexuals, heroin addicts, Haitians, and hemophiliacs. Only the last group might be "blameless" in the eyes of some popular moralities. Homosexuals and heroin addicts both did things which in many places were illegal, and in many more were thought immoral. Haitians were poor, and in both Europe and North America seemed representatives of a brutal and superstitious society. And while few blamed hemophiliacs for their infection with AIDS, or attributed its spread to them, hemophiliacs themselves feared stigmatization and even one another. Enrollment in an American summer camp for hemophiliac children fell 75 percent in a year, perhaps because parents feared their children would be infected, perhaps because identification as "hemophiliac" was to be avoided.[39]

As long as the "cause" of the disease had not been named and so "known," until it received a clear biomedical configuration, other groups—especially Haitians and above all homosexuals—fell under suspicion simply because they were members of those groups. Haitians were relatively invisible in their North American settlements (such as New York, Miami, and Montreal) among other poor black residents, and so received relatively little attention from the popular media. But Haitians, and Haiti, were feared nonetheless. In the winter of 1981–82, 75,000 United States tourists visited that country; in 1982–83 the number plummeted to 10,000.[40]

Much the greatest burden of initial stigmatization in the Western world fell on homosexuals. AIDS broke into public consciousness at a time when male homosexuals, especially in the United States, had moved into a new period of political and social assertiveness. Gay activities had achieved a high profile in the public mind, which proved something of a two-edged sword; a backlash of homophobia, often but not only or always associated with a revived traditional or fundamental religion, appeared in reaction to homosexual assertion and publicity. Such opinion quickly seized on AIDS as the outcome of the gay lifestyle, perhaps sent by the Almighty as punishment. An American physician suggested that "homosexuality is not 'alternative' behavior at all, but as the ancient wisdom of the Bible states, most certainly pathologic," and the American political xenophobe Patrick Buchanan wrote newspaper articles under the heading "AIDS Disease: It's Nature Striking Back." Authorities in Tulsa drained and disinfected a swimming pool after a gay group used it; in San Francisco some employers required gay employees to produce what amounted to a sixteenth-century health pass whenever they missed a day of work; fear of AIDS led to the denial of child custody to gay fathers caught in divorce proceedings; Buchanan (and many others) urged that gays be prohibited from handling foods or working in child care.[41]

Of course fear of AIDS and fear of homosexuals were conflated categories, and much of the stigma suffered by homosexuals fell on all possible AIDS "carriers," or at least on those known to be infected. Dennis Altman's collection of examples of the fears of the early 1980s illustrates the terror that the disease and its unknown powers of contagion inspired: jurors who refused to serve when they discovered that the defendant suffered from AIDS; the proposal by Delta Airlines (in the United States) to ban AIDS sufferers from its flights; the refusal of Sydney police to administer breathalyzer tests to those suspected of AIDS. (And such popular fears of AIDS contagion did not disappear after the mid-1980s. In July 1995 a letter carrier in Charleston, West Virginia, refused to deliver mail to a couple suffering from AIDS. Saying "It's not a matter of ignorance, it's a matter of safety," the postman feared cutting himself on the couple's metal mail slot and touching envelopes and stamps that they had licked.) More serious were the widespread cases of hospitals and medical personnel avoiding or refusing treatment, or even of a pathologist refusing to perform an autopsy.[42] In the early years of the epidemic the homosexual communities of the Western world bore the brunt of these experiences, which together with the stresses of sickness and death themselves generated great tension within those communities.

Were Western reactions to the first period of the AIDS epidemic consistent with reactions to earlier "plagues"? In some ways they were, but some of the parallels quickly broke down. Certainly fear and attempts to stigmatize the victims were rampant. Quarantines—much easier, as David Musto notes, if clear distinctions can be drawn between innocent sheep and dangerous goats—were discussed in some places, but remained politically too difficult to implement, especially while etiological possibilities were so open-ended.[43] Should homosexuals be confined to islands, as some Australian letter-writers urged in 1984?[44] Regardless of how stigmatized homosexuals or drug users might have been, no Western regime undertook such a sweeping exercise of state power. The conditions for some form of isolation were certainly right, as Musto points out: AIDS is a very serious disease with no cure, associated with groups already in low social esteem, apparently transmitted through some means that were illegal or believed immoral; its sufferers enjoyed periods of remission, but whether they were ever "safe" for others was not known.[45] In some or all of those ways the history of AIDS echoed that of medieval leprosy or modern tuberculosis, diseases that had been "solved" by heavy doses of isolation for their victims. To be sure, the addicts who took drugs intravenously could be imprisoned for illegal behavior, and many of them were, but homosexuals or Haitians were not imprisoned as a class. The medicalization of AIDS—especially its association with a specific virus, and the development of blood-screening tests for that virus—made such segregation or isolation more feasible, but it also meant that the social-factor explanations that stigmatized groups lost some of their force. In 1985 Great Britain allowed local authorities to isolate AIDS patients within hospitals, but the moment of maximum peril for such groups as homosexuals or Haitian nationals had passed.

The possibility of testing posed more serious problems than did quarantine, if only because behind it lay social (as distinct from physical) isolation. As was true of previous blood testing (for syphilis, for example), questions persisted about the reliability of the test; "false positives" might brand people who were in fact free of the infection. But even if the test proved infallible, its use once again threatened the delicate balance between public health and individual liberty. Would a negative result be a requirement for employment, for insurance, or for the establishment of credit? How could both public health imperatives and the confidentiality of the doctor-patient relationship be satisfied? Would people hesitate to seek medical help for fear of being "listed" positive or for fear of learning that they had an incurable disease? Would public health demand that all positive results be made available to a central recording authority? If so, might such a list be used for darker political purposes, such as the preventive incarceration of homosexuals or drug users ("identified" as such by seropositivity) as well as the actively "sick"? In any case, it is also likely that arguments over the legitimacy of testing slowed the purging of blood supplies and hence contributed to the persistence of transfusion as an agent in the spread of the virus.

Earlier epidemic episodes had also been marked by attempts to change the personal habits of individuals when those habits were related to the disease. Perhaps the most revealing analyses draw parallels between the AIDS epidemic and nineteenth-century cholera. In the early histories of both diseases some held the Almighty to be the ultimate and perhaps even the immediate cause of the disease, but more naturalistic explanations soon appeared as well: the environment, or a "miasma," in the case of cholera; a virus, in the case of AIDS. Once that "natural" theory gained wide acceptance, explanations of predisposition emerged to show why some got the disease and others did not. At first these predisposition ideas focused on who the sick person was: an immigrant, a poor slum dweller; a homosexual, a Haitian. Belonging to that category might itself be a sufficient contingent explanation, just as, for the Nazis, being a Jew was sufficient explanation of "disease." All immigrants, all homosexuals, might be either at risk or positively dangerous. More important in both the nineteenth century and the twentieth, however, was the predisposing cause that focused on what you did, rather than who you were: the lazy slacker who drank and womanized and violated maxims to save and not spend; the homosexual (or the heterosexual) who practiced "unsafe" sex, the intravenous drug user.[46] Were such people violating God's ordinances? Or was their sin that of stupidity or ignorance, flouting not so much divine law as the laws of nature and reason?

In either case the remedy was clear: the reformation of individual habits. If you contracted cholera, or AIDS, you individually had done something wrong. (Of course in the case of AIDS those who made that argument conveniently forgot about hemophiliacs and others infected by blood transfusions, or about infants infected as fetuses through the placenta.) In both cases—AIDS and cholera—a chain of reasoning placed individual responsibility at the center of disease prevention. In both cases some argued that social conditions, notably poverty, should be addressed. But it was consistently easier—and cheaper for public expenditure—to focus on the individual responsibility of the victim. In 1995 the conservative American senator Jesse Helms urged that less government money be appropriated for the care of AIDS patients, because AIDS was "a disease transmitted by people deliberately engaging in unnatural acts." Their "deliberate, disgusting, revolting conduct" had resulted in their disease.[47]

Thus prevention emphasized the reformation of personal habits. Late twentieth-century teachings were usually more sophisticated than nineteenth-century advice to the poor about public health, which often did not rise much above Guizot's reputed *Enrichez vous*. Instead, twentieth-century homosexuals especially received (and generated themselves) much specific advice about sex practices, including abstention, that would prevent the passage of dangerous body fluids. Such advice was inevitably freighted with sociopolitical implications. Especially in the United States, such urgings appeared just as many homosexuals began to enjoy a sexual freedom that went hand in hand with self-legitimation. "Safe sex" ideas therefore bitterly divided homosexuals between those who felt the imperatives of public health (which meant in many cases staying alive) outweighed the rights of personal free expression, and those who maintained, in effect, give me liberty or give me death. It was an old argument, cast in somewhat new terms; personal expression was the late twentieth-century equivalent of freedom of trade, disrupted by quarantines and health passes. In 1983–84 San Francisco bathhouses became the loci of such old-new struggles. Other advice—directed at homosexual and heterosexual populations alike—replayed some of the themes of earlier venereal disease episodes, especially the use and morality of condoms. Should they be distributed widely—including among the young—in the name of disease prevention, or does that act amount to a licensure of promiscuity? Should AIDS—a more terrible version of syphilis—be left like syphilis as a punishment for the wicked, and as a spur to proper behavior? The same questions surrounded the distribution of free disposable syringes for drug addicts: was disease prevention the overriding goal, or should an attack on drug use take precedence?

As Dennis Altman put it," [t]here is a fine line between education and control."[48] Some attempt at the reformation of habits, whether of the poor, the homosexual, or the drug user, meant the imposition of morality from "outside," arguing (for example) that "safe sex" meant monogamy or celibacy, that safe drug use meant no drug use, or that escaping poverty meant working harder. It should not be surprising, therefore, that some of the stigmatized groups of the late twentieth century reacted as did their nineteenth-century predecessors: by denying the menace of the disease altogether, and/or by seeing it as an excuse for the extension of the tyranny of a dominant majority over them. Recall the nineteenth-century urban crowds that cried "cholera humbug," and saw a medical plot to gain more specimens for dissection. In the early history of AIDS some homosexuals denied its seriousness, or denied its association with their sexual habits; in some African-American communities the belief persisted that AIDS was a genocidal plot hatched by the white power structure.

By the late 1980s, however, the configuration of AIDS began to change in several important respects. The global incidence of the epidemic drew some attention away from the themes of homosexuality and intravenous drug use that had dominated Western discourse. By early 1991 the number of AIDS cases reported in sub-Saharan Africa reached 800,000; a year later it was estimated that 6.5 million sub-Saharan Africans were HIV-positive, when the number of seropositives in the developed worlds of Europe and North America had reached only 1.5 million. Infection rates in some African cities were simply frightening. In 1991 one in forty of all sub-Saharan women of child-bearing age (between fifteen and forty-nine) may have been HIV-infected, but in some cities the proportion may have reached one in three. As early as 1988 between 16 and 19 percent of pregnant women in Blantyre, and 12 percent in Lusaka, were HIV-positive; in the same year in Kampala between 5 and 12 percent of all newborns were infected, over half of them expected to die before their fifth birthday. In Abidjan 43 percent of hospital patients were HIV-positive. But the most remarkable rates appeared among populations of urban prostitutes: as early as 1986, 86 percent of the prostitutes of Nairobi were found to be HIV-positive, while Blantyre recorded a "modest" 55 percent infection rate.[49]

Although precise figures were scarce, no one doubted that the most important mode of transmission of AIDS in Africa (and elsewhere in the non-Western world) was heterosexual contact, and that AIDS affected women as well as men. The African experience dismissed the construct of AIDS as a disease of homosexual or drug-using males. As this chapter has already suggested, many sub-Saharan African situations created unusually rich opportunities for sexually transmitted disease among men and women alike. Other modes of transmission entered into the African picture as well as sex. Needles used for medical procedures (including blood transfusions), when economic hardship made their disposal or careful sterilization less likely, undoubtedly accounted for some infections. Non-sterile injections, either medical or in illicit drug use, remain important in the spread of HIV-AIDS in some African states, including Mauritius and Kenya.[50]

Between 1992 and 2007 the number of sub-Saharan Africans infected by AIDS rose from 6.5 million to 22.5 million, which then accounted for about two-thirds of the world total. By 2005 roughly 13 million sub-Saharan Africans had died as a result of AIDS. The scale of the African pandemic was thus gigantic, but its incidence fell very unevenly on the continent. The countries of southern Africa bore the heaviest burden: in 2007, South Africa had more people infected with HIV (about 5.5 million) than anywhere else in the world, while in Swaziland about 26 percent of adults between the ages of 15 and 49 were infected, the world's highest such infection rate. That infection rate exceeded 15 percent in other southern African states as well. In general, east African states have somewhat lower infection rates than their southern neighbors, and west African states are lower yet.[51]

Many different circumstances contribute to regional and national differences. Some states—notably Uganda, beginning in 1992—confronted the epidemic with unusual openness and with efforts at behavioral education, enlisting their population's cooperation. That approach apparently paid dividends, especially in contrast to the experiences of other states. Congo (then Zaire) under Mobutu Sese Seko in effect forbade discussion of the subject in the crucial years in the 1980s when the new disease spread through the population. In South Africa, the government (especially under President Thabo Mbeki) chose to emphasize the broad-scale provision of general health care to the population, itself perhaps a justifiable policy, but one that was combined with ambiguous statements that seemed to deny the seriousness of the AIDS situation. And the fact that male circumcision reduces the chance of HIV transmission and infection has benefited states with large Muslim populations, especially in west Africa, and thus has contributed to the lower infection rates in states such as Senegal, Mali, and Niger.[52]

At this time it is difficult to predict the future trend of the world-wide AIDS pandemic. In sub-Saharan Africa evidence suggests that the disease may have peaked sometime between 2001 and 2005 in at least some places. It seems certain, however, that the disease will have significant demographic consequences. In five southern African countries (Botswana, Lesotho, Swaziland, Zambia, and Zimbabwe) life expectancies for people born in 2005 had fallen below 40 years; as recently as the mid-1990s those life expectancies had been above 50.[53] In some of those countries (and in South Africa as well) death rates exceeded birth rates, and (unlike the situation of many European states where birth rates fell below death rates) those birth rates were already high. Human populations have considerable power to rebound from such demographic disaster, but in the interval the prospects for economic and social advance are daunting. The fact that the disease's incidence is heaviest among what should be the most productive segment of the population—urban peoples between ages 15 and 45—will surely cripple economic development. The costs of health care are inflated, and resources (already scarce) are diverted from other serious health menaces. AIDS by its very nature works synchronistically with other infections; more syphilis means more opportunities for HIV infection, which in turn weakens a body's ability to resist the ravages of syphilis.

A particularly disturbing relationship has developed between the new disease and that nineteenth-century classic, tuberculosis. In 2005, over 600,000 people in the world were infected with both AIDS and tuberculosis; in South Africa, somewhere between 50 and 80 percent of tuberculosis patients were also HIV-positive. In that AIDS-wracked country the incidence of tuberculosis rose from 169 per 100,000 in 1998 to 645 per 100,000 in 2005.[54] On some level the cause of tuberculosis remains a complex tangle (see Chapter Eight), but certainly the body's immune system has much to do with the difference between infection by the tubercle bacillus (very common) and the full-blown clinical symptoms of tuberculosis. AIDS is therefore a logical partner of tuberculosis. The connections between HIV and tuberculosis infections announced themselves in the developed world as early as the mid-1980s. For example, between 1982 and 1987 tuberculosis cases in Chicago declined by 39 percent, only to rise by 23 percent in the period from 1987 to 1993. Between those two years the percentage of coincident cases of tuberculosis and AIDS rose from 8 to 15 percent. The proportion of tuberculosis cases was higher in the African-American population than in other groups; the proportion of coincident cases was higher yet, suggesting the importance of poverty and access to medical services as related issues. And while the surge (between 1988 and 1992) in U.S. tuberculosis infections has since receded, the disease persists in states with large pockets of urban poverty.[55]

African experiences also illustrated that women might be even more likely victims than men. Women in Africa generally have suffered higher incidence rates of AIDS and have hence been at greater risk, owing to their poverty and frequent dependence on the wishes of men. The high rates of infection experienced by pregnant women have resulted in a distressing spread of the disease to newborns. Realization of that vulnerability of women only dawned slowly in the West, where the disease had so strongly imprinted itself as a plague of male homosexuals and drug addicts. As long as the disease seemed conveyed by needles and penises, women might be either innocent or ignored, despite the long and strong cultural associations of sexually transmitted diseases with women. Western states had repeatedly attempted to control syphilis by regulating prostitutes, not their male customers; an American propaganda poster of World War II had pictured venereal disease as a woman walking arm in arm with Hitler and Tojo, and the caption named her the "Worst of the Three."[56] But when in late 1986 the American mass media began calling AIDS a "threat to us all," the position of women in the epidemic began to be reevaluated. At first confined to traditional (and largely benign) roles ("loving mother, loyal spouse, wronged lover, philanthropic celebrity," as Paula Treichler puts it), women could now assume the role of threats as well as that of victims.[57]

In addition to its heterosexual and worldwide faces, AIDS has also become a chronic problem more than an acute one. In part that has happened as the passage of time revealed the indeterminate span of latency in the HIV-infected. But biomedical intervention—from pharmacology—played a role as well. In 1986 the drug azidothymidine (AZT) was shown to prolong the period of HIV latency, and it was approved for American use in 1987. The introduction of a therapy (although it was not a "cure") changed some of the dimensions of the AIDS problem.[58] Blood testing now had a point apart from surveillance and the general "public good"; an individual might benefit from early detection if a treatment existed that prolonged life.

In the 1990s further antiretroviral drugs appeared, especially the so-called protease inhibitors, increasingly administered together with AZT. The application of these "cocktails" contributed to a dramatic decline in European and North American death rates from AIDS; between 1997 and 2001 that rate fell 84 percent. However, the benefits of these new life-prolonging therapies were slower to reach the developing world, especially sub-Saharan Africa. Their staggering initial costs far exceeded the abilities of most Africans (and their governments) to pay. Only in 2000–2001 did those costs fall, as generic drug manufacturers (particularly in India) entered the world market. But in the meanwhile the reductions in Western mortalities were not duplicated in Africa, and so AIDS "was becoming another Third World disease."[59]

The new therapies had some curious political effects in both the West and in Africa. Some Western AIDS activists welcomed the therapies, but resisted the "chronic" reconfiguration that accompanied them. The activists feared—with some reason—that the "normalization" of the disease would lessen interest in it and imperil funds mobilized against it. In the West and in Africa alike those interested in AIDS complained bitterly about the seeming reluctance of governments to spend money on AIDS research and treatment. In the West governments were faulted for indifference to the plight of the disadvantaged populations most affected by the disease; in Africa, where resources were usually limited, painful choices might have to be made between the expense of retroviral AIDS drugs and the provision of basic health care to the population. And Western activists in other health "wars," notably those against cancer, have resented the brash newcomer that has taken funds from work on diseases that still affect far more people in Western societies than AIDS.

Issues of cost have been exacerbated by the chronic character of AIDS. The long-term care of people who may be intermittently too ill to work or to care for themselves is by its nature very expensive. The majority of the sufferers from AIDS are often already among the economically (and/or socially) disadvantaged in Western societies, those least able to afford such expenses. The costs therefore fall heavily on state health systems and private insurance provisions.

Especially in the United States, these problems have illustrated two particular weaknesses in both public and private health insurance systems. The American public health system is most effective for those over the age of sixty-five; the overwhelming majority of AIDS patients is considerably younger. And in a more general way Western health care systems have had greater difficulty providing for the needs of the chronically ill, a problem that increasing Western life expectancies have magnified. The conquests of epidemic disease, in this respect as in others, have had unforeseen and not always welcome consequences; in many respects biomedicine has run ahead of both moral and social consensus about its powers. The long-term AIDS sufferer now fights for resources with other beneficiaries of biomedicine's successes. And because AIDS remains primarily a disease of the poor and socially outcast, that sufferer's position—like his or her body—remains vulnerable and weak.

Poverty as the Greatest Killer

The incidence of AIDS, falling most heavily on the poor fraction of the developed world and on the poor nations of the world as a whole, reminds us that the modern Western historiographic concern with disease as a cultural construct may be a luxury in which only a relative few can indulge. Charles Rosenberg has noticed that early twentieth-century American enthusiasm for public health, stemming from a conviction that "[s]ickness was . . . connected with poverty and deprivation," which held that "an enlightened society should purify its water, provide pure milk for its children, inspect its food, and clean its streets and tenements," lost its appeal as a comprehensive view of sickness and health later in this century.[60] Biomedicine had done its job too well. Questions began to arise about the costs of continued application of high-powered medical technology to situations of marginal social utility. Biomedicine's conception of disease—as a discrete, most often acutely acting, external to the body entity—proved less efficacious in explaining the troubles of the elderly, the chronically ill, and the parturient. The apparent conquest of epidemics left the field open for concern with ailments more easily conceived in terms of social deviance and hence cultural construction (especially mental illness), and for situations where the intervention of biomedical technology raised issues of values and the quality of life above and beyond its simple preservation.

The developed Western world has therefore moved beyond thinking of disease in purely objective, biological terms, and we have applied our broadened cultural conceptions to disease's past as well as to its present. Undoubtedly many examples can be shown of ways in which past Western societies have configured disease in cultural terms; such examples are dotted throughout this book. But this recognition of the cultural past of disease may lead us to forget those dimensions of disease recognized by scientific biomedicine, dimensions that still have primary meaning in many parts of the world, especially in those parts called "developing." Our understanding of the relationship of disease and poverty in the past may have relevance in the present, particularly in those societies that do not yet have the luxury of forgetting acute epidemics in order to concentrate on the more value-laden, problematic, chronic ailments, conditions of aging, and mental illnesses. To many in the developing world (and to poor subsocieties in wealthy industrial states as well) that view of disease which connected it with poverty and deprivation, and which proposed to eradicate it with efficient curative and preventive biomedicine, should still be taken seriously.

Poverty, declared the World Health Organization's annual report in 1995, was "the world's deadliest disease," "the world's most ruthless killer and the greatest cause of suffering on earth."[61] That statement still holds, for the social circumstances that have always allowed disease to flourish still characterize the poorer parts of the world. In twenty-nine states belonging to the World Health Organization, less than half of the rural population had access to safe drinking water in 2004; and while improved drinking water then reached about 83 percent of India's rural population, the number of rural Indians without safe water remained in the many millions. Unsafe water and poor sanitation, especially the inadequate disposal of human wastes, still mean—as they did for the newly industrializing cities of nineteenth-century Europe—higher rates of dysentery, diarrhea, intestinal parasites, and the greater risk of cholera. About 20 percent of the deaths of Indian children under the age of five were (in 2000) caused by diarrheal diseases. Overcrowded living and working spaces still mean more opportunity for airborne germs and viruses such as tuberculosis and influenza. Tuberculosis incidence in 2005 in the United States and Canada was about 5 per 100,000 people; in Kenya, South Africa and Zimbabwe it was over 500.[62] High birth rates remain associated with higher levels of infant and maternal mortality.

In many ways these old social breeding grounds of disease persist in the early twenty-first century. The number (although perhaps not the percentage) of the absolutely poor in the world continues to rise. While some developing nations escape the trap of extreme poverty, the gap still widens between them and those that have not done so. In both developed and developing countries changing family patterns disrupt traditional health support systems: marriages lose their permanence, economic necessity (however perceived) drives family members to different cities or regions, and extended networks of kin give way to nuclear families and atomistic individuals. Political, social, and economic change in the developing world often extracts a dangerous health cost: cities grow (surrounded by shanty towns) in a rapid and unplanned fashion in twenty-first-century Africa and Latin America as they once did in early nineteenth-century Britain; political conflicts generate swarms of refugees, exacerbating urban crowding; economic change brings new roads and irrigation schemes that create new opportunities for the movement of disease vectors (for instance those of malaria and schistosomiasis); and the world's seemingly inexhaustible demand for raw materials disrupts ecological balances across whole continents.

But poor nations and peoples suffer not only from their environment. Poverty also interferes with their ability to utilize the strengths of modern biomedicine. One 1996 estimate claimed that 800 million people had no access to health care at all.[63] Access to physicians and nurses varies immensely between the developed and the developing worlds. Italy in 2004 had 420 physicians for each 100,000 people; Ethiopia had 3. Great Britain (in 1997) had 1,212 nurses for each 100,000 people; Haiti (in 1998) had 11.[64] Preventive vaccines are dependent on resources; even if their cost per head is minuscule, aggregate costs for a nation of several million may be out of reach of that state's fragile finances. The infant vaccine sometimes called DPT (protecting against diphtheria, pertussis, and tetanus) is very widely used in many parts of world, but less than half of the infants in nine states (seven in Africa) receive it.[65] The same cost problems may slow the use of insecticides, allowing the spread of malaria and dengue fever, or of therapeutic remedies. Poverty means the re-use of syringes that spread AIDS and hepatitis B; poverty means that antibiotics, like vaccines, may be too costly for whole populations even when the cost of a single dose is very small. Antibiotic treatments of such widespread poverty diseases as tuberculosis and leprosy are further frustrated by the lack of a "basic health care infrastructure," for such treatment's prolonged character assumes a convenient network of dispensaries, monitoring personnel, and general popular acceptance of the dictates of medicalization.[66] Meanwhile organisms more resistant to chemotherapy and antibiotics evolve, as has happened with malaria, tuberculosis, cholera, leishmaniasis, and plague; only those countries whose biomedical resources can afford a swift response may be able to stay ahead of natural selection.

These inequalities, and their relation to disease environments, manifest themselves in huge variations in life expectancies. For example, women in many of the developed states of the world now enjoy life expectancies over 80, while in twenty-three African countries women's life expectancy is under 50. Infant mortality rates in the developed world are roughly 5 per 1,000 live births; in Liberia, Mali, Niger, Rwanda, Sierra Leone and Somalia infant mortality rates range from 203 to 282 per 1,000.[67] Contributing to these discrepancies are three colossal contemporary epidemics: HIV-AIDS, tuberculosis, and malaria. All three have had a world-wide reach, but by far their most serious inroads have been in the developing worlds of sub-Saharan Africa and southern Asia. AIDS deaths in 2007 have been put at 2.1 million, with the number of people living with the disease in the vicinity of 33 million.[68] Tuberculosis has claimed perhaps 1.6 million, of whom about 195,000 were infected with HIV as well; 8.8 million new cases of tuberculosis were identified in 2005.[69] The World Health Organization has recently estimated an annual death toll from malaria at 880,000, but as many as 250 million people worldwide are infected by malaria, whose debilitating effects on the sufferers result in an incalculable perpetuation of poverty.[70]

Some Western governments and philanthropists have begun to recognize the gravity of these epidemics, and some efforts to combat them have been extensively funded. But the political priorities of the developed world have not always accepted the reality of the problem, or addressed the underlying poverty of developing societies. Perhaps in their societies, biomedicine has worked its wonders and so the health problems of the others seem unreal. In 1995 the World Health Organization phrased it thus:

> The concept of health for all has changed the world's thinking about how health should be provided. Placing equity of access to health at the heart of health-care delivery and giving greater emphasis to achieving this goal through primary health care has become a global blueprint. However, sustaining both the belief in the concept and its practical implementation has been difficult, partly because of the economic recession, cost implications, resistance to change and political problems in diverting resources from other areas towards health. The fundamental reason is that there is still little recognition at the political and policy levels of the close interrelationship between poverty and ill-health.[71]

Perhaps in the light of the history of disease in the West we should not be surprised at the "little recognition . . . of the close interrelationship between poverty and ill-health"; perhaps that history may suggest that Western societies have perceived that relationship only too well, the better to turn their backs on it. Lepers were expected to furnish their own coffin nails, so not finding public money for vaccines is hardly new. Fifteenth-century Florence located plague in its poorer quarters as a defining excuse to marginalize those quarters. Nineteenth-century tuberculosis was interesting when Keats, Chopin, the king of Rome, and Thérèse de Lisieux suffered from it; when the extent of its ravages of poorer populations became clearer some middle and professional classes decided its incidence stemmed from the moral fiber (or lack thereof) of its sufferers. Many of the past Western cultural configurations of disease have associated it with the social margins. In doing so the confident elites of the West have created something of a self-fulfilling prophecy: the marginalized groups live in social conditions that make disease more likely, and when their disease rates soar the elite can nod knowingly while further isolating themselves from the dangers that the diseased represent. Will our insistence that disease is a cultural construct (however convincingly founded) now blind us, once again, to the physical reality of disease among the less favored?

Notes

Introduction

1. Henry E. Sigerist, *Civilization and Disease* (1943; reprint, Chicago: University of Chicago Press, 1962), 1.
2. Erwin H. Ackerknecht, *A Short History of Medicine*, rev. ed. (Baltimore: Johns Hopkins University Press, 1982), 3.
3. Robert P. Hudson, *Disease and Its Control: The Shaping of Modern Thought* (Westport, Conn.: Greenwood Press, 1983), x.
4. Claudine Herzlich and Janine Pierret, *Illness and Self in Society* (Baltimore: Johns Hopkins University Press, 1987), xiii.
5. Roy Porter, *Mind-forg'd Manacles: A History of Madness in England from the Restoration to the Regency* (Cambridge, Mass.: Harvard University Press, 1987), 2.
6. Donald F. Austin and S. Benson Werner, *Epidemiology for the Health Sciences* (Springfield, Ill.: Charles C. Thomas, 1974), 60; Leon Gordis, *Epidemiology* (Philadelphia: W. B. Saunders, 1996), 17.
7. Charles E. Rosenberg, *Explaining Epidemics and Other Studies in the History of Medicine* (Cambridge: Cambridge University Press, 1992), 278–280; Gary D. Friedman, *Primer of Epidemiology* (New York: McGraw-Hill, 1974), 75.
8. William H. McNeill, *Plagues and Peoples* (Garden City, N.Y.: Anchor Press/Doubleday, 1976), 13.

One   The Western Inheritance

1. Mirko D. Grmek, *Diseases in the Ancient Greek World*, trans. Mireille Muellner and Leonard Muellner (Baltimore: Johns Hopkins University Press, 1989), 277.
2. *Hippocratic Writings*, ed. G.E.R Lloyd, trans. J. Chadwick and W. N. Mann (London: Penguin Books, 1978), 237.
3. Ibid., 214, 240–241.
4. Ibid., 262.

5. Ralph Jackson, *Doctors and Diseases in the Roman Empire* (Norman: University of Oklahoma Press, 1988), 64.

6. Owsei Temkin, *Galenism: Rise and Decline of a Medical Philosophy* (Ithaca, N.Y.: Cornell University Press, 1973).

7. G.E.R. Lloyd, *Science, Folklore, and Ideology: Studies in the Life Sciences in Ancient Greece* (Cambridge: Cambridge University Press, 1983), 214n30.

8. Erwin H. Ackerknecht, *A Short History of Medicine*, rev. ed. (Baltimore: Johns Hopkins University Press, 1982), 61.

9. Jackson, *Doctors and Diseases*, 138.

10. *Joshua* 22: 16–18.

11. *Leviticus* 13: 46.

12. Timothy S. Miller, *The Birth of the Hospital in the Byzantine Empire* (Baltimore: Johns Hopkins University Press, 1985), 41.

13. Peregrine Horden, "Saints and Doctors in the Early Byzantine Empire: The Case of Theodore of Sykeon," in W. J. Sheils, ed., *The Church and Healing* (Oxford: Basil Blackwell, 1982), 6.

14. Aline Rousselle, "From Sanctuary to Miracle Worker: Healing in Fourth-Century Gaul," in Robert Forster and Orest Ranum, eds., *Ritual, Religion, and the Sacred* (Baltimore: Johns Hopkins University Press, 1982), 95–127. (Originally published in French in *Annales E.S.C.* 31 [1976]: 1085–1107.)

15. Peter Brown, *The Cult of the Saints: Its Rise and Function in Latin Christianity* (Chicago: University of Chicago Press, 1981), 113–119.

Two   Medieval Diseases and Responses

1. Vilhelm Møller-Christensen, "Evidence of Leprosy in Earlier Peoples," in Don Brothwell and A.T. Sandison, eds., *Diseases in Antiquity* (Springfield, Ill.: Charles C. Thomas, 1967), 295–306.

2. Peter Richards, *The Medieval Leper and His Northern Heirs* (Cambridge: D. S. Brewer, 1977), esp. 98–120; S. R. Ell, "Reconstructing the Epidemiology of Medieval Leprosy: Preliminary Efforts with Regard to Scandinavia," *Perspectives in Biology and Medicine* 31 (1988): 496–506; Luke Demaitre, "The Description and Diagnosis of Leprosy by Fourteenth-Century Physicians," *Bulletin of the History of Medicine* 59 (1985): 327–344. The most recent authoritative historical discussions are Luke Demaitre, *Leprosy in Premodern Medicine: A Malady of the Whole Body* (Baltimore: Johns Hopkins University Press, 2007), and Carole Rawcliffe, *Leprosy in Medieval England* (Woodbridge: Boydell Press, 2006).

3. E. V. Hulse, "The Nature of Biblical 'Leprosy' and the Use of Alternative Medical Terms in Modern Translations of the Bible," *Palestine Exploration Quarterly* 107 (1975): 87–105. These arguments are well summarized in Richards, *The Medieval Leper*, 9.

4. Saul Nathaniel Brody, *The Disease of the Soul: Leprosy in Medieval Literature* (Ithaca, N.Y.: Cornell University Press, 1974), 110–111.

5. Quoted in ibid, 66–67. Another (and longer) version is quoted in Richards, *The Medieval Leper*, 123–124.

6. Richards, *The Medieval Leper*, 54–56.

7. Brody, *Disease of the Soul*, esp. 51–53; Richard Palmer, "The Church, Leprosy and Plague in Medieval and Early Modern Europe," in W. J. Sheils, ed., *The Church and Healing* (Oxford: Basil Blackwell, 1982), 79–99.

8. Demaitre, *Leprosy*, 172.

9. M. W. Dols, "Leprosy in Medieval Arabic Medicine," *Journal of the History of Medicine and Allied Sciences* 34 (1979): 314–333.

10. Richards, *The Medieval Leper*, 59.

11. Ibid., 69.

12. Richard Mortimer, "The Prior of Butley and the Lepers of West Somerton," *Bulletin of the Institute of Historical Research* 53 (1980): 99–103.

13. Richards, *The Medieval Leper*, 62–67.

14. Malcolm Barber, "Lepers, Jews, and Moslems: the Plot to Overthrow Christendom in 1321," *History* 66 (1981): 1–17.

15. Mortimer, "Prior of Butley," 101.

16. F. Henschen, *Gründzuge einer historischen und geographischen Pathologie* (Berlin: Springer-Verlag, 1966), 118.

17. Rotha Mary Clay, *The Medieval Hospitals of England* (1909; reprint, New York: Barnes and Noble, 1966), 277–337, contains a tabulated list.

18. S. R. Ell, "Plague and Leprosy in the Middle Ages: A Paradoxical Cross-Immunity?" *International Journal of Leprosy and Other Mycobacterial Diseases* 55 (1987): 345–350.

19. William H. McNeill, *Plagues and Peoples* (Garden City, N.Y.: Anchor Books/Doubleday, 1976), 176–180.

20. Keith Manchester, "Tuberculosis and Leprosy in Antiquity: An Interpretation," *Medical History* 28 (1984): 162–173.

21. K. J. Leyser, *Medieval Germany and Its Neighbors, 900–1250* (London: Hambledon Press, 1982), 244.

22. Michel Rouche, "The First Stirrings of Europe: Seventh to Mid-Tenth Centuries," in Robert Fossier, ed., *The Cambridge Illustrated History of the Middle Ages*, vol. 1, *350–950* (Cambridge: Cambridge University Press, 1989), 402.

23. Horst Fuhrmann, *Germany in the High Middle Ages, c. 1050–1200* (Cambridge: Cambridge University Press, 1986), 38–40.

24. Carolly Erickson, *The Medieval Vision: Essays in History and Perception* (New York: Oxford University Press), 134.

25. Leyser, *Medieval Germany*, 245.

26. Frank Barlow, "The King's Evil," *English Historical Review* 95 (1980): 15.

27. Marc Bloch, *The Royal Touch: Sacred Monarchy and Scrofula in England and France*, trans. J. E. Anderson (1961; London: Routledge and Kegan Paul, 1973).

28. Barlow, "The King's Evil," 3–27.

29. Ibid., 25.

30. Georges Vigarello, *Concepts of Cleanliness: Changing Attitudes in France since the Middle Ages*, trans. Jean Birrell (Cambridge: Cambridge University Press, 1988), 28–37.

Three The Great Plague Pandemic

1. Especially Samuel K. Cohn, *The Black Death Transformed: Disease and Culture in Early Renaissance Europe* (London: Arnold, 2002). Also Susan Scott and Christopher J. Duncan, *Biology of Plagues: Evidence from Historical Populations* (Cambridge: Cambridge University Press, 2001); Graham Twigg, *The Black Death: A Biological Reappraisal* (New York: Schocken, 1984); J.F.D. Shrewsbury, *A History of Bubonic Plague in the British Isles* (Cambridge: Cambridge University Press, 1970).

2. Rosemary Horrox, ed. and trans., *The Black Death* (Manchester: Manchester University Press, 1994), and John Aberth, *The Black Death: The Great Mortality of 1348–1350, A Brief History with Documents* (Boston: Bedford/St. Martin's, 2005), are convenient collections of contemporary documents.

3. Recent important discussions of bubonic plague and the pandemic include: Ole J. Benedictow, *The Black Death, 1346–1353: The Complete History* (Woodbridge: Boydell Press, 2004), and Robert Sallares, "Ecology, Evolution, and Epidemiology of Plague," in Lester K. Little, ed., *Plague and the End of Antiquity: The Pandemic of 541–750* (Cambridge: Cambridge University Press, 2007), 231–289.

4. For example, Ann G. Carmichael, "Universal and Particular: The Language of Plague, 1348–1500," in *Pestilential Complexities: Understanding Medieval Plague* (*Medical History*, supplement 27), ed. Vivian Nutton (London: Wellcome Trust Centre for the History of Medicine at UCL, 2008), 17–52.

5. *Pestilential Complexities*, ed. Nutton, contains a good collection of discussions of the *Yersinia pestis* controversy.

6. Benedictow, *Black Death*, especially emphasizes this point.

7. David Herlihy, *Medieval and Renaissance Pistoia: The Social History of an Italian Town, 1200–1430* (New Haven, Conn.: Yale University Press, 1967), esp. 55–148.

8. Among many articles by McKeown: "Food, Infection, and Population," in Robert I. Rotberg and Theodore K. Rabb, eds., *Hunger and History: The Impact of Changing Food and Consumption Patterns on Society* (Cambridge: Cambridge University Press, 1985), 29–49.

9. Ann G. Carmichael, "Infection, Hidden Hunger, and History," in Rotberg and Rabb, *Hunger and History*, 51–66.

10. Jean-Noël Biraben, *Les hommes et la peste en France et dans les pays européens et méditerranéens*, vol. 2, *Les hommes face à la peste* (Paris: Mouton, 1976), 16.

11. Ibid., 19–20.

12. Richard W. Emery, "The Black Death of 1348 in Perpignan," *Speculum* 42 (1967): 618.

13. William M. Bowsky, "The Impact of the Black Death upon Sienese Government and Society," *Speculum* 39 (1964): 21.

14. Elisabeth Carpentier, *Une ville devant la peste: Orvieto et la Peste Noire* (Paris: S.E.V.P.E.N., 1962), esp. 165–198.

15. P. D. A. Harvey, *A Medieval Oxfordshire Village: Cuxham, 1240 to 1400* (Oxford: Oxford University Press, 1965), 72–73.

16. John Hatcher, *Rural Economy and Society in the Duchy of Cornwall, 1300–1500* (Cambridge: Cambridge University Press, 1970), 103.

17. Zvi Razi, *Life, Marriage, and Death in a Medieval Parish: Economy, Society and Demography in Halesowen, 1270–1400* (Cambridge: Cambridge University Press, 1980), 101–102.

18. Harvey, *Medieval Oxfordshire Village*, 135.

19. Jean-Noël Biraben, *Les hommes et la peste en France et dans les pays européens et méditerranéens*, vol. 1, *La peste dans l'histoire* (Paris: Mouton, 1975), 363–449.

20. J. M. W. Bean, "The Black Death: The Crisis and Its Social and Economic Consequences," in Daniel Williman, ed., *The Black Death: The Impact of the Fourteenth-Century Plague* (Binghamton, N.Y.: Center for Medieval and Early Renaissance Studies, 1982), 32.

21. Emmanuel LeRoy Ladurie, *The Peasants of Languedoc*, trans. John Day (Urbana: University of Illinois Press, 1974), esp. 44.

22. Harry A. Miskimin, *The Economy of Early Renaissance Europe, 1300–1460* (Cambridge: Cambridge University Press, 1975), 32–72.

23. Norman Cohn, *The Pursuit of the Millennium: Revolutionary Millenarians and Mystical Anarchists of the Middle Ages* (New York: Oxford University Press, 1970), 131–141.

24. Giovanni Boccaccio, *The Decameron*, trans. G. H. McWilliam (Harmondsworth: Penguin Books, 1972), 52.

25. J. Huizinga, *The Waning of the Middle Ages* (Garden City, N.Y.: Anchor Books, 1954), 27. A more recent edition: *The Autumn of the Middle Ages* (Chicago: University of Chicago Press, 1996); the book was originally published in Dutch in 1924.

26. Millard Meiss, *Painting in Florence and Siena after the Black Death: The Arts, Religion, and Society in the Mid-Fourteenth Century* (Princeton, N.J.: Princeton University Press, 1951), 64–73.

27. Michael W. Dols, *The Black Death in the Middle East* (Princeton, N.J.: Princeton University Press, 1977), esp. his conclusions, 281–302.

28. Robert E. Lerner, "The Black Death and Western Eschatological Mentalities," in Williman, *The Black Death*, 77–105.

29. Nancy Siraisi, "Introduction," in Williman, *The Black Death*, 17.

30. Carlo M. Cipolla, *Public Health and the Medical Profession in the Renaissance* (Cambridge: Cambridge University Press, 1976).

31. Guilia Calvi, *Histories of a Plague Year: The Social and Imaginary in Baroque Florence*, trans. Dario Biocca and Bryant T. Ragan, Jr. (Berkeley: University of California Press, 1989), esp. chap. 1.

32 Quoted in Cipolla, *Public Health*, 37.

33. Calvi, *Histories of a Plague Year*, esp. chap. 4.

34. Ann G. Carmichael, *Plague and the Poor in Renaissance Florence* (Cambridge: Cambridge University Press, 1986).

35. Paul Slack, *The Impact of Plague in Tudor and Stuart England* (London: Routledge and Kegan Paul, 1985).

36. Dorset Record Office (Dorchester) DC/BTB: H6, document 218. Rosalind Hays called this example to my attention.

37. Cipolla, *Public Health*, 53.

38. Slack, *Impact of Plague*, 187.

39. Biraben, *Les hommes et la peste*, 1: 370.

40. Andrew B. Appleby, "The Disappearance of Plague: A Continuing Puzzle," *Economic History Review*, 2d ser., 33 (1980): 161–173.

41. Sallares, "Ecology," 262.

42. Paul Slack, "The Disappearance of Plague: An Alternative View," *Economic History Review*, 2d ser., 34 (1981): 469–476.

43. Karl F. Helleiner, "The Population of Europe from the Black Death to the Eve of the Vital Revolution," in E. E. Rich and C. H. Wilson, eds., *The Cambridge Economic History of Europe*, vol. 4, *The Economy of Expanding Europe in the Sixteenth and Seventeenth Centuries* (Cambridge: Cambridge University Press, 1967), 84–85.

44. Appleby, "The Disappearance of Plague," 167.

45. Elisabeth Carniel, "Plague Today," in *Pestilential Complexities*, 119.

46. Slack, "The Disappearance of Plague," 473–475.

47. Cipolla, *Public Health*, 53–66.

48. Appleby, "The Disappearance of Plague," 168–169.

Four   New Diseases and Transatlantic Exchanges

1. Mary Lucas Powell and Della Collins Cook, "Treponematosis: Inquiries into the Nature of a Protean Disease," in *The Myths of Syphilis: The Natural History of Treponematosis*

in North America, ed. Mary Lucas Powell and Della Collins Cook (Gainesville: University Press of Florida, 2005), 10.

2. E. H. Hudson, "Treponematosis in Perspective," *Bulletin of the World Health Organization* 32 (1965): 735–748.

3. Modifications of a basic "unitary" position are suggested by T. A. Cockburn, "The Origin of the Treponematoses," *Bulletin of the World Health Organization* 24 (1961): 221–228; C. J. Hackett, "On the Origin of the Human Treponematoses," *Bulletin of the World Health Organization* 29 (1963): 7–41; and—somewhat more critical of the unitary theory—Alfred W. Crosby, Jr., "The Early History of Syphilis: A Reappraisal," *American Anthropologist* 71 (1969): 218–227.

4. Della Collins Cook and Mary Lucas Powell, "Piecing the Puzzle Together: North American Treponematosis in Overview," in *The Myths of Syphilis,* 476.

5. Anna Foa, "Il nuovo e il vecchio: l'insorgere della sifilide (1494–1530)," *Quaderni storici* 19 (1984): 11–34, discusses the "newness" of syphilis to contemporaries.

6. Robert S. Munger, "Guaiacum, the Holy Wood from the New World," *Journal of the History of Medicine and Allied Sciences* 4 (1949): 196–227. Also well discussed in Claude Quétel, *History of Syphilis,* trans. Judith Braddock and Brian Pike (Baltimore: Johns Hopkins University Press, 1990), 29–30, 59–63.

7. An argument enthusiastically made by Frederick F. Cartwright and Michael D. Biddiss, *Disease in History* (New York: New American Library, 1972), 72–81.

8. Milo Keynes, "The Personality and Health of King Henry VIII (1491–1547)," *Journal of Medical Biography* 13 (2005): 174–183; Eric Ives, *The Life and Death of Anne Boleyn: "The Most Happy"* (Oxford: Blackwell, 2004), 190–191; J. J. Scarisbrick, *Henry VIII* (Berkeley: University of California Press, 1968), 484–487.

9. Roger Williams, *The Mortal Napoleon III* (Princeton, N.J.: Princeton University Press, 1972).

10. John A. H. Wylie and Leslie H. Collier, "The English Sweating Sickness *(Sudor Anglicus)*: A Reappraisal," *Journal of the History of Medicine and Allied Sciences* 36 (1981): 431.

11. Ibid., 443.

12. Hans Zinsser, *Rats, Lice and History* (1935; reprint, New York: Basic Books, 1965), remains a a good summary of the history of typhus.

13. Friedrich Prinzing, *Epidemics Resulting from Wars* (Oxford: Clarendon Press, 1916), lugubriously summarizes such episodes; Christopher J. Friedrichs, "The War and German Society," in *The Thirty Years' War,* ed. Geoffrey Parker (2d ed., London: Routledge, 1997), 186–192.

14. Zinsser, *Rats, Lice and History,* 206.

15. Noble David Cook, *Born to Die: Disease and New World Conquest, 1492–1650* (Cambridge: Cambridge University Press, 1998), summarizes the subject clearly. Two earlier works particularly called attention to the role of disease in sixteenth-century America: Alfred W. Crosby, Jr., *The Columbian Exchange: Biological and Cultural Consequences of 1492* (Westport, Conn.: Greenwood, 1972), and William H. McNeill, *Plagues and Peoples* (Garden City, N.Y.: Anchor Press/Doubleday, 1976), 199–216. Francis J. Brooks, "Revising the Conquest of Mexico: Smallpox, Sources, and Populations," *Journal of Interdisciplinary History* 24 (1993): 1–29, disputes both the role of smallpox and the scale of the disaster; Robert McCaa, "Spanish and Nahuatl Views on Smallpox and Demographic Catastrophe in Mexico," *Journal of Interdisciplinary History* 25 (1995): 397–431, criticizes Brooks.

16. Nicolás Sánchez-Albornoz, *The Population of Latin America*, trans. W. A. R. Richardson (Berkeley: University of California Press, 1974), 28.
17. Bernard R. Ortiz de Montellano, *Aztec Medicine, Health, and Nutrition* (New Brunswick, N.J.: Rutgers University Press, 1990).
18. Alfred W. Crosby, "Virgin Soil Epidemics as a Factor in the Aboriginal Depopulation of America," *William and Mary Quarterly*, 3d ser., 33 (1976): 289–299.
19. Crosby, *The Columbian Exchange*, 35–63.
20. Cook, *Born to Die*, 206. Early attempts to estimate populations included Sherburne F. Cook and Woodrow Borah, *The Indian Population of Central Mexico, 1531–1610* (Berkeley: University of California Press, 1960), 48–51, and Woodrow Borah and Sherburne F. Cook, *The Aboriginal Population of Central Mexico on the Eve of the Spanish Conquest* (Berkeley: University of California Press, 1963), 88. Ortiz de Montellano, *Aztec Medicine*, among others, believes that Cook and Borah's initial numbers are too high.
21. Ann G. Carmichael and Arthur M. Silverstein, "Smallpox in Europe before the Seventeenth Century: Virulent Killer or Benign Disease?" *Journal of the History of Medicine and the Allied Sciences* 42 (1987): 147–168.
22. Alfred W. Crosby, *Ecological Imperialism: The Biological Expansion of Europe, 900–1900* (Cambridge: Cambridge University Press, 1986), 345.

Five Continuity and Change

1. Christopher Dyer, *Standards of Living in the Later Middle Ages: Social Change in England, c. 1200–1500* (Cambridge: Cambridge University Press, 1989), 158.
2. Jean-Claude Schmitt, *The Holy Greyhound: Guinefort, Healer of Children since the Thirteenth Century* (Cambridge: Cambridge University Press, 1983).
3. Ronald C. Finucane, *Miracles and Pilgrims: Popular Beliefs in Medieval England* (Totowa, N.J.: Rowman and Littlefield, 1977), 31.
4. R. A. Fletcher, *Saint James's Catapult: The Life and Times of Diego Gelmirez of Santiago de Compostela* (Oxford: Clarendon Press, 1984), 98–99.
5. Finucane, *Miracles and Pilgrims*, 146–151.
6. For example, Keith Thomas, *Religion and the Decline of Magic: Studies in Popular Beliefs in Sixteenth- and Seventeenth-Century England* (1971; Harmondsworth: Penguin Books, 1973), 46, adopts James Frazer's old schematic division between religion, which supplicates nature, and magic, which commands it.
7. Richard Kieckhefer, *Magic in the Middle Ages* (Cambridge: Cambridge University Press, 1989), 9.
8. Thomas, *Religion and the Decline of Magic*, 217–219, and many other examples passim.
9. Ibid., 212.
10. Barbara Kaplan, "Greatrakes the Stroker: The Interpretations of His Contemporaries," *Isis* 73 (1982): 178–185.
11. Kieckhefer, *Magic in the Middle Ages*, 65.
12. Monica Green, "Women's Medical Practice and Health Care in Medieval Europe," *Signs* 14 (1989): 472.
13. Nina Rattner Gelbart, *The King's Midwife: A History and Mystery of Madame du Coudray* (Berkeley: University of California Press, 1998).
14. Laurel Thatcher Ulrich, *A Midwife's Tale: The Life of Martha Ballard, Based on Her Diary, 1785–1812* (New York: Alfred A. Knopf, 1990).

15. Nancy G. Siraisi, *Medieval and Early Renaissance Medicine: An Introduction to Knowledge and Practice* (Chicago: University of Chicago Press, 1990), 117–118.

16. Ibid., 174.

17. Finucane, *Miracles and Pilgrims*, 73.

18. Peter Linebaugh, "The Tyburn Riot against the Surgeons," in Douglas Hay et al., *Albion's Fatal Tree: Crime and Society in Eighteenth-Century England* (New York: Random House, 1978), 65–117, esp. 102–105.

19. Thomas, *Religion and the Decline of Magic*, 249–250.

20. Much of the argument of Thomas, *Religion and the Decline of Magic*, is devoted to these points, especially 27–332.

21. William M. Ivins, Jr., *Prints and Visual Communication* (Cambridge, Mass.: Harvard University Press, 1953), 23.

22. Quoted in C. D. O'Malley, *Andreas Vesalius of Brussels, 1514–1564* (Berkeley: University of California Press, 1965), 177.

23. Quoted in Allen G. Debus, *The Chemical Philosophy: Paracelsian Science and Medicine in the Sixteenth and Seventeenth Centuries* (New York: Science History Publications, 1977), 1: 52.

24. Quoted in ibid., 1: 58–59.

25. René Descartes, *Discourse on Method*, trans. L. J. Lafleur (Indianapolis: Bobbs-Merrill, 1960), 41.

26. Isaac Newton, *Opticks* (New York: Dover, 1952; based on 1730 London edition), 369.

27. Descartes, *Discourse on Method*, 46.

28. Charles Webster, *The Great Instauration: Science, Medicine, and Reform, 1626–1660* (New York: Holmes and Meier, 1976).

Six   Disease and the Enlightenment

1. The city populations are from Karl F. Helleiner, "The Population of Europe from the Black Death to the Eve of the Vital Revolution," in E. E. Rich and C. H. Wilson, eds., *The Cambridge Economic History of Europe*, vol. 4, *The Economy of Expanding Europe in the Sixteenth and Seventeenth Centuries* (Cambridge: Cambridge University Press, 1967), 81–84.

2. Andrew D. Cliff and Peter Haggett, *The Spread of Measles in Fiji and the Pacific: Spatial Components in the Transmission of Epidemic Waves through Island Communities* (Canberra: Australian National University, Research School of Pacific Studies, Department of Human Geography Publication, 1985), 12.

3. The "subsistence crisis" idea has been especially treated in the works of John D. Post: *The Last Great Subsistence Crisis in the Western World* (Baltimore: Johns Hopkins University Press, 1977), and *Food Shortage, Climatic Variability, and Epidemic Disease in Preindustrial Europe: The Mortality Peak in the Early 1740s* (Ithaca, N.Y.: Cornell University Press, 1985).

4. Stephen J. Kunitz, "Speculations on the European Mortality Decline," *Economic History Review*, 2d ser., 36 (1983): 349–364.

5. Lloyd G. Stevenson, " 'New Diseases' in the Seventeenth Century," *Bulletin of the History of Medicine* 39 (1965): 1–21.

6. Georges Vigarello, *Concepts of Cleanliness: Changing Attitudes in France since the Middle Ages* (Cambridge: Cambridge University Press, 1988), 112–163.

7. Alain Corbin, *The Foul and the Fragrant: Odor and the French Social Imagination* (Cambridge, Mass.: Harvard University Press, 1986).

8. James C. Riley, *The Eighteenth-Century Campaign to Avoid Disease* (New York: St. Martin's Press, 1987).

9. Erwin H. Ackerknecht, "Anti-Contagionism between 1821 and 1867," *Bulletin of the History of Medicine* 22 (1948): 562–593, esp. 567.

10. Johanna Geyer-Kordesch, "Fevers and Other Fundamentals: Dutch and German Medical Explanations c. 1680 to 1730," in William F. Bynum and Vivian Nutton, eds., *Theories of Fever from Antiquity to the Enlightenment* (*Medical History*, supplement 1, 1981), 100.

11. Stevenson, " 'New Diseases,' " 10–13.

12. Joseph A. Gagliano, "Coca and Popular Medicine in Peru: An Historical Analysis of Attitudes," in Francis X. Grollig and Harold B. Haley, eds., *Medical Anthropology* (The Hague: Mouton, 1976), 49–66.

13. L. J. Bruce-Chwatt and J. de Zulueta, *The Rise and Fall of Malaria in Europe: A Historico-Epidemiological Study* (Oxford: Oxford University Press, 1980), surveys the subject. A more detailed regional study: Mary J. Dobson, *Contours of Death and Disease in Early Modern England* (Cambridge: Cambridge University Press, 1997), 287–367.

14. Ibid.

15. Isaac Newton, *Opticks* (New York: Dover Publications, 1952; based on 1730 London edition), 375–376.

16. Isaac Newton, *Mathematical Principles of Natural Philosophy*, rev. trans. Florian Cajori (Berkeley: University of California Press, 1966), 547.

17. Robert Darnton, *Mesmerism and the End of Enlightenment in France* (Cambridge, Mass.: Harvard University Press, 1968), 8. My discussion of Mesmer is greatly indebted to Darnton's work.

18. Erwin H. Ackerknecht, *Medicine at the Paris Hospital, 1794–1848* (Baltimore: Johns Hopkins University Press, 1967), and David M. Vess, *Medical Revolution in France, 1789–1796* (Gainesville: University Presses of Florida, 1975). Among those taking a more evolutionary view are Toby Gelfand, *Professionalizing Modern Medicine: Paris Surgeons and Medical Sciences and Institutions in the Eighteenth Century* (Westport, Conn.: Greenwood Press, 1980), and Matthew Ramsey, *Professional and Popular Medicine in France, 1770–1830* (Cambridge: Cambridge University Press, 1988).

19. Stevenson, " 'New Diseases,' " 19.

20. Ramsey, *Professional and Popular Medicine*, 111–115.

21. W. F. Bynum, "Physicians, Hospitals and Career Structures in Eighteenth-Century London," in W. F. Bynum and Roy Porter, eds., *William Hunter and the Eighteenth-Century Medical World* (Cambridge: Cambridge University Press, 1985), 121.

22. Roy Porter, "William Hunter: A Surgeon and a Gentleman," in Bynum and Porter, *William Hunter*, 7–34; Ramsey, *Professional and Popular Medicine*.

23. Quoted in Ackerknecht, *Medicine at the Paris Hospital*, 31–32.

24. Especially relevant here are Michel Foucault, *The Birth of the Clinic: An Archaeology of Medical Perception* (1963; New York: Vintage, 1978), and *Madness and Civilization: A History of Insanity in the Age of Reason* (New York: Pantheon, 1965).

25. Roy Porter, *Mind-Forg'd Manacles: a History of Madness in England from the Restoration to the Regency* (Cambridge, Mass.: Harvard University Press, 1987).

26. Ann G. Carmichael and Arthur M. Silverstein, "Smallpox in Europe before the Seventeenth Century: Virulent Killer or Benign Disease?" *Journal of the History of Medicine and Allied Sciences* 42 (1987): 162.

27. Derrick Baxby, *Jenner's Smallpox Vaccine: The Riddle of Vaccinia Virus and Its Origin* (London: Heinemann, 1981), 12.

28. Donald R. Hopkins, *Princes and Peasants: Smallpox in History* (Chicago: University of Chicago Press, 1983), 35–72.

29. Ben Jonson, "An Epigram: To the Small Poxe," in William B. Hunter, Jr., ed., *The Complete Poetry of Ben Jonson* (Garden City, N.Y.: Doubleday Anchor, 1963), 172.

30. Oliver Goldsmith, "The Double Transformation: A Tale," in Arthur Friedman, ed., *Collected Works of Oliver Goldsmith* (Oxford: Clarendon Press, 1966), 4: 370–371.

31. Joseph Needham and Lu Gwei-Djen, *Science and Civilisation in China*, vol. 6, *Biology and Biological Technology*, part VI: *Medicine* (Cambridge: Cambridge University Press, 2000), 124–126.

32. Quoted in Robert Halsband, *The Life of Mary Wortley Montagu* (Oxford: Clarendon Press, 1956), 80–81.

33. S. J. Gendzier, ed., *Denis Diderot's The Encyclopedia: Selections* (New York: Harper, 1967), 150.

34. Peter Razzell, *The Conquest of Smallpox: The Impact of Inoculation on Smallpox Mortality in Eighteenth Century Britain* (Firle: Caliban Books, 1977).

35. Ibid., 16.

36. Maisie May, "Inoculating the Urban Poor in the Late Eighteenth Century," *British Journal for the History of Science* 30 (1997): 291–305.

37. Philip H. Clendenning, "Dr. Thomas Dimsdale and Smallpox Inoculation in Russia," *Journal of the History of Medicine and Allied Sciences* 28 (1973): 117, 123.

38. Thomas McKeown, "Fertility, Mortality and Causes of Death: An Examination of Issues Related to the Modern Rise of Population," *Population Studies* 32 (1978): 535–542, esp. 539.

39. Quoted in Baxby, *Jenner's Smallpox Vaccine*, 41.

40. Baxby, *Jenner's Smallpox Vaccine*, esp. 1–5.

41. Peter Razzell, *Edward Jenner's Cowpox Vaccine: The History of a Medical Myth* (Firle: Caliban Books, 1977). Jenner's claims had been systematically attacked by Charles Creighton in his *Jenner and Vaccination* (London: Swan Sonnenschein, 1889).

42. Baxby, *Jenner's Smallpox Vaccine*, 179–196.

43. O.H.K. Spate, *The Pacific since Magellan*, vol. 3, *Paradise Found and Lost* (Minneapolis: University of Minnesota Press, 1988), 191.

44. Kenneth J. Carpenter, *The History of Scurvy and Vitamin C* (Cambridge: Cambridge University Press, 1986), 1–2.

45. Carpenter, *History of Scurvy*, 51–63.

46. Spate, *Paradise Found and Lost*, 195.

47. Even if its diagnostic conclusions remain controversial, Ida MacAlpine and Richard Hunter, *George III and the Mad Business* (New York: Pantheon Books, 1970), contains a thorough clinical summary of the king's illness. Alternative diagnostic suggestions are advanced in critical reviews of MacAlpine and Hunter's work by A. H. T. Robb-Smith in *English Historical Review* 84 (1969): 805–806, and 85 (1970): 808–810.

48. J. H. Powell, *Bring Out Your Dead: The Great Plague of Yellow Fever in Philadelphia in 1793* (Philadelphia: University of Pennsylvania Press, 1949), is a good narrative of the episode. These particular points are on 49 and 234. Powell's narrative may be supplemented by the essays in J. Worth Estes and Billy G. Smith, eds., *A Melancholy Scene of Devastation: The Public Response to the 1793 Philadelphia Yellow Fever Epidemic* (Canton, Mass. Science History Publications, 1997).

49. Powell, *Bring Out Your Dead*, 220.

50. Dumas Malone, *Jefferson and His Time*, vol. 3, *Jefferson and the Ordeal of Liberty* (Boston: Little, Brown, 1962), 142; Harry Ammon, "The Genêt Mission and the Development of Political Parties," *Journal of American History* 52 (1966): 725–741.

51. Eve Kornfeld, "Crisis in the Capital: The Cultural Significance of Philadelphia's Great Yellow Fever Epidemic," *Pennsylvania History* 51 (1984): 189–205.

52. E.M. Sigsworth, "Gateways to Death? Medicine, Hospitals and Mortality, 1700–1850," in Peter Mathias, ed., *Science and Society, 1600–1900* (Cambridge: Cambridge University Press, 1972), 97–110.

Seven   Cholera and Sanitation

1. Paris figures from Catherine J. Kudlick, *Cholera in Post-Revolutionary Paris: A Cultural History* (Berkeley: University of California Press, 1996), 1, 15. Kudlick's book thoroughly discusses the uncertainties surrounding cholera mortality and morbidity figures. Hamburg figures from Richard J. Evans, *Death in Hamburg: Society and Politics in the Cholera Years, 1830–1910* (Oxford: Oxford University Press, 1987), 52, 445.

2. E. H. Ackerknecht, "Anticontagionism between 1821 and 1867," *Bulletin of the History of Medicine* 22 (1948): 562–593.

3. Roderick E. McGrew, *Russia and the Cholera, 1823–1832* (Madison: University of Wisconsin Press, 1965), 111–112.

4. Peter Baldwin, *Contagion and the State in Europe, 1830–1930* (Cambridge: Cambridge University Press, 1999), esp. chapter 3, 123–243.

5. Charles E. Rosenberg, *The Cholera Years: The United States in 1832, 1849, and 1866* (Chicago: University of Chicago Press, 1962), 59–64.

6. Quoted in R. J. Morris, *Cholera 1832: The Social Response to an Epidemic* (New York: Holmes and Meier, 1976), 135.

7. Owen Chadwick, *The Victorian Church*, 3d ed. (London: A. and C. Black, 1971), 1:36.

8. William Coleman, *Death Is a Social Disease: Public Health and Political Economy in Early Industrial France* (Madison: University of Wisconsin Press, 1982), 241–247.

9. Morris, *Cholera 1832*, 109–110.

10. McGrew, *Russia and the Cholera*, 100–102.

11. Norman Howard-Jones, "Cholera Therapy in the Nineteenth Century," *Journal of the History of Medicine and Allied Sciences* 27 (1972): 373.

12. Margaret Pelling, *Cholera, Fever and English Medicine, 1825–1865* (Oxford: Oxford University Press, 1978).

13. Hans Zinsser, *Rats, Lice and History* (1935; reprint, New York: Basic Books, 1965), 206.

14. Anthony S. Wohl, *Endangered Lives: Public Health in Victorian Britain* (Cambridge, Mass.: Harvard University Press, 1983), esp. 257–284.

15. Coleman, *Death Is a Social Disease*, 292–302.

16. Barbara G. Rosenkrantz, *Public Health and the State: Changing Views in Massachusetts, 1842–1936* (Cambridge, Mass.: Harvard University Press, 1972), 18.

17. S. E. Finer, *The Life and Times of Sir Edwin Chadwick* (London: Methuen, 1952), 154–163, 209–229; Anthony Brundage, *England's "Prussian Minister": Edwin Chadwick and the Politics of Government Growth, 1832–1854* (University Park: Pennsylvania State University Press, 1988), 79–99.

18. G. M. Young and W. D. Handcock, eds., *English Historical Documents, 1833–1874* (New York: Oxford University Press, 1956), 791. This work contains a convenient

selection from Chadwick's 1842 report (772–793). The report itself has been reprinted: Edwin Chadwick, *The Sanitary Condition of the Labouring Population of Great Britain*, ed. M. W. Flinn (Edinburgh: Edinburgh University Press, 1965).

19. G. M. Young, *Victorian England: Portrait of an Age* (London: Oxford University Press, 1936; reprint, 1960), 11.

20. Christopher Hamlin, *Public Health and Social Justice in the Age of Chadwick: Britain, 1800–1854* (Cambridge: Cambridge University Press, 1998), 13.

21. Bill Luckin, *Pollution and Control: A Social History of the Thames in the Nineteenth Century* (Bristol: Adam Hilger, 1986).

22. Evans, *Death in Hamburg*, 118–120, 133–134, 145–146.

23. Royston Lambert, *Sir John Simon, 1816–1904, and English Social Administration* (London: MacGibbon and Kee, 1963).

24. Evans, *Death in Hamburg*, 205.

25. Rosenberg, *Cholera Years*, 191–212.

26. The subsequent discussion of the 1892 Hamburg epidemic relies on Evans, *Death in Hamburg*.

27. Frank M. Snowden, *Naples in the Time of Cholera, 1884–1911* (Cambridge: Cambridge University Press, 1995).

Eight   Tuberculosis and Poverty

1. Lilian R. Furst, *The Contours of European Romanticism* (Lincoln: University of Nebraska Press, 1979), 5.

2. H. G. Schenk, *The Mind of the European Romantics: An Essay in Cultural History* (New York: Frederick Ungar, 1967), 49, 50, 63; see esp. 49–65.

3. Hermione de Almeida, *Romantic Medicine and John Keats* (New York: Oxford University Press, 1991), 139.

4. René and Jean Dubos, *The White Plague: Tuberculosis, Man, and Society* (1952; reprint, New Brunswick, N.J.: Rutgers University Press, 1987), 45–46.

5. John Warrack, *Carl Maria von Weber*, 2d ed. (Cambridge: Cambridge University Press, 1976), 359.

6. Dubos and Dubos, *The White Plague*, 56–57.

7. de Almeida, *Romantic Medicine*, 211.

8. Dubos and Dubos, *The White Plague*, 58–59.

9. Ibid., 65.

10. Mortality rates are summarized from tables in Godias J. Drolet, "Epidemiology of Tuberculosis," in Benjamin Goldberg, ed., *Clinical Tuberculosis*, 4th ed. (Philadelphia: F. A. Davis, 1944), A5–A12.

11. David S. Barnes, *The Making of a Social Disease: Tuberculosis in Nineteenth-Century France* (Berkeley: University of California Press, 1995), 48–73.

12. Sidney W. Mintz, *Sweetness and Power: The Place of Sugar in Modern History* (New York: Penguin Books, 1985), 126–150.

13. Brian Harrison, *Drink and the Victorians: The Temperance Question in England, 1815–1872* (London: Faber and Faber, 1971), 37.

14. E.P. Thompson, "Time, Work Discipline and Industrial Capitalism," in *Customs in Common* (New York: New Press, 1993; originally published in *Past and Present* in 1967), 352–403, gives a vivid statement of disorientation; Michael Anderson, *Family Structure in Nineteenth-Century Lancashire* (Cambridge: Cambridge University Press, 1971), 171, is more coldly sociological.

15. M. J. Daunton, *Progress and Poverty: An Economic and Social History of Britain, 1700–1850* (Oxford: Oxford University Press, 1995), 436.

16. Contrast the pessimism of Phyllis Deane, *The First Industrial Revolution*, 2d ed. (Cambridge: Cambridge University Press, 1979), 268–269, with Peter M. Lindert and Jeffrey G. Williamson, "English Workers' Standards of Living during the Industrial Revolution," *Economic History Review*, 2d ser., 36 (1983): 1–25, and N. F. R. Crafts, "English Workers' Real Wages during the Industrial Revolution: Some Remaining Problems," *Journal of Economic History* 45 (1985): 139–144.

17. Roderick Floud and Bernard Harris, "Health, Height, and Welfare: Britain, 1700–1980," in *Health and Welfare during Industrialization*, ed. Richard H. Steckel and Roderick Floud (Chicago: University of Chicago Press, 1997), 97.

18. Maxine Berg and Pat Hudson, "Rehabilitating the Industrial Revolution," *Economic History Review* 45 (1992): 40; E. H. Hunt, "Industrialization and Regional Inequality: Wages in Britain, 1760–1914," *Journal of Economic History* 46 (1986): 935–966, an attempt to maintain the optimist case while taking regional wage variations into account.

19. Henry E. Sigerist, *Civilization and Disease* (1943; reprint, Chicago: University of Chicago Press, 1962), 56.

20. Drolet, "Epidemiology of Tuberculosis," A13; David McBride, *From TB to AIDS: Epidemics among Urban Blacks since 1900* (Albany: State University of New York Press, 1991), 46–47.

21. André Armengaud, "Population in Europe, 1700–1914," in Carlo M. Cipolla, ed., *The Fontana Economic History of Europe*, vol. 3, *The Industrial Revolution* (London: Collins, 1973), 37.

22. Walter Minchinton, "Patterns of Demand, 1750–1914," in Cipolla, *Fontana Economic History*, 3:149.

23. For instance, Thomas McKeown, *The Modern Rise of Population* (New York: Academic Press, 1976), and *The Role of Medicine: Dream, Mirage or Nemesis?* (Princeton, N.J.: Princeton University Press, 1979), esp. 92–96.

24. Richard H. Steckel and Roderick Floud in *Health and Welfare*, 423–449.

25. Minchinton, "Patterns of Demand," 120.

26. F. B. Smith, *The Retreat of Tuberculosis 1850–1950* (London: Croom Helm, 1988), 9, 244. In contrast Anne Hardy, *The Epidemic Streets: Infectious Disease and the Rise of Preventive Medicine, 1856–1900* (Oxford: Clarendon Press, 1993), 211–266, while critical of McKeown's emphasis on diet, urges the importance of the social ameliorations promoted by local health officers.

27. Armengaud, "Population in Europe," 55.

28. Dubos and Dubos, *The White Plague*, 34–42.

29. Allan Mitchell, "Obsessive Questions and Faint Answers: The French Response to Tuberculosis in the Belle Epoque," *Bulletin of the History of Medicine* 62 (1988): 215–235; Claude Quétel, *History of Syphilis* (Baltimore: Johns Hopkins University Press, 1990), esp. 198–199, and Bruno Latour, *The Pasteurization of France* (Cambridge, Mass.: Harvard University Press, 1988), esp. 16–18.

30. Smith, *Retreat of Tuberculosis*, 37–38.

31. Dubos and Dubos, *The White Plague*, 175.

32. Barbara Bates, *Bargaining for Life: A Social History of Tuberculosis, 1876–1938* (Philadelphia: University of Pennsylvania Press, 1992), 78.

33. Mitchell, "Obsessive Questions," 226–231.

34. Linda Bryder, *Below the Magic Mountain: A Social History of Tuberculosis in Twentieth-Century Britain* (Oxford: Clarendon Press, 1988), 57.
35. Ibid., 210.
36. Ruth G. Hodgkinson, *The Origins of the National Health Service: The Medical Services of the New Poor Law* (Berkeley: University of California Press, 1967).
37. Bates, *Bargaining for Life*, 70.
38. Leonard G. Wilson, "The Historical Decline of Tuberculosis in Europe and America: Its Causes and Significance," *Journal of the History of Medicine and Allied Sciences* 45 (1990): 366–396.
39. Anne Digby, *Pauper Palaces* (London: Routledge and Kegan Paul, 1978), 167,169.
40. Charles Singer and E. Ashworth Underwood, *A Short History of Medicine*, 2d ed. (Oxford: Clarendon Press, 1962), 425.
41. Drolet, "Epidemiology of Tuberculosis," A20–A21.
42. Bates, *Bargaining for Life*, 322–324.
43. Smith, *Retreat of Tuberculosis*, 153–154.
44. Roger Kervan, *Albert Calmette et le B.C.G.* (Paris: Hachette, 1962), 184.
45. Barbara G. Rosenkrantz, "The Trouble with Bovine Tuberculosis," *Bulletin of the History of Medicine* 59 (1985): 155–175.
46. John Francis, *Bovine Tuberculosis* (London: Staples Press, 1947), 170.
47. Rosenkrantz, "Trouble with Bovine Tuberculosis," 167.
48. Smith, *Retreat of Tuberculosis*, 187, 189.
49. Gillian Cronje, "Tuberculosis and Mortality Decline in England and Wales, 1851–1910," in Robert Woods and John Woodward, eds., *Urban Disease and Mortality in Nineteenth-Century England* (New York: St. Martin's Press, 1984), 79–101.

Nine   Disease, Medicine, and Western Imperialism

1. Numbers from André Armengaud, "Population in Europe, 1700–1914," in Carlo M. Cipolla, ed., *The Fontana Economic History of Europe*, vol. 3, *The Industrial Revolution* (London: Collins, 1973), 28–29.
2. William Woodruff, "The Emergence of an International Economy, 1700–1914," in Carlo M. Cipolla, ed., *The Fontana Economic History of Europe*, vol. 4, *The Emergence of Industrial Societies* (London: Collins, 1973), 690.
3. Daniel R. Headrick, *The Tools of Empire: Technology and European Imperialism in the Nineteenth Century* (New York: Oxford University Press, 1981), 148.
4. Examples from David Budlong Tyler, *Steam Conquers the Atlantic* (New York: D. Appleton-Century, 1939), 50–52, 370, and William Woodruff, *Impact of Western Man: A Study of Europe's Role in the World Economy, 1750–1960* (New York: St. Martin's Press, 1967), 237.
5. Bernard Porter, *The Lion's Share: A Short History of British Imperialism, 1850–2004*, 4th ed. (London: Pearson/Longman, 2004), 14, 20.
6. Figures from Woodruff, *Impact of Western Man*, 154–156, 255, 313.
7. Philip D. Curtin, *Death by Migration: Europe's Encounter with the Tropical World in the Nineteenth Century* (Cambridge: Cambridge University Press, 1989), 104 (title of Curtin's chap. 5).
8. David Arnold, "Introduction: Disease, Medicine, and Empire," in David Arnold, ed., *Imperial Medicine and Indigenous Societies* (Manchester: Manchester University Press, 1988), 7.

9. Nancy E. Gallagher, *Medicine and Power in Tunisia, 1780–1900* (Cambridge: Cambridge University Press, 1983), 83–96.

10. Carol Benedict, "Bubonic Plague in Nineteenth-Century China," *Modern China* 14 (1988): 108.

11. Ibid., 132–136.

12. James C. Mohr, *Plague and Fire: Battling Black Death and the 1900 Burning of Honolulu's Chinatown* (New York: Oxford University Press, 2005).

13. Charles T. Gregg, *Plague: An Ancient Disease in the Twentieth Century*, rev. ed. (Albuquerque: University of New Mexico Press, 1985), 40, 43. For San Francisco, see also Susan Craddock, *City of Plagues: Disease, Poverty, and Deviance in San Francisco* (Minneapolis: University of Minnesota Press, 2000), and Nayam Shah, *Contagious Divides: Epidemics and Race in San Francisco's Chinatown* (Berkeley: University of California Press, 2001).

14. Ibid., 144.

15. Ann Bowman Jannetta, *Epidemics and Mortality in Early Modern Japan* (Princeton, N.J.: Princeton University Press, 1987), 194.

16. For the spread of disease in the Pacific: Norma McArthur, *Island Populations of the Pacific* (Canberra: Australian National University Press, 1968); Andrew D. Cliff and Peter Haggett, *The Spread of Measles in Fiji and the Pacific: Spatial Components in the Transmission of Epidemic Waves through Island Communities* (Canberra: Australian National University Research School of Pacific Studies, 1985); Raeburn Lange, "European Medicine in the Cook Islands," and Wolfgang U. Eckart, "Medicine and German Colonial Expansion in the Pacific: The Caroline, Mariana, and Marshall Islands," in Roy MacLeod and Milton Lewis, eds., *Disease, Medicine, and Empire: Perspectives on Western Medicine and the Experience of European Expansion* (London: Routledge, 1988), 61–79, 80–102; David E. Stannard, *Before The Horror: the Population of Hawai'i on the Eve of Western Contact* (Honolulu: University of Hawaii Social Science Research Institute, 1989).

17. Gordon Harrison, *Mosquitoes, Malaria, and Man: A History of the Hostilities since 1880* (New York: E. P. Dutton, 1978), 199, 213.

18. John Farley, *Bilharzia: A History of Imperial Tropical Medicine* (Cambridge: Cambridge University Press, 1991), 45–51.

19. Monica Wilson and Leonard Thompson, eds., *The Oxford History of South Africa*, vol. 1, *South Africa to 1870* (New York: Oxford University Press, 1969), 132.

20. Ken De Bevoise, "Until God Knows When: Smallpox in the Late-Colonial Philippines," *Pacific Historical Review* 59 (1990): 153.

21. Gwyn Prins, "But What Was the Disease? The Present State of Health and Healing in African Studies," *Past and Present*, no. 124 (1989): 167–171; the argument summarized by Prins was first put forward in John Ford, *The Role of the Trypanosomiases in African Ecology: A Study of the Tsetse Fly Problem* (Oxford: Clarendon Press, 1971).

22. Terence Ranger, "The Influenza Pandemic in Southern Rhodesia: A Crisis of Comprehension," in Arnold, *Imperial Medicine*, 172–188.

23. Anne Marcovich, "French Colonial Medicine and Colonial Rule: Algeria and Indochina," in MacLeod and Lewis, *Disease, Medicine, and Empire*, 103–117.

24. Eckart, "Medicine and German Colonial Expansion," 91–96.

25. Maryinez Lyons, *The Colonial Disease: A Social History of Sleeping Sickness in Northern Zaire, 1900–1940* (Cambridge: Cambridge University Press, 1992), esp. 40–51.

26. For the African reference: Megan Vaughan, *Curing their Ills: Colonial Power and African Illness* (Stanford, Calif: Stanford University Press, 1991), 38–39.
27. Prins, "But What Was the Disease?" 165.
28. De Bevoise, "Until God Knows When," 152.
29. Marcovich, "French Colonial Medicine," 107.
30. General sources for this discussion of the Fiji measles epidemic are Cliff and Haggett, *The Spread of Measles in Fiji*, and McArthur, *Island Populations*.
31. Cliff and Haggett, *The Spread of Measles in Fiji*, 32–34.
32. Population estimate from McArthur, *Island Populations*, 5–11.
33. *Hansard Parliamentary Debates*, 3d ser., vol. 224 (1875), cols. 1618–19.
34. Quoted by McArthur, *Island Populations*, 9; Cliff and Haggett, *The Spread of Measles in Fiji*, 55.
35. Cliff and Haggett, *The Spread of Measles in Fiji*, 60–64.
36. Especially useful for this discussion have been: De Bevoise, "Until God Knows When," and Ken De Bevoise, *Agents of Apocalypse: Epidemic Disease in the Colonial Philippines* (Princeton, N.J.: Princeton University Press, 1995); Reynaldo Ileto, "Cholera and the Origins of the American Sanitary Order in the Philippines," in Arnold, *Imperial Medicine*, 125–148; and Rodney Sullivan, "Cholera and Colonialism in the Philippines, 1899–1903," in MacLeod and Lewis, *Disease, Medicine, and Empire*, 284–300.
37. O.H.K. Spate, *Monopolists and Freebooters* (Minneapolis: University of Minnesota Press, 1983), 280.
38. Ileto, "Cholera and the Origins," 144; Sullivan, "Cholera and Colonialism," passim.
39. Quoted by Sullivan, "Cholera and Colonialism," 288, from *Manila Times*, March 6, 1903.
40. Sullivan, "Cholera and Colonialism," 285.
41. De Bevoise, "Until God Knows When," passim, and De Bevoise, *Agents of Apocalypse*, 94–117.
42. This discussion relies heavily on David Arnold, *Colonizing the Body: State Medicine and Epidemic Disease in Nineteenth-Century India* (Berkeley: University of California Press, 1993); Mark Harrison, *Public Health in British India: Anglo-Indian Preventive Medicine, 1859–1914* (Cambridge: Cambridge University Press, 1994), and *Climates and Constitutions: Health, Race, Environment and British Imperialism in India, 1600–1850* (Oxford: Oxford University Press, 1999); Ira Klein, "Death in India, 1871–1921," *Journal of Asian Studies* 32 (1973): 639–659; I. J. Catanach, "Plague and the Tensions of Empire: India, 1896–1918," in Arnold, *Imperial Medicine*, 45–65, 149–171; Rajnarayan Chandavarkar, "Plague Panic and Epidemic Politics in India, 1896–1914," in *Epidemics and Ideas: Essays on the Historical Perception of Pestilence*, ed. Terence Ranger and Paul Slack (Cambridge: Cambridge University Press, 1992), 203–240; and Radhika Ramasubbin, "Imperial Health in British India, 1857–1900," in MacLeod and Lewis, *Disease, Medicine, and Empire*, 38–60.
43. Harrison, *Public Health in British India*, 1.
44. Ramasubbin, "Imperial Health," 44.
45. Porter, *Lion's Share*, 52.
46. Quoted in Klein, "Death in India," 647.
47. Quoted in Harrison, *Public Health in British India*, 125.
48. Harrison, *Public Health in British India*, chap. 1, 6–35. For critical views of British cholera policies and motives, see Sheldon Watts, "From Rapid Change to Stasis: Official Responses to Cholera in British-Ruled India and Egypt, 1860 to c. 1921," *Journal of World History* 12 (2001): 321–374, and Biswamoy Pati, "Ordering Disorder in the Holy City: Colonial Health Intervention in Puri during the Nineteenth Century," in *Health,*

Medicine and Empire: Perspectives on Colonial India, ed. Biswamoy Pati and Mark Harrison (Hyderabad: Orient Longman, 2001), 270–298.

49. Chandavarkar, "Plague Panic and Epidemic Politics."

50. Gregg, *Plague*, 57.

51. On Haffkine: Catanach, "Plague and the Tensions," 154–160.

52. Ramasubbin, "Imperial Health," 54–55.

53. Catanach, "Plague and the Tensions," 160.

54. Harrison, *Public Health in British India*, 221.

55. This discussion relies heavily on Randall M. Packard, *White Plague, Black Labor: Tuberculosis and the Political Economy of Health and Disease in South Africa* (Berkeley: University of California Press, 1989); Shula Marks and Neil Andersson, "Typhus and Social Control: South Africa, 1917–1950," in MacLeod and Lewis, *Disease, Medicine, and Empire*, 257–283; Maynard W. Swanson, "The Sanitation Syndrome: Bubonic Plague and Urban Native Policy in the Cape Colony, 1900–1909," *Journal of African History* 18 (1977): 387–410.

56. Populations from Wilson and Thompson, *Oxford History of South Africa*, 1:274, 425, and Monica Wilson and Leonard Thompson, eds., *The Oxford History of South Africa*, vol. 2, *South Africa, 1870–1966* (New York: Oxford University Press, 1971), 2.

57. Wilson and Thompson, *Oxford History of South Africa*, 1:68,184.

58. Marks and Andersson, "Typhus and Social Control," 266.

59. The significance of these migrations is discussed in Packard, *White Plague, Black Labor*, 38–40.

60. Marks and Andersson, "Typhus and Social Control," 262.

61. Quoted in Robert I. Rotberg, *The Founder: Cecil Rhodes and the Pursuit of Power* (New York: Oxford University Press, 1988), 187.

62. Packard, *White Plague, Black Labor*, 68–73.

63. Ibid., 34–35.

64. Quoted in Swanson, "Sanitation Sydrome," 398.

65. Headrick, *The Tools of Empire*, 59–62.

66. From tables in Curtin, *Death by Migration*, 7–8.

67. Joel A. Tarr et al., "Water and Wastes: A Retrospective Assessment of Wastewater Technology in the United States, 1800–1932," *Technology and Culture* 25 (1984): 226–263, esp. 239.

68. Randall Packard, *The Making of a Tropical Disease: A Short History of Malaria* (Baltimore: Johns Hopkins University Press, 2007), esp. chap. 4, 84–110.

69. François Delaporte, *The History of Yellow Fever: An Essay on the Birth of Tropical Medicine*, trans. Arthur Goldhammer (Cambridge, Mass.: MIT Press, 1991), esp. 82.

70. According to tables in Sergio Díaz-Briquet, *The Health Revolution in Cuba* (Austin: University of Texas Press, 1983), 58, the death rates from malaria in Havana fell from 58.2 to 7.6 (per 100,000 population) between 1901 and 1907.

71. The figures are from Harrison, *Mosquitoes, Malaria, and Man*, 167.

72. David McCullough, *The Path between the Seas: The Creation of the Panama Canal, 1870–1914* (New York: Simon and Schuster, 1977), 573.

73. These examples are collected from Harrison, *Mosquitoes, Malaria, and Man*, 123–135.

74. Daniel R. Headrick, *The Tentacles of Progress: Technology Transfer in the Age of Imperialism, 1850–1940* (New York: Oxford University Press, 1988), 159–167.

75. Swanson, "Sanitation Syndrome," passim.

76. Harrison, *Mosquitoes, Malaria, and Man*, 17.

77. Vaughan, *Curing their Ills*, 24.

Ten   The Scientific View

1. Quoted in Walter E. Houghton, *The Victorian Frame of Mind, 1830–1870* (New Haven, Conn.: Yale University Press, 1957), 35–36.
2. This summary of the French medical situation relies most heavily on Matthew Ramsey, *Professional and Popular Medicine in France, 1770–1830: The Social World of Medical Practice* (Cambridge: Cambridge University Press, 1988).
3. This summary of the German medical situation relies most heavily on Charles E. McClelland, *The German Experience of Professionalization: Modern Learned Professions and Their Organizations* (New York: Cambridge University Press, 1991).
4. Among the sources used for the British medical situation: M. Jeanne Peterson, *The Medical Profession in Mid-Victorian London* (Berkeley: University of California Press, 1978), and Hilary Marland, *Medicine and Society in Wakefield and Huddersfield, 1780–1870* (Cambridge: Cambridge University Press, 1987).
5. Among the sources for the American medical situation: Samuel Haber, *The Quest for Authority and Honor in the American Professions, 1750–1900* (Chicago: University of Chicago Press, 1991); Paul Starr, *The Social Transformation of American Medicine* (New York: Basic Books, 1982). The quotation is from Starr, 104.
6. John E. Lesch, *Science and Medicine in France: The Emergence of Experimental Physiology, 1790–1855* (Cambridge, Mass.: Harvard University Press, 1984), 76.
7. Quoted in George A. Foote, "Sir Humphry Davy and His Audience at the Royal Institution," *Isis* 43 (1952): 9.
8. In 1846 the index to the British medical journal *Lancet* contained only one reference to "ether," that to a note describing ill effects following its inhalation. The January 2, 1847, issue of the journal contained a letter from Boston, dated November 28, 1846, describing ether's surgical use; the index for the first six months of the *Lancet* for 1847 contains nearly an entire column of entries about "ether."
9. Quoted in Elizabeth Longford, *Queen Victoria: Born to Succeed* (1965; reprint, New York: Pyramid, 1966), 234.
10. Charles Singer and E. Ashworth Underwood, in *A Short History of Medicine*, 2d ed. (Oxford: Clarendon Press, 1962), 341, suggest that the great increase in surgical operations spurred by anesthesia in turn stimulated interest in discovering antiseptic techniques.
11. McClelland, *The German Experience of Professionalization*, 34.
12. Ibid., 118.
13. Kenneth Ludmerer, *Learning to Heal: The Development of American Medical Education* (New York: Basic Books, 1985), especially 47–101.
14. Starr, *The Social Transformation of American Medicine*, 51.
15. Ruth Richardson, *Death, Dissection and the Destitute* (1987; reprint, London: Penguin, 1989).
16. Anne Digby, *Pauper Palaces* (London: Routledge and Kegan Paul, 1978), 176.
17. Jane Donegan, *"Hydropathic Highway to Health": Women and Water-Cure in Antebellum America* (Westport, Conn.: Greenwood Press, 1986).
18. Sarah Stage, *Female Complaints: Lydia Pinkham and the Business of Women's Medicine* (New York: W. W. Norton, 1979), 80–81.
19. Quoted in Patricia A. Vertinsky, *Eternally Wounded Woman: Women, Doctors, and Exercise in the Late Nineteenth Century* (New York: St. Martin's Press, 1991), 113.
20. James Keown, *Abortion, Doctors, and the Law: Some Aspects of the Legal Regulation of Abortion in England from 1803 to 1982* (Cambridge: Cambridge University Press, 1988), esp. 35–48; J. C. Mohr, *Abortion in America: The Origins and Evolution of*

National Policy, 1800–1900 (New York: Oxford University Press, 1978); Leslie J. Reagan, *When Abortion Was a Crime: Women, Medicine, and the Law in the United States, 1867–1973* (Berkeley: University of California Press, 1997), 80–112.

21. D. V. Glass, *Population Policies and Movements* (Oxford: Oxford University Press, 1940), 281.

22. Regina Morantz, "The Lady and Her Physician," in Mary S. Hartman and Lois Banner, eds., *Clio's Consciousness Raised: New Perspectives on the History of Women* (New York: Harper and Row, 1974), 47.

23. Judith Walzer Leavitt, *Brought to Bed: Childbearing in America, 1750–1950* (New York: Oxford University Press, 1986), esp. 116–141.

24. Daniel Scott Smith, "Family Limitation, Sexual Control, and Domestic Feminism in Victorian America," in Hartman and Banner, *Clio's Consciousness Raised*, 119–136.

25. Ann Oakley, *The Captured Womb: A History of the Medical Care of Pregnant Women* (Oxford: Basil Blackwell, 1984), 28.

26. Leavitt, *Brought to Bed*, esp. 87–115.

27. Starr, *The Social Transformation of American Medicine*, esp. 79–144.

28. Ramsey, *Professional and Popular Medicine*, 132.

29. James Harvey Young, *The Toadstool Millionaires: A Social History of Patent Medicines in America before Federal Regulation* (Princeton, N.J.: Princeton University Press, 1961), 32, 67.

30. Stage, *Female Complaints*, 32, 168–170.

31. Young, *The Toadstool Millionaires*, 157.

32. Erwin H. Ackerknecht, *A Short History of Medicine*, rev. ed. (Baltimore: Johns Hopkins University Press, 1982), 176.

33. This discussion relies heavily on René Dubos, *Louis Pasteur: Free Lance of Science* (Boston: Little, Brown, 1950).

34. Quoted in Bruno Latour, *The Pasteurization of France* (Cambridge, Mass.: Harvard University Press, 1988), 87.

35. Claude E. Dolman, "Robert Koch," in *Dictionary of Scientific Biography*, 7: 427.

36. Kathleen Kete, "*La rage* and the Bourgeoisie: The Cultural Context of Rabies in the French Nineteenth Century," *Representations* 22 (1988): 89–107.

37. Neil Pemberton and Michael Worboys, *Mad Dogs and Englishmen: Rabies in Britain, 1830–2000* (Basingstoke: Palgrave Macmillan, 2007); John K. Walton, "Mad Dogs and Englishmen: The Conflict over Rabies in Late Victorian England," *Journal of Social History* 13 (1979): 219–239.

38. Gerald L. Geison, "Louis Pasteur," in *Dictionary of Scientific Biography*, 10:405.

39. Theodore Zeldin, *France, 1848–1945*, vol. 1, *Ambition, Love, and Politics* (Oxford: Clarendon Press, 1973), 390.

40. Quoted in Harold Malkin, "Louis Pasteur and 'Le rage'—100 Years Ago," *Perspectives in Biology and Medicine* 30 (1986): 44.

41. Gerald L. Geison, "Pasteur, Roux, and Rabies: Scientific *versus* Clinical Mentalities," *Journal of the History of Medicine* 45 (1990): 341–365, and his *The Private Science of Louis Pasteur* (Princeton, N.J.: Princeton University Press, 1995), 145–176, 206–256.

42. Latour, *The Pasteurization of France*; quotations from 20–21 and 48.

43. Ibid., 76.

44. Michael Worboys, *Spreading Germs: Disease Theories and Medical Practice in Britain, 1865–1900* (Cambridge: Cambridge University Press, 2000); Nancy Tomes, *The Gospel of Germs: Men, Women, and the Microbe in American Life* (Cambridge, Mass.: Harvard University Press, 1999).

Eleven   The Apparent End of Epidemics

1. *U.S. News and World Report* 38, no. 21 (April 29, 1955): 29, 32; Richard Harrison Shryock, *The Development of Modern Medicine: An Interpretation of the Social and Scientific Factors Involved* (1947; reprint, Madison: University of Wisconsin Press, 1979), 456. Writing in 1976, William H. McNeill could still reasonably refer to "fundamentally altered disease patterns in nearly all the inhabited world since 1948": *Plagues and Peoples* (Garden City, N.Y: Anchor Press/Doubleday, 1976), 287.

2. R. Schofield, D. Reher, and A. Bideau, eds., *The Decline of Mortality in Europe* (Oxford: Clarendon Press, 1991), has been generally helpful for this section; its initial chapter, Roger Schofield and David Reher, "The Decline of Mortality in Europe," 1–17, is an especially concise summary of recent arguments. Also helpful have been Simon Szreter, "The Importance of Social Intervention in Britain's Mortality Decline, c. 1850–1914: A Reinterpretation of the Role of Public Health," *Social History of Medicine* 1 (1988): 1–37; Stephen J. Kunitz, "Speculations on the European Mortality Decline," *Economic History Review*, 2d ser., 36 (1983): 349–364.

3. Thomas McKeown, *The Modern Rise of Population* (New York: Academic Press, 1976), and *The Role of Medicine: Dream, Mirage or Nemesis* (Princeton, N.J.: Princeton University Press, 1979), among many other works.

4. James C. Riley, *The Eighteenth-Century Campaign to Avoid Disease* (New York: St. Martin's Press, 1987).

5. Marie-France Morel, "The Care of Children: The Influence of Medical Innovation and Medical Institutions on Infant Mortality, 1750–1914," in Schofield et al., *The Decline of Mortality*, 196–219. Alfred Perrenoud, "The Attenuation of Mortality Crises and the Decline of Mortality," in Schofield et al., 18–37, offers Genevan evidence that confirms Morel's argument.

6. Perrenoud, "The Attenuation of Mortality Crises," 37.

7. Morel, "The Care of Children," 218–219.

8. Robert Woods, "Public Health and Public Hygiene: The Urban Environment in the Late Nineteenth and Early Twentieth Centuries," in Schofield et al., *The Decline of Mortality*, 234.

9. Anne Hardy, *The Epidemic Streets: Infectious Disease and the Rise of Preventive Medicine, 1856–1900* (Oxford: Clarendon Press, 1993), 104–105 (for diphtheria) and 64–66 (for scarlet fever).

10. Graziella Caselli, "Health Transition and Cause-Specific Mortality," in Schofield et al., *The Decline of Mortality*, 68–96, esp. 95.

11. Caselli, "Health Transition," lists data, especially on 74.

12. Myron Echenberg, *Plague Ports: The Global Urban Impact of Bubonic Plague, 1894–1901* (New York: New York University Press, 2007), 236.

13. Charles T. Gregg, *Plague: An Ancient Disease in the Twentieth Century*, rev. ed. (Albuquerque: University of New Mexico Press, 1985), 150–151. Gregg also notes (209–210) that the decline in plague in the United States occurred before the development of warfarin.

14. For rabies, Kathleen Kete, "*La rage* and the Bourgeoisie: The Cultural Context of Rabies in the French Nineteenth Century," *Representations* 22 (1988): 89–107; Neil Pemberton and Michael Worboys, *Mad Dogs and Englishmen: Rabies in Britain, 1830–2000* (Basingstoke: Palgrave Macmillan, 2007).

15. Hardy, *The Epidemic Streets*, 169–172.

16. Judith Walzer Leavitt, *Typhoid Mary: Captive to the Public's Health* (Boston: Beacon Press, 1996), is much the most reliable and thoughtful account.

17. Harry F. Dowling, *Fighting Infection: Conquests of the Twentieth Century* (Cambridge, Mass.: Harvard University Press, 1977), 122. Dowling's work is a very helpful summary of its subject, and it offers modest qualifications to a generally positivist story.

18. David P. Adams, *"The Greatest Good to the Greatest Number": Penicillin Rationing on the American Home Front, 1940–1945* (New York: Peter Lang, 1991), 160.

19. This discussion owes most to Allan M. Brandt, *No Magic Bullet: A Social History of Venereal Disease in the United States since 1880* (New York: Oxford University Press, 1985), and Claude Quétel, *History of Syphilis*, trans. Judith Braddock and Brian Pike (Baltimore: Johns Hopkins University Press, 1990).

20. Quoted in Eva Le Galliene's introduction to Henrik Ibsen, *Eight Plays* (New York: Modern Library, 1951), xvii.

21. Quétel, *History of Syphilis*, 23–24.

22. Ibid., 134.

23. British policies and their meanings are thoroughly discussed in Judith R. Walkowitz, *Prostitution and Victorian Society: Women, Class, and the State* (New York: Cambridge University Press, 1980).

24. Quétel, *History of Syphilis*, 180.

25. Brandt, *No Magic Bullet*, 205–206.

26. Quoted in Arthur Marwick, *The Deluge: British Society and the First World War* (Harmondsworth: Penguin Press, 1965), 116.

27. Brandt, *No Magic Bullet*, 69.

28. Ibid., 127.

29. Quétel, *History of Syphilis*, 182.

30. Ibid., 210.

31. Ibid., 182.

32. Brandt, *No Magic Bullet*, 104, 116, 157–158; quotation from 157.

33. James H. Jones, *Bad Blood: The Tuskegee Syphilis Experiment* (New York: Free Press, 1981).

34. This discussion owes most to John R. Paul, *A History of Poliomyelitis* (New Haven, Conn.: Yale University Press, 1971), and Naomi Rogers, *Dirt and Disease: Polio before FDR* (New Brunswick, N.J.: Rutgers University Press, 1992). See also Bernard Seytre and Mary Shaffer, *The Death of a Disease: A History of the Eradication of Poliomyelitis* (New Brunswick, N.J.: Rutgers University Press, 2005).

35. This summary of early poliomyelitis history is based on Paul, *History of Poliomyelitis*, esp. 71–97, and Rogers, *Dirt and Disease*, 10–11.

36. Rogers, *Dirt and Disease*, 40.

37. Guenter B. Risse, "Revolt against Quarantine: Community Responses to the 1916 Polio Epidemic, Oyster Bay, N.Y.," *Transactions and Studies of the College of Physicians of Philadelphia* 14 (1992): 48.

38. Paul, *History of Poliomyelitis*, 221.

39. Ibid., 434.

40. Paul A. Offit, *The Cutter Incident: How America's First Polio Vaccine Led to the Growing Vaccine Crisis* (New Haven, Conn.: Yale University Press, 2005), 89.

41. Paul, *A History of Poliomyelitis*, 413.

42. Most generally helpful for this discussion have been Alfred W. Crosby, *America's Forgotten Pandemic: The Influenza of 1918* (Cambridge: Cambridge University Press, 1989; originally published as *Epidemic and Peace, 1918*, Westport, Conn.: Greenwood, 1976); Howard Phillips and David Killingray, eds., *The Spanish Influenza Pandemic of 1918–19: New Perspectives* (London: Routledge, 2003); Niall P. A. S. Johnson and

Juergen Mueller, "Updating the Accounts: Global Mortality of the 1918–1920 'Spanish' Influenza Pandemic," *Bulletin of the History of Medicine* 76 (2002): 105–115, which supplements and corrects K. David Patterson and Gerald F. Pyle, "The Geography and Mortality of the 1918 Influenza Pandemic," *Bulletin of the History of Medicine* 65 (1991): 4–21.

43. Johnson and Mueller, "Updating the Accounts," 115.

44. K. David Patterson, *Pandemic Influenza, 1700–1900: A Study in Historical Epidemiology* (Totowa, N.J.: Rowman and Littlefleld, 1986), provides helpful background.

45. Ibid., 89.

46. Patterson and Pyle, "Geography and Mortality," 8.

47. Wataru Iijima, "Spanish Influenza in China, 1918–20: A Preliminary Probe," in *Spanish Influenza Pandemic*, 101–109.

48. Martha L. Hildreth, "The Influenza Epidemic of 1918–1919 in France: Contemporary Concepts of Aetiology, Therapy, and Prevention," *Social History of Medicine* 4 (1991): 278–294.

49. The African references are from Don C. Ohadike, "Diffusion and Physiological Responses to the Influenza Pandemic of 1918–19 in Nigeria," *Social Science and Medicine* 32 (1991): 1394, and K. David Patterson, "The Influenza Epidemic of 1918–1919 in the Gold Coast," *Journal of African History* 24 (1983): 487–488, 491; the Australian reference is from Patterson and Pyle, "Geography and Mortality," 11.

50. For masks, see Crosby, *America's Forgotten Pandemic*, 101–113; for French and Nigerian responses see Hildreth, "The Influenza Epidemic," 277, and Odahike, "Diffusion and Physiological Responses," 1397.

51. Crosby, *America's Forgotten Pandemic*, 321.

52. I. D. Mills, "The 1918–1919 Influenza Pandemic—The Indian Experience," *Indian Economic and Social History Review* 23 (1986): 1–40, esp. 10; Myron Echenberg, " 'The Dog That did not Bark': Memory and the 1918 Influenza Epidemic in Senegal," in *Spanish Influenza Pandemic*, 230–238.

53. Crosby, *America's Forgotten Pandemic*, 240, 250–251.

54. Patterson and Pyle, "Geography and Mortality," 13.

55. Crosby, *America's Forgotten Pandemic*, 227–231; Mills, "The 1918–1919 Influenza Pandemic," 32–35; Patterson and Pyle, "Geography and Mortality," 13.

56. Geoffrey W. Rice, *Black November: The 1918 Influenza Pandemic in New Zealand*, 2d ed. (Christchurch: Canterbury University Press, 2005), 159–161.

57. Patterson, "The Influenza Epidemic of 1918–1919," 487, 493.

58. Ibid., 502; Howard Phillips, "South Africa's Worst Demographic Disaster: The Spanish Influenza Epidemic of 1918," *South African Historical Journal* 20 (1988), 57, 64; Mills, "The 1918–1919 Influenza Pandemic," 17–32.

59. Andrew Noymer and Michel Garenne, "Long-term Effects of the 1918 'Spanish' Influenza Epidemic on Sex Differentials of Mortality in the USA: Exploratory Findings from Historical Data," in *Spanish Influenza Pandemic*, 202–217.

60. Dowling, *Fighting Infection*, chap. 13, offers a clear discussion of these points.

Twelve   Disease and Power

1. Donald R. Hopkins, *Princes and Peasants: Smallpox in History* (Chicago: University of Chicago Press, 1983), is a generally convenient source for such facts.

2. Claudia Huerkamp, "The History of Smallpox Vaccination in Germany: A First Step in the Medicalization of the General Public," *Journal of Contemporary History* 20 (1985): 629.

3. For example, the behavior of Canadians cited by P. A Bator, "The Health Reformers versus the Common Canadian: The Controversy over Compulsory Vaccination against Smallpox in Toronto and Ontario, 1900–1920," *Ontario History* 75 (1983): 349.

4. Among many examples, ibid., 358.

5. Nadja Durbach, *Bodily Matters: The Anti-Vaccination Movement in England, 1853–1907* (Durham, N.C.: Duke University Press, 2005).

6. Huerkamp, "The History of Smallpox Vaccination," 624.

7. Naomi Williams, "The Implementation of Compulsory Health Legislation: Infant Smallpox Vaccination in England and Wales, 1840–1880," *Journal of Historical Geography* 20 (1994): 403–405.

8. R. J. Lambert, "A Victorian National Health Service: State Vaccination, 1855–1871," *Historical Journal* 5 (1962): 10. Lambert's view should be seen in the context of a historiographic controversy about the growth of government intervention in nineteenth-century Britain.

9. Hopkins, *Princes and Peasants*, 303. This paragraph and the next rely to a large measure on Hopkins's account.

10. Contributors to the discussion of "national decline" include: Robert A. Nye, *Crime, Madness, and Politics in Modern France: The Medical Concept of National Decline* (Princeton, N.J.: Princeton University Press, 1984); Daniel Pick, *Faces of Degeneration: Aspects of a European Disorder, c. 1848–1918* (Cambridge: Cambridge University Press, 1989); William H. Schneider, *Quality and Quantity: The Quest for Biological Regeneration in Twentieth Century France* (Cambridge: Cambridge University Press, 1990); Richard A. Soloway, *Demography and Degeneration: Eugenics and the Declining Birthrate in Twentieth-Century Britain* (Chapel Hill: University of North Carolina Press, 1990).

11. Bentley B. Gilbert, *The Evolution of National Insurance in Great Britain: The Origins of the Welfare State* (London: Michael Joseph, 1966), 85.

12. Cynthia R. Comacchio, *"Nations Are Built of Babies": Saving Ontario's Mothers and Children, 1900–1940* (Montreal: McGill-Queen's University Press, 1993), 15. Other discussions of infant health policies include Rima D. Apple, *Mothers and Medicine: A Social History of Infant Feeding, 1890–1950* (Madison: University of Wisconsin Press, 1988); Alisa Klaus, *Every Child a Lion: the Origins of Maternal and Infant Health Policy in the United States and France, 1890–1920* (Ithaca, N.Y.: Cornell University Press, 1993); Richard A. Meckel, *"Save the Babies": American Public Health Reform and the Prevention of Infant Mortality, 1850–1929* (Baltimore: Johns Hopkins University Press, 1990).

13. Helpful discussions of eugenics include Daniel J. Kevles, *In the Name of Eugenics: Genetics and the Uses of Human Heredity* (Berkeley: University of California Press, 1986); Pauline Mazumdar, *Eugenics, Human Genetics, and Human Failings* (New York: Routledge, 1992); G. R. Searle, *Eugenics and Politics in Britain, 1900–1914* (Leiden: Noordhoff, 1976).

14. Jean Webster, *Dear Enemy* (New York: Grosset and Dunlap, 1915), 75. Rosalind Hays called this reference to my attention.

15. Philip R. Reilly, *The Surgical Solution: A History of Involuntary Sterilization in the United States* (Baltimore: Johns Hopkins University Press, 1991), 26. See also Mark A. Largent,

Breeding Contempt: The History of Coerced Sterilization in the United States (New Brunswick, N.J.: Rutgers University Press, 2008).

16. Reilly, *Surgical Solution*, 103.

17. Paul Weindling, *Health, Race, and German Politics between National Unification and Nazism, 1870–1945* (Cambridge: Cambridge University Press, 1989), 7. Other helpful discussions of the medical aspects of the Nazi period include Götz Aly, Peter Chroust, and Christian Pross, *Cleansing the Fatherland: Nazi Medicine and Racial Hygiene* (Baltimore: Johns Hopkins University Press, 1994); Michael H. Kater, *Doctors under Hitler* (Chapel Hill: University of North Carolina Press, 1989); Robert N. Proctor, *Racial Hygiene: Medicine under the Nazis* (Cambridge, Mass.: Harvard University Press, 1988). Useful perspective can be gained from Reilly, *The Surgical Solution*; James H. Jones, *Bad Blood: The Tuskegee Syphilis Experiment* (New York: Free Press, 1981); Edward J. Larson, *Sex, Race, and Science: Eugenics in the Deep South* (Baltimore: Johns Hopkins University Press, 1995); and Susan E. Lederer, *Subjected to Science: Human Experimentation in America before the Second World War* (Baltimore: Johns Hopkins University Press, 1995).

18. Proctor, *Racial Hygiene*, 233–234. In another work Proctor discusses ways in which some Nazi attitudes toward disease and health could be seen as progressive: Robert N. Proctor, *The Nazi War on Cancer* (Princeton, N.J.: Princeton University Press, 1999).

19. Weindling, *Health, Race, and German Politics*, 533.

20. Reilly, *The Surgical Solution*, 16–17.

21. Aly et al., *Cleansing the Fatherland*, 22.

22. Ibid., 55–56.

23. Kater, *Doctors under Hitler*, 181.

24. Proctor, *Racial Hygiene*, 198.

25. Aly et al., *Cleansing the Fatherland*, 23.

26. Ibid., 92.

27. Kater, *Doctors under Hitler*, 182.

28. David F. Musto, *The American Disease: Origins of Narcotic Control*, exp. ed. (New York: Oxford University Press, 1987), shows the equations of addiction and marginal social groups; Laura Engelstein, "Morality and the Wooden Spoon: Russian Doctors View Syphilis, Social Class, and Sexual Behavior, 1890–1905," *Representations* 14 (1986): 169–208, discusses Russian linkages of disease and social class; Linda Bryder, *Below the Magic Mountain: A Social History of Tuberculosis in Twentieth-Century Britain* (Oxford: Clarendon Press, 1988), and F. B. Smith, *The Retreat of Tuberculosis, 1850–1950* (London: Croom Helm, 1988), both clearly illustrate the class associations of the disease; and Susan Sontag, *Illness as Metaphor and AIDS and Its Metaphors* (New York: Doubleday, 1990) examines the different uses made by modern culture of tuberculosis, cancer, and (now) AIDS.

29. Different aspects of this complex issue are discussed by Linda Gordon, *Women's Body, Women's Right: A Social History of Birth Control in America* (New York: Grossman, 1976); Judith Walzer Leavitt, *Brought to Bed: Childbearing in America, 1750–1950* (New York: Oxford University Press, 1986); Elizabeth Lunbeck, *The Psychiatric Persuasion: Knowledge, Gender, and Power in Modern America* (Princeton, N.J.: Princeton University Press, 1994); Ann Oakley, *The Captured Womb: A History of the Medical Care of Pregnant Women* (Oxford: Blackwell, 1984); Yannick Ripa, *Women and Madness: The Incarceration of Women in Nineteenth-Century France* (Minneapolis: University of Minnesota Press, 1991); Elaine Showalter, *The Female Malady: Women,*

Madness, and English Culture, 1830–1980 (New York: Pantheon, 1985); Sarah Stage, *Female Complaints: Lydia Pinkham and the Business of Women's Medicine* (New York: W. W. Norton, 1979); Patricia A. Vertinsky, *Eternally Wounded Woman: Women, Doctors, and Exercise in the Late Nineteenth Century* (New York: St. Martin's, 1991).

30. Joan Jacobs Brumberg, *Fasting Girls: The Emergence of Anorexia Nervosa as a Modern Disease* (Cambridge, Mass.: Harvard University Press, 1988).

31. James T. Patterson, *The Dread Disease: Cancer and Modern American Culture* (Cambridge, Mass.: Harvard University Press, 1987), esp. 111–112, 152–153. In the latter pages Patterson discusses the cancer cases of American baseball hero Babe Ruth (1948) and American political leader Robert Taft (1953), both illustrating the general reticence about mentioning the word "cancer."

32. This discussion of the early history of AIDS in the West relies particularly heavily on the essays in Elizabeth Fee and Daniel M. Fox, eds., *AIDS: The Burdens of History* (Berkeley: University of California Press, 1988) and Elizabeth Fee and Daniel M. Fox, eds., *AIDS: The Making of a Chronic Disease* (Berkeley: University of California Press, 1992), and on Mirko D. Grmek, *History of AIDS: Emergence and Origin of a Modern Pandemic* (Princeton, N.J.: Princeton University Press, 1990). Useful for different aspects of the early chronology are Dennis Altman, *AIDS in the Mind of America* (Garden City, N.Y.: Anchor Press, 1986); Jacques Leibowitch, *A Strange Virus of Unknown Origin*, trans. Richard Howard (New York: Ballantine Books, 1985); and Randy Shilts, *And the Band Played On: Politics, People, and the AIDS Epidemic* (New York: Penguin Books, 1988).

33. Grmek, *History of AIDS*, 33.

34. Figures are from James Chin, Maria-Antonia Remenyi, Florence Morrison, and Rudolfo Bulatao, "The Global Epidemiology of the HIV/AIDS Pandemic and Its Projected Demographic Impact on Africa," *World Health Statistics Quarterly* 45 (1992): 220–227; Centers for Disease Control, *Morbidity and Mortality Weekly Report* 43, no. 9 (1994): 155–161, and 43, no. 35 (1994): 644–648; and Peter Piot, "AIDS, an Epidemic in Search of a Vaccine," *Manchester Guardian Weekly*, December 8,1996, p. 12.

35. John Iliffe, *The African AIDS Epidemic: A History* (Athens: Ohio University Press, 2006), provides an excellent summary of the subject.

36. Ibid., 1.

37. Population figures from B. R. Mitchell, *International Historical Statistics: Africa and Asia* (New York: New York University Press, 1982), 66, and *The World Almanac and Book of Facts, 2006* (New York: World Almanac Books, 2006).

38. The phrase comes from Leibowitch, *A Strange Virus*; the point about transfusions from William H. Schneider and Ernest Drucker, "Blood Transfusions in the Early Years of AIDS in Sub-Saharan Africa," *American Journal of Public Health* 96 (2006): 984–994.

39. Altman, *AIDS in the Mind of America*, 70.

40. Ibid., 72.

41. Examples from ibid., 59–61, 65–66, 68.

42. Ibid., 60; *Chicago Tribune*, July 13, 1995, sec. 1, p. 6.

43. David Musto, "Quarantine and the Problem of AIDS," in Fee and Fox, *AIDS: The Burdens of History*, 81.

44. Altman, *AIDS in the Mind of America*, 63–64.

45. Musto, "Quarantine," 82.

46. Said the executive director of a Washington AIDS organization in 1985: "AIDS is not transmitted because of who you *are*, but because of what you *do*"; quoted in

Paula A. Treichler, "AIDS, Gender, and Biomedical Discourse: Current Contests for Meaning," in Fee and Fox, *AIDS: The Burdens of History*, 204.

47. *New York Times*, July 5, 1995, A12.

48. Altman, *AIDS in the Mind of America*, 166.

49. A. Rossi-Espagnet, G. B. Goldstein, and I. Tabibzadeh, "Urbanization and Health in Developing Countries: A Challenge for Health for All," *World Health Statistics Quarterly* 44 (1991): figures from 224–226.

50. UNAIDS, "2007 AIDS Epidemic Update," http://data.unaids.org/pub/Report/2008, "Sub-Saharan Africa," 14.

51. Ibid., passim.

52. Ibid.; Helen Epstein, *The Invisible Cure: Africa, the West, and the Fight against AIDS* (London: Viking/Penguin, 2007); Iliffe, *African AIDS Epidemic*, 13 (Mobutu), 144–147 (Mbeki).

53. World Health Organization, *World Health Statistics: 2007* (Geneva: World Health Organization, 2008), 22–31.

54. UNAIDS, "Sub-Saharan Africa," 10.

55. Centers for Disease Control, *Morbidity and Mortality Weekly Report* 44, no. 11 (1994): 227–231; *Chicago Tribune*, March 25,1997, sec. 1, p. 3.

56. The poster is reproduced in Allan M. Brandt, *No Magic Bullet: A Social History of Venereal Disease in the United States since 1880* (New York: Oxford University Press, 1985), 165.

57. Treichler, "AIDS, Gender, and Biomedical Discourse," 212, 217.

58. Daniel M. Fox, "The Politics of HIV Infection: 1989–1990 as Years of Change," in Fee and Fox, *AIDS: The Making of a Chronic Disease*, 125–143.

59. Iliffe, *African AIDS Epidemic*, 148.

60. Charles E. Rosenberg, "Disease and Social Order in America: Perceptions and Expectations," in Fee and Fox, *AIDS: The Burdens of History*, 22–23.

61. World Health Organization, *The World Health Report 1995: Bridging the Gaps* (Geneva: World Health Organization, 1995), v, 1.

62. WHO, *World Health Statistics*, 32–35.

63. *Manchester Guardian Weekly*, May 5, 1996, p. 5.

64. WHO, *World Health Statistics*, 58–63.

65. WHO, *World Health Statistics*.

66. WHO, *World Health Report 1995*, 24.

67. WHO, *World Health Statistics*, 22–31.

68. UNAIDS, "2007 AIDS Epidemic Update," Global Summary, 1.

69. WHO, *World Health Statistics*, 18.

70. *New York Times*, September 23, 2008, D5, D7.

71. WHO, *World Health Report 1995*, 42.

Suggestions for Further Reading

The following lists do not constitute a comprehensive bibliography of the histories of disease and medicine. They are intended rather as suggestions for those readers who wish to pursue topics more thoroughly. Their order follows the chapters of this book; some works may appear on the list more than once.

General Works

Ackerknecht, Erwin H. *A Short History of Medicine*, rev. ed. Baltimore: Johns Hopkins University Press, 1982.

Burnet, Macfarlane, and David O. White. *Natural History of Infectious Disease*, 4th ed. Cambridge: Cambridge University Press, 1972.

Cliff, Andrew D., and Peter Haggett. *Atlas of Disease Distributions: Analytic Approaches to Epidemiological Data*. Oxford: Blackwell Publishers, 1988.

Conrad, Lawrence I., Michael Neve, Roy Porter, Vivian Nutton, and Andrew Wear. *The Western Medical Tradition, 800 B.C-1800 A.D.* Cambridge: Cambridge University Press, 1995.

Davis, Audrey B. *Medicine and Its Technology: An Introduction to the History of Medical Instrumentation*. Westport, Conn.: Greenwood Press, 1981.

Diamond, Jared. *Guns, Germs, and Steel: The Fates of Human Societies*. New York: W. W. Norton, 1997.

Gilman, Sander L. *Picturing Health and Illness: Images of Identity and Difference*. Baltimore: Johns Hopkins University Press, 1995.

Grob, Gerald N. *The Deadly Truth: A History of Disease in America*. Cambridge, Mass.: Harvard University Press, 2002.

Hahn, Robert A. *Sickness and Healing: An Anthropological Perspective*. New Haven, Conn.: Yale University Press, 1995.

Kiple, Kenneth F., ed. *The Cambridge World History of Human Disease*. Cambridge: Cambridge University Press, 1993.

Kleinman, Arthur. *The Illness Narratives: Suffering, Healing, and the Human Condition.* New York: Basic Books, 1988.

McKeown, Thomas. *The Origins of Human Disease.* Oxford: Basil Blackwell, 1988.

McNeill, William H. *Plagues and Peoples.* Garden City, N.Y.: Anchor/Doubleday, 1976.

Numbers, Ronald L., and Judith Walzer Leavitt, eds. *Sickness and Health in America: Readings in the History of Medicine and Public Health,* 2d ed. Madison: University of Wisconsin Press, 1985.

Porter, Roy, ed. *The Cambridge Illustrated History of Medicine.* Cambridge: Cambridge University Press, 1996.

————. *The Greatest Benefit to Mankind: A Medical History of Humanity.* New York: W. W. Norton, 1998.

————. *Madness: A Brief History.* Oxford: Oxford University Press, 2002.

Ranger, Terence, and Paul Slack, eds. *Epidemics and Ideas: Essays on the Historical Perception of Pestilence.* Cambridge: Cambridge University Press, 1992.

Rey, Roselyne. *The History of Pain.* Cambridge, Mass.: Harvard University Press, 1995.

Risse, Guenter B. *Mending Bodies, Saving Souls: A History of Hospitals.* New York: Oxford University Press, 1999.

Rosenberg, Charles E. *Explaining Epidemics, and Other Studies in the History of Medicine.* Cambridge: Cambridge University Press, 1992.

Rothman, David J., Steven Marcus, and Stephanie A. Kiceluk, eds. *Medicine and Western Civilization.* New Brunswick, N.J.: Rutgers University Press, 1995.

Wear, Andrew, ed. *Medicine in Society: Historical Essays.* Cambridge: Cambridge University Press, 1992.

Web Sites of General Interest

Centers for Disease Control and Prevention: http://www.cdc.gov

National Library of Medicine: http://www.nlm.nih.gov

Wellcome Library, London: http://library.wellcome.ac.uk

World Health Organization: http://www.who.int

One   The Western Inheritance

Amundsen, Darrel W. *Medicine, Society, and Faith in the Ancient and Medieval Worlds.* Baltimore: Johns Hopkins University Press, 1995.

Grmek, Mirko D. *Diseases in the Ancient Greek World.* Baltimore: Johns Hopkins University Press, 1989.

Jackson, Ralph. *Doctors and Diseases in the Roman Empire.* Norman: University of Oklahoma Press, 1988.

Lloyd, G.E.R. *In the Grip of Disease: Studies in the Greek Imagination.* Oxford: Oxford University Press, 2003.

————. *Science, Folklore, and Ideology: Studies in the Life Sciences in Ancient Greece.* Cambridge: Cambridge University Press, 1983.

Miller, Timothy S. *The Birth of the Hospital in the Byzantine Empire.* Baltimore: Johns Hopkins University Press, 1985.

Nutton, Vivian. *Ancient Medicine.* London: Routledge, 2004.

Sallares, Robert. *The Ecology of the Ancient Greek World.* Ithaca, N.Y.: Cornell University Press, 1991.

————. *Malaria and Rome: A History of Malaria in Ancient Italy*. Oxford: Oxford University Press, 2002.

Temkin, Owsei. *Galenism: Rise and Decline of a Medical Philosophy*. Ithaca, N.Y: Cornell University Press, 1973.

————. *Hippocrates in a World of Pagans and Christians*. Baltimore: Johns Hopkins University Press, 1991.

Two   Medieval Diseases and Responses

Bloch, Marc. *The Royal Touch: Sacred Monarchy and Scrofula in England and France*. London: Routledge and Kegan Paul, 1973.

Brody, Saul Nathaniel. *The Disease of the Soul: Leprosy in Medieval Literature*. Ithaca, N.Y.: Cornell University Press, 1974.

Demaitre, Luke. *Leprosy in Premodern Medicine: A Malady of the Whole Body*. Baltimore: Johns Hopkins University Press, 2007.

Kealey, Edward J. *Medieval Medicus: A Social History of Anglo-Norman Medicine*. Baltimore: Johns Hopkins University Press, 1981.

Little, Lester K., ed. *Plague and the End of Antiquity: The Pandemic of 541–750*. Cambridge: Cambridge University Press, 2007.

Rawcliffe, Carole. *Leprosy in Medieval England*. Woodbridge: Boydell, 2006.

Richards, Peter. *The Medieval Leper and His Northern Heirs*. Cambridge: D. S. Brewer, 1977.

Sheils, W. J., ed. *The Church and Healing*. Oxford: Basil Blackwell, 1982.

Siraisi, Nancy G. *Medieval and Early Renaissance Medicine: An Introduction to Knowledge and Practice*. Chicago: University of Chicago Press, 1990.

Three   The Great Plague Pandemic

Aberth, John. *The Black Death: The Great Mortality of 1348–1350: A Brief History with Documents*. Boston: Bedford/St. Martin's, 2005.

Alexander, John T. *Bubonic Plague in Early Modern Russia: Public Health and Urban Disaster*. Baltimore: Johns Hopkins University Press, 1980.

Benedictow, Ole J. *The Black Death, 1346–1353: The Complete History*. Woodbridge: Boydell, 2004.

Biraben, Jean-Noël. *Les hommes et la peste en France et dans les pays européens et mediterranéens*. Paris: Mouton, 1975–76.

Calvi, Guilia. *Histories of a Plague Year: The Social and the Imaginary in Baroque Florence*. Berkeley: University of California Press, 1989.

Campbell, Anna M. *The Black Death and Men of Learning*. New York: AMS Press, 1966; originally published in 1931.

Carmichael, Ann G. *Plague and the Poor in Renaissance Florence*. Cambridge: Cambridge University Press, 1986.

Cipolla, Carlo M. *Christofano and the Plague: A Study in the History of Public Health in the Age of Galileo*. Berkeley: University of California Press, 1973.

————. *Public Health and the Medical Profession in the Renaissance*. Cambridge: Cambridge University Press, 1976.

Cohn, Samuel K., Jr. *The Black Death Transformed: Disease and Culture in Early Renaissance Europe*. New York: Oxford University Press, 2002.

Dols, Michael W. *The Black Death in the Middle East*. Princeton, N.J.: Princeton University Press, 1977.

Getz, Faye M. "Black Death and Silver Lining: Meaning, Continuity, and Revolutionary Change in Histories of Medieval Plague." *Journal of the History of Biology* 24 (1991): 265–289.

Hatcher, John. *Plague, Population and the English Economy, 1348–1530*. London: Macmillan, 1977.

Horrox, Rosemary, ed. *The Black Death*. Manchester: Manchester University Press, 1994.

Moote, A. Lloyd, and Dorothy C. Moote. *The Great Plague: The Story of London's Most Deadly Year*. Baltimore: Johns Hopkins University Press, 2004.

Nutton, Vivian, ed. "Pestilential Complexities: Understanding Medieval Plague." Supplement 27, *Medical History* (2008).

Platt, Colin. *King Death: The Black Death and Its Aftermath in Late-Medieval England*. London: UCL Press, 1996.

Shrewsbury, J.F.D. *A History of Bubonic Plague in the British Isles*. Cambridge: Cambridge University Press, 1970.

Slack, Paul. *The Impact of Plague in Tudor and Stuart England*. London: Routledge and Kegan Paul, 1985.

Steel, David. "Plague Writing: From Boccaccio to Camus." *Journal of European Studies* 11 (1981): 88–110.

Williman, Daniel, ed. *The Black Death: The Impact of the Fourteenth-Century Plague*. Binghamton, N.Y.: Center for Medieval and Early Renaissance Studies, 1982.

Ziegler, Philip. *The Black Death*. New York: Harper and Row, 1969.

Four   New Diseases and Transatlantic Exchanges

Arrizabalaga, Jon, John Henderson, and Roger French. *The Great Pox: The French Disease in Renaissance Europe*. New Haven, Conn.: Yale University Press, 1997.

Cook, Noble David. *Born to Die: Disease and New World Conquest, 1492–1650*. Cambridge: Cambridge University Press, 1998.

Cook, N. D., and W. G. Lovell, eds. *"Secret Judgments of God": Old World Disease in Colonial Spanish America*. Norman: University of Oklahoma Press, 1992.

Crosby, Alfred W., Jr. *The Columbian Exchange: Biological and Cultural Consequences of 1492*. Westport, Conn.: Greenwood Press, 1972.

———. *Ecological Imperialism: The Biological Expansion of Europe, 900–1900*. Cambridge: Cambridge University Press, 1986.

Dobyns, Henry F. *Their Number Became Thinned: Native American Population Dynamics in Eastern North America*. Knoxville: University of Tennessee Press, 1983.

Hopkins, Donald R. *The Greatest Killer: Smallpox in History*. Chicago: University of Chicago Press, 2002. (Originally published 1983 as *Princes and Peasants: Smallpox in History*.)

Jones, David S. *Rationalizing Epidemics: Meanings and Uses of American Indian Mortality Since 1600*. Cambridge, Mass.: Harvard University Press, 2004.

McNeill, William H. *Plagues and Peoples*. Garden City, N.Y.: Anchor/Doubleday, 1976.

Ortiz de Montellano, Bernard R. *Aztec Medicine, Health, and Nutrition*. New Brunswick, N.J.: Rutgers University Press, 1990.

Powell, Mary Lucas, and Della Collins Cook, eds. *The Myth of Syphilis: The Natural History of Treponematosis in North America*. Gainesville: University Press of Florida, 2005.

Prinzing, Friedrich. *Epidemics Resulting from Wars*. Oxford: Clarendon Press, 1916.

Quétel, Claude. *History of Syphilis*. Baltimore: Johns Hopkins University Press, 1990.

Ramenofsky, Ann F. *Vectors of Death: The Archaeology of European Contact*. Albuquerque: University of New Mexico Press, 1987.

Zinsser, Hans. *Rats, Lice and History*. New York: Basic Books, 1965; originally published in 1935.

Five   Continuity and Change

Cook, Harold J. *The Decline of the Old Medical Regime in Stuart London*. Ithaca, N.Y.: Cornell University Press, 1986.

———. *Matters of Exchange: Commerce, Medicine, and Science in the Dutch Golden Age*. New Haven, Conn.: Yale University Press, 2007.

Debus, Allen G. *The Chemical Philosophy: Paracelsian Science and Medicine in the Sixteenth and Seventeenth Centuries*. New York: Science History Publications, 1977.

———. *Man and Nature in the Renaissance*. Cambridge: Cambridge University Press, 1978.

Finucane, Ronald C. *Miracles and Pilgrims: Popular Beliefs in Medieval England*. Totowa, N.J.: Rowman and Littlefield, 1977.

French, Roger. *Medicine before Science: The Rational and Learned Doctor from the Middle Ages to the Enlightenment*. Cambridge: Cambridge University Press, 2003.

French, Roger, and Andrew Wear, eds. *The Medical Revolution of the Seventeenth Century*. Cambridge: Cambridge University Press, 1989.

Hall, A. R. *The Scientific Revolution, 1500–1800*. Boston: Beacon Press, 1954.

Kieckhefer, Richard. *Magic in the Middle Ages*. Cambridge: Cambridge University Press, 1989.

Koyré, Alexandre. *From the Closed World to the Infinite Universe*. Baltimore: Johns Hopkins University Press, 1957.

Kuhn, Thomas S. *The Copernican Revolution*. Cambridge, Mass.: Harvard University Press, 1957.

Lindberg, David C., and Ronald L. Numbers, eds. *God and Nature: Historical Essays on the Encounter between Christianity and Science*. Berkeley: University of California Press, 1986.

McVaugh, Michael R. *Medicine before the Plague: Practitioners and Their Patients in the Crown of Aragon, 1285–1345*. Cambridge: Cambridge University Press, 1993.

Merchant, Carolyn. *The Death of Nature: Women, Ecology, and the Scientific Revolution*. San Francisco: Harper and Row, 1980.

O'Malley, C. D. *Andreas Vesalius of Brussels, 1514–1564*. Berkeley: University of California Press, 1965.

Pagel, Walter. *Paracelsus: An Introduction to Philosophical Medicine in the Era of the Renaissance*. Basel: S. Karger, 1958.

———. *William Harvey's Biological Ideas*. Basel: S. Karger, 1967.

Park, Katharine. *Doctors and Medicine in Early Renaissance Florence*. Princeton, N.J.: Princeton University Press, 1985.

Siraisi, Nancy G. *Medieval and Early Renaissance Medicine: An Introduction to Knowledge and Practice*. Chicago: University of Chicago Press, 1990.

Thomas, Keith. *Religion and the Decline of Magic: Studies in Popular Beliefs in Sixteenth- and Seventeenth-Century England*. Harmondsworth: Penguin Books, 1973; originally published in 1971.

Webster, Charles. *The Great Instauration: Science, Medicine, and Reform, 1626–1660*. New York: Holmes and Meier, 1976.

Westfall, Richard S. *The Construction of Modern Science: Mechanisms and Mechanics*. New York: John Wiley, 1971.

———. *Never at Rest: a Biography of Isaac Newton*. Cambridge: Cambridge University Press, 1980.

Whitteridge, Gweneth. *William Harvey and the Circulation of the Blood*. London: Macdonald, 1971.

Yates, Frances. *Giordano Bruno and the Hermetic Tradition*. Chicago: University of Chicago Press, 1964.

Six Disease and the Enlightenment

Ackerknecht, Erwin H. *Medicine at the Paris Hospital, 1794–1848*. Baltimore: Johns Hopkins University Press, 1967.

Baxby, Derrick. *Jenner's Smallpox Vaccine: The Riddle of Vaccinia Virus and Its Origin*. London: Heinemann, 1981.

Broman, Thomas H. *The Transformation of German Academic Medicine, 1750–1820*. Cambridge: Cambridge University Press, 1996.

Bruce-Chwatt, L. J., and J. de Zulueta. *The Rise and Fall of Malaria in Europe: A Historico-Epidemiological Study*. Oxford: Oxford University Press, 1980.

Bynum, William F., and Vivian Nutton, eds. *Theories of Fever from Antiquity to the Enlightenment*. Supplement 1 to *Medical History*, 1981.

Bynum, William F., and Roy Porter, eds. *William Hunter and the Eighteenth-Century Medical World*. Cambridge: Cambridge University Press, 1985.

Carpenter, Kenneth J. *The History of Scurvy and Vitamin C*. Cambridge: Cambridge University Press, 1986.

Corbin, Alain. *The Foul and the Fragrant: Odor and the French Social Imagination*. Cambridge, Mass.: Harvard University Press, 1986.

Cunningham, Andrew, and Roger French, eds. *The Medical Enlightenment of the Eighteenth Century*. Cambridge: Cambridge University Press, 1990.

Darnton, Robert. *Mesmerism and the End of Enlightenment in France*. Cambridge, Mass.: Harvard University Press, 1968.

Dobson, Mary J. *Contours of Death and Disease in Early Modern England*. Cambridge: Cambridge University Press, 1997.

Estes, J. Worth, and Billy G. Smith, eds. *A Melancholy Scene of Devastation: The Public Response to the 1793 Philadelphia Yellow Fever Epidemic*. Canton, Mass.: Science History Publications, 1997.

Fissell, Mary E. *Patients, Power, and the Poor in Eighteenth-Century Bristol*. Cambridge: Cambridge University Press, 1991.

Foucault, Michel. *The Birth of the Clinic: An Archaeology of Medical Perception*. New York: Vintage, 1978; originally published in 1963.

Gelfand, Toby. *Professionalizing Modern Medicine: Paris Surgeons and Medical Sciences and Institutions in the Eighteenth Century*. Westport, Conn.: Greenwood Press, 1980.

Hopkins, Donald R. *The Greatest Killer: Smallpox in History*. Chicago: University of Chicago Press, 2002. (Originally published in 1983 as *Princes and Peasants: Smallpox in History*.)

Jarcho, Saul. *Quinine's Predecessor: Francesco Torti and the Early History of Cinchona*. Baltimore: Johns Hopkins University Press, 1993.

Landers, John. *Death and the Metropolis: Studies in the Demographic History of London, 1670–1830*. Cambridge: Cambridge University Press, 1993.

Lindemann, Mary. *Health and Healing in Eighteenth-Century Germany*. Baltimore: Johns Hopkins University Press, 1996.

Loudon, Irvine. *Medical Care and the General Practitioner, 1750–1850*. Oxford: Clarendon Press, 1986.

MacAlpine, Ida, and Richard Hunter. *George III and the Mad Business*. New York: Pantheon, 1970.

Matossian, Mary K. *Poisons of the Past: Molds, Epidemics, and History*. New Haven, Conn.: Yale University Press, 1989.

Miller, Genevieve. *The Adoption of Inoculation for Smallpox in England and France*. Philadelphia: University of Pennsylvania Press, 1957.

Porter, Roy. *Mind-Forg'd Manacles: A History of Madness in England from the Restoration to the Regency*. Cambridge, Mass.: Harvard University Press, 1987.

Post, John D. *Food Shortage, Climatic Variability, and Epidemic Disease in Preindustrial Europe: the Mortality Peak in the Early 1740s*. Ithaca, N.Y.: Cornell University Press, 1985.

Powell, J. H. *Bring Out Your Dead: The Great Plague of Yellow Fever in Philadelphia in 1793*. Philadelphia: University of Pennsylvania Press, 1949.

Ramsey, Matthew. *Professional and Popular Medicine in France, 1770–1830*. Cambridge: Cambridge University Press, 1988.

Razzell, Peter. *The Conquest of Smallpox: The Impact of Inoculation on Smallpox Mortality in Eighteenth Century Britain*. Firle: Caliban Books, 1977.

Riley, James C. *The Eighteenth-Century Campaign to Avoid Disease*. New York: St. Martin's, 1987.

Vess, David M. *Medical Revolution in France, 1789–1796*. Gainesville: University Press of Florida, 1975.

Vigarello, Georges. *Concepts of Cleanliness: Changing Attitudes in France since the Middle Ages*. Cambridge: Cambridge University Press, 1988.

Seven   Cholera and Sanitation

Ackerknecht, E. H. "Anticontagionism between 1821 and 1867." *Bulletin of the History of Medicine* 22 (1948): 562–593.

Baldwin, Peter. *Contagion and the State in Europe, 1830–1930*. Cambridge: Cambridge University Press, 1999.

Briggs, Asa. "Cholera and Society in the Nineteenth Century. " *Past and Present* no. 19 (1961): 76–96.

Coleman, William. *Death Is a Social Disease: Public Health and Political Economy in Early Industrial France*. Madison: University of Wisconsin Press, 1982.

Duffy, John. *A History of Public Health inNew York City, 1625–1866*. New York: Russell Sage Foundation, 1968.

Durey, Michael. *The Return of the Plague: British Society and the Cholera, 1831–32*. Dublin: Gill and Macmillan, 1979.

Evans, Richard J. *Death in Hamburg: Society and Politics in the Cholera Years, 1830–1910*. Oxford: Oxford University Press, 1987; reprint, London: Penguin Books, 1990.

———. "Epidemics and Revolutions: Cholera in Nineteenth-Century Europe." *Past and Present* no. 120 (1988): 123–146.

Goubert, Jean-Pierre. *The Conquest of Water: The Advent of Health in the Industrial Age*. Princeton, N.J.: Princeton University Press, 1989.

Hamlin, Christopher. *Public Health and Social Justice in the Age of Chadwick*. Cambridge: Cambridge University Press, 1998.

Hardy, Anne. *The Epidemic Streets: Infectious Disease and the Rise of Preventive Medicine, 1856–1900*. Oxford: Clarendon Press, 1993.

Kudlick, Catherine J. *Cholera in Post-Revolutionary Paris: A Cultural History*. Berkeley: University of California Press, 1996.

Luckin, Bill. *Pollution and Control: A Social History of the Thames in the Nineteenth Century*. Bristol: Adam Hilger, 1986.

McGrew, Roderick. *Russia and the Cholera, 1823–1832*. Madison: University of Wisconsin Press, 1965.

Morris, R. J. *Cholera 1832: The Social Response to an Epidemic*. New York: Holmes and Meier, 1976.

Pelling, Margaret. *Cholera, Fever and English Medicine, 1825–1865*. Oxford: Oxford University Press, 1978.

Rosenberg, Charles E. *The Cholera Years: The United States in 1832, 1849, and 1866*. Chicago: University of Chicago Press, 1962.

Rosenkrantz, Barbara G. *Public Health and the State: Changing Views in Massachusetts, 1842–1936*. Cambridge, Mass.: Harvard University Press, 1972.

Snowden, Frank M. *Naples in the Time of Cholera, 1884–1911*. Cambridge: Cambridge University Press, 1995.

Wohl, Anthony S. *Endangered Lives: Public Health in Victorian Britain*. Cambridge, Mass.: Harvard University Press, 1983.

Woodham-Smith, Cecil. *Florence Nightingale, 1820–1910*. London: Constable, 1950.

Eight   Tuberculosis and Poverty

Barnes, David S. *The Making of a Social Disease: Tuberculosis in Nineteenth-Century France*. Berkeley: University of California Press, 1995.

Bates, Barbara. *Bargaining for Life: A Social History of Tuberculosis, 1876–1938*. Philadelphia: University of Pennsylvania Press, 1992.

Bryder, Linda. *Below the Magic Mountain: A Social History of Tuberculosis in Twentieth-Century Britain*. Oxford: Clarendon Press, 1988.

Dubos, René, and Jean Dubos. *The White Plague: Tuberculosis, Man, and Society*. New Brunswick, N.J.: Rutgers University Press, 1987; originally published in 1952.

Feldberg, Georgina D. *Disease and Class: Tuberculosis and the Shaping of Modern North American Society*. New Brunswick, N.J.: Rutgers University Press, 1996.

Hardy, Anne. *The Epidemic Streets: Infectious Disease and the Rise of Preventive Medicine, 1856–1900*. Oxford: Clarendon Press, 1993.

Rothman, Sheila M. *Living in the Shadow of Death: Tuberculosis and the Social Experience of Illness in American History*. New York: Basic Books, 1994.

Smith, F. B. *The Retreat of Tuberculosis, 1850–1950*. London: Croom Helm, 1988.

Teller, Michael E. *The Tuberculosis Movement: A Public Health Campaign in the Progressive Era*. New York: Greenwood Press, 1988.

Wohl, Anthony S. *Endangered Lives: Public Health in Victorian Britain*. Cambridge, Mass.: Harvard University Press, 1983.

Woods, Robert, and John Woodward, eds. *Urban Disease and Mortality in Nineteenth-Century England*. New York: St. Martin's, 1984.

Nine   Disease, Medicine, and Western Imperialism

Anderson, Warwick. *Colonial Pathologies: American Tropical Medicine, Race and Hygiene in the Philippines*. Durham, N.C.: Duke University Press, 2006.

Arnold, David. *Colonizing the Body: State Medicine and Epidemic Disease in Nineteenth-Century India*. Berkeley: University of California Press, 1993.

Arnold, David, ed. *Imperial Medicine and Indigenous Societies*. Manchester: Manchester University Press, 1988.

Benedict, Carol. *Bubonic Plague in Nineteenth-Century China*. Stanford, Calif.: Stanford University Press, 1996.

Bewell, Alan. *Romanticism and Colonial Disease*. Baltimore: Johns Hopkins University Press, 1999.

Cliff, A. D., P. Haggett, and M. R. Smallman-Raynor. *Island Epidemics*. Oxford: Oxford University Press, 2000.

Coleman, William. *Yellow Fever in the North: The Methods of Early Epidemiology*. Madison: University of Wisconsin Press, 1987.

Craddock, Susan. *City of Plagues: Disease, Poverty, and Deviance in San Francisco*. Minneapolis: University of Minnesota Press, 2000.

Crosby, Alfred W. *Ecological Imperialism: The Biological Expansion of Europe, 900–1900*. Cambridge: Cambridge University Press, 1986.

Curson, Peter, and Kevin McCracken. *Plague in Sydney: The Anatomy of an Epidemic*. Kensington, NSW: New South Wales University Press, 1989.

Curtin, Philip F. *Death by Migration: Europe's Encounter with the Tropical World in the Nineteenth Century*. Cambridge: Cambridge University Press, 1989.

De Bevoise, Ken. *Agents of Apocalypse: Epidemic Disease in the Colonial Philippines*. Princeton, N.J.: Princeton University Press, 1995.

Delaporte, François. *The History of Yellow Fever: An Essay on the Birth of Tropical Medicine*. Cambridge, Mass.: MIT Press, 1991.

Echenberg, Myron. *Plague Ports: The Global Urban Impact of Bubonic Plague, 1894–1901*. New York: New York University Press, 2007.

Farley, John. *Bilharzia: A History of Imperial Tropical Medicine*. Cambridge: Cambridge University Press, 1991.

Ford, John. *The Role of the Trypanosomiases in African Ecology: A Study of the Tsetse Fly Problem*. Oxford: Clarendon Press, 1971.

Gallagher, Nancy E. *Medicine and Power in Tunisia, 1780–1900*. Cambridge: Cambridge University Press, 1983.

Gregg, Charles T. *Plague: An Ancient Disease in the Twentieth Century*. Albuquerque: University of New Mexico Press, 1985.

Harrison, Gordon. *Mosquitoes, Malaria, and Man: A History of the Hostilities since 1880*. New York: E. P. Dutton, 1978.

Harrison, Mark. *Climates and Constitutions: Health, Race, Environment and British Imperialism in India, 1600–1850*. New Delhi: Oxford University Press, 1999.

———. *Public Health in British India: Anglo-Indian Preventive Medicine, 1859–1914*. Cambridge: Cambridge University Press, 1994.

Hartwig, G. W., and K. D. Patterson, eds. *Disease in African History*. Durham, N.C.: Duke University Press, 1978.

Haynes, Douglas M. *Imperial Medicine: Patrick Manson and the Conquest of Tropical Disease*. Philadelphia: University of Pennsylvania Press, 2001.

Headrick, Daniel F. *The Tools of Empire: Technology and European Imperialism in the Nineteenth Century.* New York: Oxford University Press, 1981.

Jannetta, Ann Bowman. *Epidemics and Mortality in Early Modern Japan.* Princeton, N.J.: Princeton University Press, 1987.

Kiple, Kenneth F. *The Caribbean Slave: A Biological History.* Cambridge: Cambridge University Press, 1984.

———. ed. *The African Exchange: Toward a Biological History of Black People.* Durham, N.C.: Duke University Press, 1987.

Kuhnke, LaVerne. *Lives at Risk: Public Health in Nineteenth-Century Egypt.* Berkeley: University of California Press, 1990.

Kunitz, Stephen J. *Disease and Social Diversity: The European Impact on the Health of Non-Europeans.* Oxford: Oxford University Press, 1994.

Lyons, Maryinez. *The Colonial Disease: A Social History of Sleeping Sickness in Northern Zaire, 1900–1940.* Cambridge: Cambridge University Press, 1992.

McArthur, Norma. *Island Populations of the Pacific.* Canberra: Australian National University Press, 1968.

MacLeod, Roy, and Milton Lewis, eds. *Disease, Medicine, and Empire: Perspectives on Western Medicine and the Experience of European Expansion.* London: Routledge, 1988.

MacPherson, Kerrie L. "Cholera in China, 1820–1930: An Aspect of the Internationalization of Infectious Disease." In *Sediments of Time: Environment and Society in Chinese History,* ed. Mark Elvin and Liu Ts'ui-jung, 487–519. Cambridge: Cambridge University Press, 1998.

———. *A Wilderness of Marshes: The Origins of Public Health in Shanghai, 1843–1893.* Oxford: Oxford University Press, 1987.

Manderson, Lenore. *Sickness and the State: Health and Illness in Colonial Malaya, 1870–1940.* Cambridge: Cambridge University Press, 1996.

Mohr, James C. *Plague and Fire: Battling Black Death and the 1900 Burning of Honolulu's Chinatown.* New York: Oxford University Press, 2005.

Owen, Norman G., ed. *Death and Disease in Southeast Asia: Explorations in Social, Medical and Demographic History.* Singapore: Oxford University Press, 1987.

Packard, Randall M. *The Making of a Tropical Disease: A Short History of Malaria.* Baltimore: Johns Hopkins University Press, 2007.

———. *White Plague, Black Labor: Tuberculosis and the Political Economy of Health and Disease in South Africa.* Berkeley: University of California Press, 1989.

Patterson, K. David. *Health in Colonial Ghana: Disease, Medicine, and Socio-Economic Change, 1900–1955.* Waltham, Mass.: Crossroads Press, 1981.

Rogaski, Ruth. *Hygienic Modernity: Meanings of Health and Disease in Treaty-Port China.* Berkeley: University of California Press, 2004.

Shah, Nayan. *Contagious Divides: Epidemics and Race in San Francisco's Chinatown.* Berkeley: University of California Press, 2001.

Sheridan, Richard B. *Doctors and Slaves: A Medical and Demographic History of Slavery in the British West Indies, 1680–1834.* Cambridge: Cambridge University Press, 1985.

Sutphen, Mary P., and Bridie Andrews, eds. *Medicine and Colonial Identity.* London: Routledge, 2003.

Turshen, Meredeth. *The Political Ecology of Disease in Tanzania.* New Brunswick, N.J.: Rutgers University Press, 1984.

Vaughan, Megan. *Curing Their Ills: Colonial Power and African Illness.* Stanford, Calif.: Stanford University Press, 1991.

Watts, Sheldon. *Epidemics and History: Disease, Power and Imperialism*. New Haven: Yale University Press, 1997.

Ten   The Scientific View

Ackerman, Evelyn B. *Health Care in the Parisian Countryside, 1800–1914*. New Brunswick, N.J.: Rutgers University Press, 1990.

Bonner, Thomas N. *American Doctors and German Universities: A Chapter in International Intellectual Relations, 1870–1914*. Lincoln: University of Nebraska Press, 1963.

Borst, Charlotte. *Catching Babies: The Professionalization of Childbirth, 1870–1920*. Cambridge, Mass.: Harvard University Press, 1995.

Brock, Thomas D. *Robert Koch: A Life in Medicine and Bacteriology*. Madison, Wis.: Science Tech Publishers, 1988.

Bynum, W. F. *Science and the Practice of Medicine in the Nineteenth Century*. Cambridge: Cambridge University Press, 1994.

Cassedy, James H. *Medicine in America: A Short History*. Baltimore: Johns Hopkins University Press, 1991.

Cherry, Steven. *Medical Services and the Hospitals in Britain, 1860–1939*. Cambridge: Cambridge University Press, 1996.

Digby, Anne. *Making a Medical Living: Doctors and Their Patients in English Society, 1720–1911*. Cambridge: Cambridge University Press, 1994.

Donegan, Jane. *"Hydropathic Highway to Health": Women and Water-Cure in Antebellum America*. Westport, Conn.: Greenwood Press, 1986.

Dowbiggin, Ian. *Inheriting Madness: Professionalization and Psychiatric Knowledge in Nineteenth-Century France*. Berkeley: University of California Press, 1991.

Dubos, René. *Louis Pasteur: Free Lance of Science*. Boston: Little, Brown, 1950.

Geison, Gerald L. *The Private Science of Louis Pasteur*. Princeton, N.J.: Princeton University Press, 1995.

Gevitz, Norman. *The D.O.'s: Osteopathic Medicine in America*. Baltimore: Johns Hopkins University Press, 1982.

Goldstein, Jan. *Console and Classify: The French Psychiatric Profession in the Nineteenth Century*. Cambridge: Cambridge University Press, 1987.

Gordon, Linda. *Woman's Body, Woman's Right: A Social History of Birth Control in America*. New York: Grossman, 1976.

Grob, Gerald N. *Mental Illness and American Society, 1875–1940*. Princeton, N.J.: Princeton University Press, 1983.

Haber, Samuel. *The Quest for Authority and Honor in the American Professions, 1750–1900*. Chicago: University of Chicago Press, 1991.

Keown, James. *Abortion, Doctors, and the Law: Some Aspects of the Legal Regulation of Abortion in England from 1803 to 1982*. Cambridge: Cambridge University Press, 1988.

Latour, Bruno. *The Pasteurization of France*. Cambridge, Mass.: Harvard University Press, 1988.

Leavitt, Judith Walzer. *Brought to Bed: Childbearing in America, 1750–1950*. New York: Oxford University Press, 1986.

Leavitt, Judith Walzer, ed. *Women and Health in America*. Madison: University of Wisconsin Press, 1984.

Lesch, John E. *Science and Medicine in France: The Emergence of Experimental Physiology, 1790–1855*. Cambridge, Mass.: Harvard University Press, 1984.

Litoff, Judy B. *American Midwives: 1860 to the Present*. Westport, Conn.: Greenwood Press, 1978.

Ludmerer, Kenneth. *Learning to Heal: The Development of American Medical Education*. New York: Basic Books, 1985.

——. *Time to Heal: American Medical Education from the Turn of the Century to the Era of Managed Care*. New York: Oxford University Press, 1999.

McClelland, Charles E. *The German Experience of Professionalization: Modern Learned Professions and Their Organizations*. New York: Cambridge University Press, 1991.

McGuire, Meredith B., and Debra Kantor. *Ritual Healing in Suburban America*. New Brunswick, N.J.: Rutgers University Press, 1988.

Marks, Harry M. *The Progress of Experiment: Science and Therapeutic Reform in the United States, 1900–1990*. Cambridge: Cambridge University Press, 1997.

Marland, Hilary. *Medicine and Society in Wakefield and Huddersfield, 1780–1870*. Cambridge: Cambridge University Press, 1987.

Matthews, J. Rosser. *Quantification and the Quest for Medical Certainty*. Princeton, N.J.: Princeton University Press, 1995.

Maulitz, Russell C. *Morbid Appearances: The Anatomy of Pathology in the Early Nineteenth Century*. Cambridge: Cambridge University Press, 1987.

Mohr, James C. *Doctors and the Law: Medical Jurisprudence in Nineteenth-Century America*. New York: Oxford University Press, 1993.

Moore, J. Stuart. *Chiropractic in America: The History of a Medical Alternative*. Baltimore: Johns Hopkins University Press, 1993.

Moore, Judith. *A Zeal for Responsibility: The Struggle for Professional Nursing in Victorian England, 1868–1883*. Athens: University of Georgia Press, 1988.

Oakley, Ann. *The Captured Womb: A History of the Medical Care of Pregnant Women*. Oxford: Basil Blackwell, 1984.

Pemberton, Neil, and Michael Worboys. *Mad Dogs and Englishmen: Rabies in Britain, 1830–2000*. Basingstoke: Palgrave Macmillan, 2007.

Pernick, Martin S. *A Calculus of Suffering: Pain, Professionalism, and Anesthesia in Nineteenth-Century America*. New York: Columbia University Press, 1985.

Peterson, M. Jeanne. *The Medical Profession in Mid-Victorian London*. Berkeley: University of California Press, 1978.

Ramsey, Matthew. *Professional and Popular Medicine in France, 1770–1830: The Social World of Medical Practice*. Cambridge: Cambridge University Press, 1988.

Reagan, Leslie J. *When Abortion Was a Crime: Women, Medicine, and the Law in the United States, 1867–1973*. Berkeley: University of California Press, 1997.

Reverby, Susan. *Ordered to Care: The Dilemma of American Nursing, 1850–1945*. Cambridge: Cambridge University Press, 1987.

Richardson, Ruth. *Death, Dissection and the Destitute*. London: Routledge and Kegan Paul, 1987.

Rosenberg, Charles E. *The Care of Strangers: The Rise of America's Hospital System*. New York: Basic Books, 1987.

Stage, Sarah. *Female Complaints: Lydia Pinkham and the Business of Women's Medicine*. New York: W.W.Norton, 1979.

Starr, Paul. *The Social Transformation of American Medicine*. New York: Basic Books, 1982.

Tomes, Nancy. *The Gospel of Germs: Men, Women, and the Microbe in American Life*. Cambridge, Mass.: Harvard University Press, 1998.

Warner, John H. *The Therapeutic Perspective: Medical Practice, Knowledge, and Identity in America, 1820–1885*. Cambridge, Mass.: Harvard University Press, 1986.

Weisz, George. *Divide and Conquer: A Comparative History of Medical Specialization*. New York: Oxford University Press, 2006.

Worboys, Michael. *Spreading Germs: Disease Theories and Medical Practice in Britain, 1865–1900*. Cambridge: Cambridge University Press, 2000.

Young, James Harvey. *The Toadstool Millionaires: A Social History of Patent Medicines in America before Federal Regulation*. Princeton, N.J.: Princeton University Press, 1961.

Eleven   The Apparent End of Epidemics

Adams, David P. *"The Greatest Good to the Greatest Number": Penicillin Rationing on the American Home Front, 1940–1945*. New York: Peter Lang, 1991.

Baeumler, Ernest. *Paul Ehrlich: Life Scientist*. New York: Holmes and Meier, 1983.

Brandt, Allan M. *No Magic Bullet: A Social History of Venereal Disease in the United States since 1880*. New York: Oxford University Press, 1985.

Cliff, Andrew, Peter Haggett, and Matthew Smallman-Raynor. *Deciphering Global Epidemics: Analytical Approaches to the Disease Records of World Cities, 1888–1912*. Cambridge: Cambridge University Press, 1998.

Crosby, Alfred W. *America's Forgotten Pandemic: The Influenza of 1918*. Cambridge: Cambridge University Press, 1989. Originally published as *Epidemic and Peace, 1918*. Westport, Conn.: Greenwood Press, 1976.

Dowling, Harry F. *Fighting Infection: Conquests of the Twentieth Century*. Cambridge, Mass.: Harvard University Press, 1977.

Floud, Roderick, Kenneth Wachter, and Annabel Gregory. *Height, Health and History: Nutritional Status in the United Kingdom, 1750–1980*. Cambridge: Cambridge University Press, 1991.

Gould, Tony. *A Summer Plague: Polio and its Survivors*. New Haven, Conn.: Yale University Press, 1995.

Hammonds, Evelynn Maxine. *Childhood's Deadly Scourge: The Campaign to Control Diphtheria in New York City, 1880–1930*. Baltimore: Johns Hopkins University Press, 1999.

Hardy, Anne. *The Epidemic Streets: Infectious Disease and the Rise of Preventive Medicine, 1856–1900*. Oxford: Clarendon Press, 1993.

Hobby, Gladys L. *Penicillin: Meeting the Challenge*. New Haven, Conn.: Yale University Press, 1985.

Hughes, Sally Smith. *The Virus: A History of the Concept*. London: Heinemann, 1977.

Kolata, Gina. *Flu: The Story of the Great Influenza Pandemic of 1918 and the Search for the Virus that Caused It*. New York: Touchstone Books, 2001. (Originally publ.: New York: Farrar, Straus & Giroux, 1999).

Leavitt, Judith Walzer. *Typhoid Mary: Captive to the Public's Health*. Boston: Beacon Press, 1996.

Livi-Bacci, Massimo. *Population and Nutrition: An Essay on European Demographic History*. Cambridge: Cambridge University Press, 1991.

Macfarlane, Gwyn. *Alexander Fleming: The Man and the Myth*. London: Chatto and Windus, 1984.

McKeown, Thomas. *The Modern Rise of Population*. New York: Academic Press, 1976.

————. *The Role of Medicine: Dream, Mirage or Nemesis?* Princeton, N.J.: Princeton University Press, 1979.

Offit, Paul A. *The Cutter Incident: How America's First Polio Vaccine Led to the Growing Vaccine Crisis.* New Haven, Conn.: Yale University Press, 2005.

Patterson, K. David. *Pandemic Influenza, 1700–1900: A Study in Historical Epidemiology.* Totowa, N.J.: Rowman and Littlefield, 1986.

Paul, John R. *A History of Poliomyelitis.* New Haven, Conn.: Yale University Press, 1971.

Phillips, Howard, and David Killingray, eds. *The Spanish Influenza Pandemic of 1918–19: New Perspectives.* London: Routledge, 2003.

Poirier, Suzanne. *Chicago's War on Syphilis, 1937–1940: The Times, the "Trib," and the Clap Doctor.* Urbana: University of Illinois Press, 1995.

Preston, Samuel H., and Michael R. Haines. *Fatal Years: Child Mortality in Late Nineteenth-Century America.* Princeton, N.J.: Princeton University Press, 1991.

Quétel, Claude. *History of Syphilis.* Baltimore: Johns Hopkins University Press, 1990.

Rogers, Naomi. *Dirt and Disease: Polio before FDR.* New Brunswick, N.J.: Rutgers University Press, 1992.

Rosen, George. *Preventive Medicine in the United States, 1900–1975.* New York: Science History Publications, 1975.

Schofield, R., D. Reher, and A. Bideau, eds. *The Decline of Mortality in Europe.* Oxford: Clarendon Press, 1991.

Seytre, Bernard, and Mary Shaffer. *The Death of a Disease: A History of the Eradication of Poliomyelitis.* New Brunswick, N.J.: Rutgers University Press, 2005.

Silverstein, Arthur M. *A History of Immunology.* San Diego: Academic Press, 1989.

Smith, Jane S. *Patenting the Sun: Polio and the Salk Vaccine.* New York: William Morrow, 1990.

Snell, Marc. *Polio and its Aftermath: The Paralysis of Culture.* Cambridge, Mass.: Harvard University Press, 2005.

Williams, Trevor I. *Howard Florey: Penicillin and After.* New York: Oxford University Press, 1984.

Twelve   Disease and Power

Aly, Götz, Peter Chroust, and Christian Pross. *Cleansing the Fatherland: Nazi Medicine and Racial Hygiene.* Baltimore: Johns Hopkins University Press, 1994.

Armstrong, David. *Political Anatomy of the Body: Medical Knowledge in Britain in the Twentieth Century.* Cambridge: Cambridge University Press, 1983.

Berridge, Virginia, and Philip Strong, eds. *AIDS and Contemporary History.* Cambridge: Cambridge University Press, 1993.

Brumberg, Joan Jacobs. *Fasting Girls: The Emergence of Anorexia Nervosa as a Modern Disease.* Cambridge, Mass.: Harvard University Press, 1988.

Burleigh, Michael. *Death and Deliverance: "Euthanasia" in Germany, c. 1900–1945.* Cambridge: Cambridge University Press, 1994.

Colgrove, James. *State of Immunity: The Politics of Immunization in Twentieth-Century America.* Berkeley: University of California Press, 2006.

Cowan, Ruth Schwartz. *Heredity and Hope: The Case for Genetic Screening.* Cambridge, Mass.: Harvard University Press, 2008.

Durbach, Nadja. *Bodily Matters: The Anti-Vaccination Movement in England, 1853–1907.* Durham, N.C.: Duke University Press, 2005.

Etheridge, Elizabeth W. *Sentinel for Health: A History of the Centers for Disease Control*. Berkeley: University of California Press, 1992.

Farmer, Paul. *AIDS and Accusation: Haiti and the Geography of Blame*. Berkeley: University of California Press, 1992.

Fee, Elizabeth, and Daniel Fox, eds. *AIDS: The Burdens of History*. Berkeley: University of California Press, 1988.

———. *AIDS: The Making of a Chronic Disease*. Berkeley: University of California Press, 1992.

Fox, Daniel M. *Health Policies, Health Politics: The British and American Experience, 1911–1965*. Princeton, N.J.: Princeton University Press, 1986.

Friedlander, Henry. *The Origins of Nazi Genocide: From Euthanasia to the Final Solution*. Chapel Hill: University of North Carolina Press, 1995.

Garrett, Laurie. *The Coming Plague: Newly Emerging Diseases in a World out of Balance*. New York: Farrar, Straus & Giroux, 1994.

Gostin, Lawrence O. *The AIDS Pandemic: Complacency, Injustice, and Unfulfilled Expectations*. Chapel Hill: University of North Carolina Press, 2004.

Grmek, Mirko D. *History of AIDS: Emergence and Origin of a Modern Pandemic*. Princeton, N.J.: Princeton University Press, 1990.

Gussow, Zachary. *Leprosy, Racism, and Public Health: Social Policy in Chronic Disease Control*. Boulder, Colo.: Westview Press, 1989.

Harden, Victoria A. *Inventing the NIH: Federal Biomedical Research Policy, 1887–1937*. Baltimore: Johns Hopkins University Press, 1986.

Harden, Victoria, and Guenter Risse, eds. *AIDS and the Historian*. Bethesda, Md.: National Institutes of Health, 1991.

Hopkins, Donald R. *Princes and Peasants: Smallpox in History*. Chicago: University of Chicago Press, 1983.

Hopkins, Jack W. *The Eradication of Smallpox: Organizational Learning and Innovation in International Health*. Boulder, Colo.: Westview Press, 1989.

Iliffe, John. *The African AIDS Epidemic: A History*. Athens: Ohio University Press, 2006.

Jacobs, Lawrence R. *The Health of Nations: Public Opinion and the Making of American and British Health Policy*. Ithaca, N.Y.: Cornell University Press, 1993.

Jones, James H. *Bad Blood: The Tuskegee Syphilis Experiment*. New York: Free Press, 1981.

Kater, Michael H. *Doctors under Hitler*. Chapel Hill: University of North Carolina Press, 1989.

Kevles, Daniel J. *In the Name of Eugenics: Genetics and the Uses of Human Heredity*. Berkeley: University of California Press, 1986.

Kinsella, James. *Covering the Plague: AIDS and the American Media*. New Brunswick, N.J.: Rutgers University Press, 1989.

Kirp, David, and Ronald Bayer, eds. *AIDS in the Industrialized Democracies*. New Brunswick, N.J.: Rutgers University Press, 1992.

Klaus, Alisa. *Every Child a Lion: The Origins of Maternal and Infant Health Policy in the United States and France, 1890–1920*. Ithaca, N.Y.: Cornell University Press, 1993.

Kraut, Alan M. *Silent Travellers: Germs, Genes, and the "Immigrant Menace"*. New York: Basic Books, 1994.

Largent, Mark A. *Breeding Contempt: The History of Coerced Sterilization in the United States*. New Brunswick, N.J.: Rutgers University Press, 2008.

Larson, Edward J. *Sex, Race, and Science: Eugenics in the Deep South*. Baltimore: Johns Hopkins University Press, 1995.

Lederer, Susan E. *Subjected to Science: Human Experimentation in America before the Second World War*. Baltimore: Johns Hopkins University Press, 1995.

McBride, David. *From TB to AIDS: Epidemics among Urban Blacks since 1900*. Albany: SUNY Press, 1991.

Mazumdar, Pauline. *Eugenics, Human Genetics, and Human Failings*. New York: Routledge, 1992.

Murray, Christopher J. L., and Alan D. Lopez, eds. *The Global Burden of Disease*. Cambridge, Mass.: Harvard School of Public Health, distributed by Harvard University Press, 1996.

Nye, Robert A. *Crime, Madness, and Politics in Modern France: The Medical Concept of National Decline*. Princeton, N.J.: Princeton University Press, 1984.

Patterson, James T. *The Dread Disease: Cancer and Modern American Culture*. Cambridge, Mass.: Harvard University Press, 1987.

Pick, Daniel. *Faces of Degeneration: Aspects of a European Disorder, c. 1848–1918*. Cambridge: Cambridge University Press, 1989.

Proctor, Robert N. *Racial Hygiene: Medicine under the Nazis*. Cambridge, Mass.: Harvard University Press, 1988.

Reilly, Philip R. *The Surgical Solution: A History of Involuntary Sterilization in the United States*. Baltimore: Johns Hopkins University Press, 1991.

Schneider, William H. *Quality and Quantity: The Quest for Biological Regeneration in Twentieth Century France*. Cambridge: Cambridge University Press, 1990.

Shilts, Randy. *And the Band Played On: Politics, People, and the AIDS Epidemic*. New York: Penguin Books, 1988.

Soloway, Richard A. *Demography and Degeneration: Eugenics and the Declining Birthrate in Twentieth-Century Britain*. Chapel Hill: University of North Carolina Press, 1990.

Sontag, Susan. *Illness as Metaphor and AIDS and Its Metaphors*. New York: Doubleday, 1990.

Stepan, Nancy Leys. *"The Hour of Eugenics": Race, Gender, and Nation in Latin America*. Ithaca, N.Y.: Cornell University Press, 1991.

UNAIDS Web site: http://www.unaids.org

Weindling, Paul. *Health, Race, and German Politics between National Unification and Nazism, 1870–1945*. Cambridge: Cambridge University Press, 1989.

World Health Organization. *The World Health Report, 1995: Bridging the Gaps*. Geneva: World Health Organization, 1995.

Index

About the Author

Jo Hays is professor emeritus of history at Loyola University of Chicago. In addition to the first edition of *The Burdens of Disease* (1998), his recent publications have included *Epidemics and Pandemics* (2005) and "Historians and Epidemics: Simple Questions, Complex Answers," in Lester K. Little, ed., *Plague and the End of Antiquity: The Pandemic of 541–750* (2007). He received his P' from the University of Chicago. Married with two children and   grandchildren, he makes his home in Oak Park, Illinois, in the Fra   Lloyd Wright Historic District but in a house of absolutely no architectu   significance.

CPSIA information can be obtained at www.ICGtesting.com
Printed in the USA
BVOW030915171111

276296BV00004B/1/P